High-Yield™

Physiology

FIRST EDITION

High-Yield™

Physiology

FIRST EDITION

Ronald W. Dudek
Brody School of Medicine
East Carolina University
Department of Anatomy and Cell Biology
Greenville, North Carolina

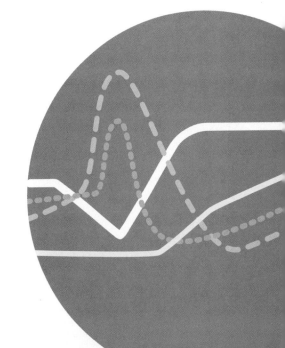

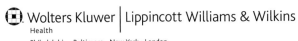 Wolters Kluwer | Lippincott Williams & Wilkins
Health
Philadelphia · Baltimore · New York · London
Buenos Aires · Hong Kong · Sydney · Tokyo

Acquisitions Editor: Nancy Duffy
Developmental Editor: Kathleen Scogna
Managing Editor: Melissa Blaney
Marketing Manager: Emilie Moyer
Production Editor: Gina Aiello
Designer: Teresa Mallon
Compositor: Nesbitt Graphics, Inc.

351 West Camden Street
Baltimore, MD 21201

530 Walnut Street
Philadelphia, PA 19106

Printed in the United States

9 8 7 6 5 4 3 2 1

Library of Congress Cataloging-in-Publication Data

Dudek, Ronald W., 1950-
  High-yield cell physiology / Ronald W. Dudek
      p. ; cm.
  ISBN-13: 978-0-7817-4587-1
  ISBN-10: 0-7817-4587-X
  1. Physiology--Outlines, syllabi, etc. I. Title.
  [DNLM: 1. Physiology. QT 104 D845h 2008]
  QP41.D77 2008
  612--dc22

                                   2007025901

DISCLAIMER

Care has been taken to confirm the accuracy of the information present and to describe generally accept-ed practices. However, the authors, editors, and publisher are not responsible for errors or omissions or for any consequences from application of the information in this book and make no warranty, expressed or implied, with respect to the currency, completeness, or accuracy of the contents of the publication. Application of this information in a particular situation remains the professional responsibility of the prac-titioner; the clinical treatments described and recommended may not be considered absolute and univer-sal recommendations.

The authors, editors, and publisher have exerted every effort to ensure that drug selection and dosage set forth in this text are in accordance with the current recommendations and practice at the time of publi-cation. However, in view of ongoing research, changes in government regulations, and the constant flow of information relating to drug therapy and drug reactions, the reader is urged to check the package insert for each drug for any change in indications and dosage and for added warnings and precautions. This is particularly important when the recommended agent is a new or infrequently employed drug.

Some drugs and medical devices presented in this publication have Food and Drug Administration (FDA) clearance for limited use in restricted research settings. It is the responsibility of the health care provider to ascertain the FDA status of each drug or device planned for use in their clinical practice.

To purchase additional copies of this book, call our customer service department at **(800) 638-3030** or fax orders to **(301) 223-2320**. International customers should call **(301) 223-2300**.

Visit Lippincott Williams & Wilkins on the Internet: http://www.lww.com. Lippincott Williams & Wilkins customer service representatives are available from 8:30 am to 6:00 pm, EST.

Preface

The training of a medical student to become a qualified physician starts with an understanding of the gross anatomical structures of the human body, the embryological formation of those structures, and the microscopic anatomy of those structures. This provides the anatomical base from which the student can launch into other subjects like physiology. Physiology is the study of the functional aspects of the anatomical structures. Structures and function go hand-in-hand. This high yield book provides a synopsis of the most important basic physiological processes that are relevant to the future physician. Hopefully, this book will provide the physiological base from which the student can launch into other subjects like pathology, where the physiology is abnormal, and pharmacology to ameliorate the pathophysiology.

In writing a High Yield Physiology book, it is clear that not all the detailed physiological aspects can be included. However, an understanding of the basic physiological processes, especially those that are most commonly affected pathologically and that can be ameliorated pharmacologically, is necessary to practice medicine.

Please send your feedback, comments, and suggestions to me at dudekr@ecu.edu for inclusion in the next edition.

Ronald W. Dudek, PhD

Contents

1

Cell Physiology

① Bioenergetics. Bioenergetics is the study of energy transformations in living cells. In living cells, biological activities occur at the molecular level and are collectively referred to as the metabolic activities of a cell or **metabolism.** Cellular metabolism requires an energy supply and mammalian cells can only use **free energy,** that is, energy left over from a chemical reaction. This free energy is transferred in two ways as indicated below:

A. Adenosine Triphosphate (ATP) and Phosphoryl Group Transfer. ATP is formed by the addition of a phosphoryl group to adenosine diphosphate (ADP) which adds **7.5 kilocalories of free energy** to the new ATP molecule. When ATP is cleaved, ADP and a phosphoryl group with 7.5 kilocalories of free energy are released. The phosphoryl group and its 7.5 kilocalories of free energy immediately attach to some other molecule, which raises it to a higher energy level so it can engage in a metabolic reaction.

B. Electron Transfer and Oxidation-Reduction Reactions. Oxidation-reductions reactions involve the loss of an electron from one molecule (i.e., oxidation) and the coupled gain of an electron by another molecule (i.e., reduction). The three principal groups of electron-transferring substances in a cell are **pyridine nucleotides (e.g., NAD, NADH), riboflavin,** and **iron-porphyrin complexes.**

② The Lipid Component of the Cell Membrane. The lipid component consists of four phospholipids: **phosphatidylcholine, sphingomyelin, phosphatidylethanolamine, and phosphatidylserine.** The four phospholipids are amphiphilic; i.e., they have a hydrophilic (polar) head and a hydrophobic (nonpolar) tail. The lipid component produces arachidonic acid which leads to the formation of eicosanoids through the following process:

A. In response to physical injury or inflammatory response, **phospholipase A_2 or C** catalyzes the breakdown of membrane lipids to **arachidonic acid.**

B. Arachidonic acid may be converted to straight-chain eicosanoids called **leukotrienes (LTB_4, LTC_4, LTD_4)** by **lipoxygenase.**

C. Arachidonic acid may be converted to cyclical eicosanoids called **prostaglandins (PGE_1, PGE_2, PGF_{2a}), prostacyclin (PGI_2),** and **thromboxane (TXA2)** by **cyclooxygenase (COX I and COX II).** COX I produces eicosanoids used in many normal physiological processes, hence it is sometimes referred to as "good COX". COX II produces eicosanoids used in the inflammatory response, hence it is sometimes referred to as "bad COX".

D. Pharmacology. Aspirin (acetylsalicylic acid, Bayer, Bufferin) is a non-steroidal anti-inflammatory drug (NSAID) that irreversibly inhibits cyclooxygenase and is used clinically to ameliorate effects of myocardial infarction, inhibit platelet aggregation, reduce pain, reduce fever, and as a general anti-inflammatory agent. **Ibuprofen (Advil, Motrin, Nuprin) and Naproxen (Aleve)** are NSAIDs (propionic acid derivatives) that reversibly inhibit cyclooxygenase and are used clinically to reduce pain, to treat rheumatoid arthritis, and to treat osteoarthritis. **Indomethacin** is a NSAID (an acetic acid derivative) that reversibly inhibits cyclooxygenase and is used clinically to treat acute gout, to treat ankylosing spondylitis, and to promote closure of the ductus arteriosus.

III **The Protein Component of the Cell Membrane.** The protein component consists of **peripheral** and **integral proteins. Peripheral proteins** can be easily disassociated from the lipid bilayer by changes in ionic strength or pH. **Integral proteins** are difficult to disassociate from the lipid bilayer unless detergents [e.g., sodium dodecyl sulfate or Triton X-100] are used. **Transmembrane proteins** are integral proteins that span the lipid bilayer, exposing the protein to both the extracellular space and the cytoplasm.

IV **Membrane Transport Proteins** allow for the passage of polar molecules (e.g., ions, sugars, amino acids, nucleotides, and metabolites) across a membrane. There are two main classes of transport proteins: carrier proteins and ion channel proteins.

A. Carrier Proteins (Transporters). Carrier proteins or transporters bind a specific molecule and undergo **conformational changes** in order to transport the molecule across the membrane. Carrier proteins that transport a single solute are called **uniporters.** Other carrier proteins function as **coupled transporters** in which the transport of one solute depends on the simultaneous transport of another solute either in the same direction **(symporters or cotransporters)** or in the opposite direction (antiporters or exchangers). Some important carrier proteins include the following: **Glucose Transporter 4 (GLUT-4), Na$^+$-K$^+$ ATPase, Ca^{2+}ATPase, H$^+$-K$^+$ ATPase, Na$^+$-glucose Cotransporter, Na$^+$-Ca^{2+} Exchanger.**

B. Ion Channel Proteins. Ion channel proteins form **hydrophilic pores** in order to transport **inorganic ions** across the cell membrane. Ion channel proteins are **ion selective** and **gated** (i.e., open briefly and then close). Stimuli that open gates include: changes in voltage across the cell membrane or the membrane potential (i.e., **voltage-gated ion channels**) and ligand binding (i.e., **ligand-gated ion channels**). Some important ion channel proteins include the following:
1. **Voltage-gated Ion Channels.** Some important voltage-gated ion channels include the following: **L-type Ca^{2+} channel protein (dihydropyridine receptor; L=long-lasting, T-type Ca^{2+} channel protein (T=transient), Slow (funny) Na+ channel protein, and the Fast Na$^+$ channel protein.**
2. **Ligand-gated Ion Channels.** In ligand-gated ion channels, the ligand may be a **hormone, second messenger,** or a **neurotransmitter**. One of the more important types of ligand-gated ion channels is the **transmitter-gated ion channels** that bind neurotransmitters and mediate ion movement. Some important transmitter-gated ion channels include the following: **Nicotinic Acetylcholine (nACh) Receptor, N-methyl-D-aspartate (NMDA) Receptor, and the Gamma-Aminobutyric acidA (GABA$_A$) Receptor.**

V # Cell Membrane Transport. (Table 1-1)

A. **Simple Diffusion.**
   1. **Characteristics.** Simple diffusion occurs down an electrochemical gradient (i.e., "downhill"), is not mediated by a carrier protein, and does not require metabolic energy (therefore it is a type of passive transport).
   2. **Permeability.** Permeability describes the ease with which a solute diffuses through a cell membrane and depends on the characteristics of both the solute and the cell membrane. The factors that play a role in permeability include the: **oil/water partition coefficient of the solute** ($\uparrow$coefficient = $\uparrow$solubility in the lipid of the membrane=$\uparrow$ diffusion); **radius of the solute** ($\uparrow$radius = $\downarrow$diffusion); thickness of the membrane ($\uparrow$thickness = $\downarrow$diffusion).
   3. Simple diffusion is calculated by the equation below:

$$J = -PA\,(C_1 - C_2)$$

where,
   J = rate of diffusion
   P = permeability
   A = area
   C = concentration
The minus sign indicates the direction of diffusion is from high to low concentration.

B. **Facilitated Diffusion.** Facilitated diffusion occurs down an electrochemical gradient (i.e., "downhill"), is mediated by a carrier protein (therefore demonstrates stereospecificity, saturation, and competition), and does not require metabolic energy (therefore it is a type of passive transport). Facilitated diffusion is faster than simple diffusion. An example of facilitated diffusion is the action of GLUT4.

C. **Primary Active Transport.** Primary active transport occurs against an electrochemical gradient (i.e., "uphill"), is mediated by a carrier protein (therefore demonstrates stereospecificity, saturation, and competition), and requires metabolic energy in the form of ATP (therefore it is a type of active transport). Examples of primary active transport are the actions of **Na^+-K^+ ATPase, Ca^{2+}ATPase, and H^+-K^+ ATPase.**

D. **Secondary Active Transport.** Secondary active transport involves the coupled transport of two or more solutes in which one solute (usually Na^+) is transported "downhill" and indirectly provides the energy for the "uphill" transport of the other solute. The metabolic energy is not supplied directly, but indirectly through the Na^+ gradient maintained by Na^+-K^+ ATPase. Thus, inhibition of Na^+-K^+ ATPase will shut down secondary active transport.
   1. **Cotransport.** Cotransport occurs when both solutes move in the same direction across the cell membrane. An example of cotransport is the action of the Na^+-glucose transporter.
   2. **Countertransport (Exchange).** Countertransport (or exchange) occurs when the solutes move in opposite directions across the cell membrane. An example of countertransport (or exchange) is the action of the Na^+-Ca^{2+} exchanger.

TABLE 1-1	CHARACTERISTICS OF CELL MEMBRANE TRANSPORT		
	Electrochemical Gradient	Carrier Protein Mediated	Metabolic Energy
Simple Diffusion Passive transport	Downhill	No	No Passive transport
Facilitated Diffusion	Downhill	Yes*	No Passive transport
Primary Active Transport	Uphill	Yes*	Yes ATP Active transport
Secondary Active Transport	Uphill	Yes*	Yes Indirect (Na+-K+ATPase) Active transport

* Carrier protein mediated transport demonstrates stereospecificity (D-glucose is transported but the L-glucose is not), saturation (transport rate increases as the solute concentration increases until the carrier protein is saturated), and competition (structurally related solutes compete for the carrier protein).

VI Osmosis.

A. **Osmolarity.** The osmolarity of a solution refers to the concentration of osmotically active particles in the solution. **Isosmotic** refers to two solutions each with the same osmolarity. If two solutions have different osmolarities, the solution with the higher osmolarity is called **hyperosmotic** and the solution with the lower osmolarity is called **hyposmotic.** Osmolarity is calculated by the equation below.

B. **Osmosis.** Osmosis is the **flow of H_2O** across a semipermeable membrane from a solution with a low solute concentration to a solution with high solute concentration.

C. **Osmotic Pressure.** The osmotic pressure depends on the concentration of osmotically active particles in solution. The osmotic pressure increases when the number of particles in solution increases. For example, a 1M $CaCl_2$ solution has a higher osmotic pressure than a 1M NaCl solution. The lower the osmotic pressure of a solution, the greater the H_2O flow out of it. The higher the osmotic pressure of a solution, the greater the H_2O flow into it. Osmotic pressure is calculated by the van't Hoff equation below:

D. **Effective Osmotic Pressure.** The effective osmotic pressure is π calculated by the van't Hoff equation multiplied by the reflection coefficient (δ). The δ is a number between zero and one that describes the permeability of a solute through a membrane. If $\delta =1$ (e.g., albumin), then the solute is impermeable which means that the solute is retained in the original solution, the solute creates an osmotic pressure, and the solute causes H_2O flow. If $\delta = 0$ (e.g., urea), then the solute is completely permeable which means that the solute is not retained in the original solution, the solute does not create an osmotic pressure, and the solute does not cause H_2O flow.

E. **Oncotic Pressure.** The oncotic pressure is the osmotic pressure caused by proteins (e.g., albumin, plasma proteins, etc.).

F. **Isotonicity**

   a.   If cells are incubated in an extracellular milieu (or solution) and the volume of the cells remains unchanged, then the extracellular milieu is called an **isotonic solution (i.e., 290 mOsm/L)** meaning that there is no movement of H_2O in or out of the cells.

   b.   If cells are incubated in an extracellular milieu (or solution) and the volume of the cells decreases (i.e., the cells shrink), then the extracellular milieu is called a **hypertonic solution (i.e., >290 mOsm/L)** meaning that there is movement of H_2O out of the cells.

   c.   If cells are incubated in an extracellular milieu (or solution) and the volume of the cells increases (i.e., the cells swell), then the extracellular milieu is called a **hypotonic solution (i.e., <290 mOsm/L)** meaning that there is movement of H_2O into the cells.

VII **Resting Membrane Potential.** The resting membrane potential is the difference in electrical potential (i.e., millivolts; mV) across the cell membrane. The resting membrane potential is expressed as the intracellular potential relative to the extracellular potential so that a resting membrane potential of -70mV means 70mV, cell negative. The resting membrane potential is established due to the concentration differences of various permeable ions. Each permeable ion tries to drive the membrane potential towards its equilibrium potential such that the ion with the **highest permeability (or highest conductance)** makes the greatest contribution to the resting membrane potential. The Na^+-K^+ ATPase pump contributes indirectly to the resting membrane potential by maintaining a Na^+ and K^+ concentration gradient across the cell membrane which produces a small potential.

VIII **Action Potential** An action potential consists of a rapid depolarization (or upstroke) followed by a repolarization of the membrane potential. An action potential is a characteristic of excitable cells (e.g., neurons, skeletal muscle, smooth muscle, and cardiac muscle) each of which has a **stereotypical size and shape**, are **propagating**, and are **all-or-none**. A **depolarization** event makes the membrane potential more positive due to an **influx of positive ions** into the cell called an **inward current.** A **hyperpolarization** event makes the membrane potential more negative due to an **efflux of positive ions** out of the cell called an **outward current.**

IX **Clinical Considerations.** **Cystic Fibrosis (CF)** is caused by production of abnormally thick mucus secretions by epithelial cells lining the respiratory and gastrointestinal tract (sweat glands and the reproductive tract are also affected). This results clinically in obstruction of airways and recurrent bacterial infections (e.g., *Staphylococcus aureus, Pseudomonas aeruginosa*). CF is caused by autosomal recessive mutations of the CFTR gene, which is located on the long arm of chromosome 7 (q7). The CFTR gene encodes for a protein called **CFTR (cystic fibrosis transporter)** which functions as a cAMP-dependent **Cl^- ion channel protein** which allows passage of Cl^- into the mucus secretion which is followed by H_2O, thereby maintaining a low viscosity mucus layer. CFTR may in turn regulate the activity of other Cl^- and Na^+ ion channel proteins. An associated finding is an increased concentration of Cl^- in sweat secretions, which constitutes a clinical method of diagnosis. In North America, 70% of CF cases are due to a three base deletion, which codes for the amino acid **phenylalanine at position #508** such that phenylalanine is missing from CFTR.

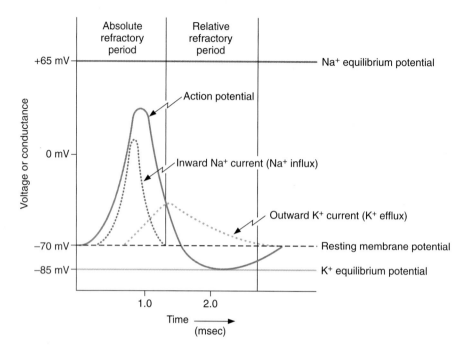

● **Figure 1-1:** Action Potential of a Neuron. The resting membrane potential of a neuron is -70mV (cell negative) due to the high resting conductance (or permeability) of K⁺ which drives the membrane potential towards the K⁺ equilibrium potential of -85mV. The upstroke of the action potential is due to the **inward Na⁺ current** (i.e., Na⁺ influx into the cell) which drives the membrane potential towards the Na⁺ equilibrium potential of +65mV. The **overshoot** is observed at the peak of the action potential when the membrane potential is positive for a brief period of time. The repolarization of the action potential involves a closure of the Na⁺ channels so that the inward Na⁺ current decreases and a slow opening of K⁺ channels so that the **outward K⁺ current** increases. The **undershoot** is observed at the nadir of the action potential when the membrane potential is driven to about -80mV because the outward K⁺ current remains high for sometime after the inward Na⁺ current returns to its resting level (i.e., -70mV). The **absolute refractory period** is the period in which another action potential cannot be elicited. The relative refractory period begins at the end of the absolute refractory period and coincides with the undershoot. An action potential can be elicited during this refractory period only if the inward Na⁺ current is greater than usual. **Tetrodotoxin** (a poison found in puffer fish) and **saxitoxin** [a poison found in dinoflagellates ("red tides")] are potent **Na⁺ channel blockers.** Tetraethylammonium (a poison) is a potent **K⁺ channel blocker.**

2

Skeletal Muscle

Ⅰ **Muscle Fiber Types (Table 2-1).** Skeletal muscle fibers can be classified mainly into **red fibers (Type I)** and **white (Type II) fibers** that have quite different characteristics based on their function.

    A. **Red fibers (Type I)** are **slow-twitch fibers** and are largely present, for example, in the long muscles of the back (antigravity muscles).

    B. **White fibers (Type II)** are **fast-twitch fibers** and are largely present, for example, in the extraocular muscles of the eye.

TABLE 2-1	MUSCLE FIBER TYPES	
	Fiber Type	
	RED Type I	WHITE Type II
Speed of contraction	Slow twitch	Fast twitch
Myoglobin content*	High	Low
Generation of ATP	Aerobic glycolysis** Oxidative Phosphorylation	Anaerobic glycolysis***
Number of Mitochondria	Many	Few
Glycogen content	Low	High
Succinate dehydrogenase NADH dehydrogenase	High	Low
Glycolytic enzymes	Low	High

* Myoglobin is an oxygen-binding protein similar to hemoglobin and accounts for the reddish appearance of red (Type I) fibers.
** Aerobic glycolysis (conversion of glucose $\rightarrow CO_2 + H_2O$) is a relatively slow process so it can meet the demands of red fibers, but yields 36–38 moles of ATP per mole of glucose.
*** Anaerobic glycolysis (conversion of glucose $\rightarrow$ lactate is a relatively fast process so it can meet the demands of white fibers, but yields only 2 moles of ATP per mole of glucose.

II Thin Myofilaments.
Thin myofilaments are composed of **F-actin, tropomyosin,** and the **troponin complex.**

A. F-actin has a myosin-binding site.

B. Tropomyosin is a filamentous protein that runs along the groove of F-actin and blocks the myosin-binding site on F-actin during relaxation.

C. The troponin complex is a complex of three globular proteins called **troponin T, troponin I,** and **troponin C.** Troponin T attaches the troponin complex to tropomyosin. Troponin I blocks the myosin-binding site on F-actin during relaxation along with tropomyosin. Troponin C is a **Ca^{2+}-binding protein** that produces a conformational change in the troponin complex that re-positions tropomyosin thereby exposing the myosin-binding site on F-actin.

III Thick Myofilaments.
Thick myofilaments are composed of **myosin** which consists of six polypeptide chains (one pair of **heavy chains** and two pairs of **light chains**). Myosin has two heads attached to a single tail. The myosin heads have an **actin-binding site** and **ATPase activity.** Myosin can be cleaved by trypsin into light meromyosin and heavy meromyosin.

IV Cross-striations.

A. The **A band** contains both thin and thick myofilaments and is the **dark band** (i.e., dark in color).

B. The **I band** contains only thin myofilaments and is the **light band** (i.e., light in color).

C. The **H band** bisects the A band and contains only thick myofilaments.

D. The **Z disk** bisects the I band. The distance between two Z disks delimits a **sarcomere,** which is the basic unit of contraction for the myofibril. The Z disk contains **a-actinin,** which anchors thin filaments to the Z disk.

V Changes in Contracted and Stretched Muscle (Figure 2-1D).
The cross-striational pattern of skeletal muscle changes when it is contracted or stretched. These changes are caused by the degree of interdigitation of the thin and thick myofilaments.

VI The Triad.
The triad consists of one T-tubule flanked by two terminal cisternae. T tubules are invaginations of the cell membrane and transmit an action potential to the depths of a muscle fiber. T tubules contain an **L-type voltage-gated Ca^{2+} channel protein** (also called the **dihydropyridine receptor**) which changes its conformation in response to an action potential and induces the action of the **fast Ca^{2+} release channel protein** (also called the **ryanodine receptor**). Terminal cisternae are dilated sacs of sarcoplasmic reticulum (SR) that store, release, and re-accumulate Ca^{2+} critical for muscle contraction. TC/SR contain a **fast Ca^{2+} release channel protein** (also called the **ryanodine receptor**) that releases Ca^{2+} from the TC/SR into the cytoplasm and a **Ca^{2+}ATPase** that pumps Ca^{2+} from the cytoplasm into the TC/SR. Ca21 is stored within the TC/SR bound to a protein called **calsequestrin.**

VII **Steps in the Skeletal Muscle Contraction.** An action potential is generated which releases stored Ca^{2+} from the TC/SR via **fast Ca^{2+} release channel proteins (ryanodine receptors)** into the cytoplasm. Note that there is no entry of extracellular Ca^{2+}.

A. Ca^{2+} binds to troponin C which allows the **myosin head–ADP–PO_4^{2-} complex** to bind actin. $ADP + PO_4^{2-}$ is released, leaving the myosin head bound to actin forming a **crossbridge.**

B. Thick and thin filaments slide past each other (i.e., **power stroke**). Repetitive action potentials may produce saturating levels of Ca^{2+} for troponin C which extends the time for crossbridge cycling, thereby causing **tetany.**

C. Due to ATP binding, the myosin head detaches from actin and is displaced towards the + end of actin. If ATP is not available, the myosin head will not detach from actin and **rigor mortis** results.

D. ATP hydrolysis by **myosin ATPase** occurs and the products ($ADP + PO_4^{2-}$) remain bound to the myosin head, thereby reforming the **myosin head–ADP–PO_4^{2-} complex** so that myosin can bind to a new site on actin towards the + end. During each crossbridge cycle, the myosin head "walks" $\approx$10nm along the actin filament.

E. Ca^{2+} is pumped from the cytoplasm back into the TC/SR by **Ca^{2+}ATPase** causing muscle relaxation.

VIII **Neuromuscular Junction** (also called **myoneural junction** or **motor endplate**). **(Figure 2-3).** The neuromuscular junction is the synapse between axons of α-motoneurons and skeletal muscle.

A. Synaptic terminals of **α-motoneurons** contain synaptic vesicles, which store **acetylcholine (ACh).** ACh is synthesized by the condensation of **acetyl CoA** and **choline,** which is catalyzed by **choline-O-acetyltransferase.** Choline is obtained by active uptake from the extracellular fluid.

B. The cell membrane of the synaptic terminal is called the **presynaptic membrane** and is where exocytotic release of ACh occurs. The cell membrane of the muscle fiber is called the **postsynaptic membrane,** and it contains the **nicotinic acetylcholine receptor (nAChR).**

C. The space between the presynaptic and postsynaptic membrane is called the **synaptic cleft,** and it contains the basal lamina associated with the enzyme **acetylcholinesterase (AChE),** which hydrolyzes ACh (ACh → acetate + choline). A Na^+-choline cotransporter transports $\approx$50% of the choline back into the synaptic terminal which is used to synthesize new ACh.

D. nAChR is a **transmitter-gated ion channel** such that when nAChR binds two molecules of ACh, the "gate" is opened and allows the influx of Na^+ and Ca^{2+} and efflux of K^+. Na^+ influx primarily causes a depolarization of the postsynaptic membrane called the **endplate potential (EPP).** Note that an EPP is NOT an action potential. The contents of one synaptic vesicle produce a miniature endplate potential (MEPP) which is the smallest possible EPP. The MEPPs summate to produce a full-fledged EPP.

E. EPPs spread to areas of the cell membrane and T tubule by **electrotonic conduction** until a threshold is reached and an action potential is generated. Note that an action potential is not generated per se at the neuromuscular junction. The generation of an action potential is followed by skeletal muscle contraction.

IX **Innervation.** A single axon of an α-motoneuron may innervate 1–5 muscle fibers (forming a **small motor unit**), or the axon may branch and innervate >150 muscle fibers (forming a **large motor unit**). **A motor unit is the functional contractile unit of a muscle** (not a muscle fiber). A small motor unit is found in muscles that require fine motor control (e.g., extraocular muscles or laryngeal muscles). A large motor unit is found in muscles that do not require fine motor control (e.g., gastrocnemius, gluteus maximus).

X **Denervation.** If a nerve to a muscle is severed, **fasciculations** (small irregular contractions) occur caused by release of ACh from the degenerating axon. Several days after denervation, **fibrillations** (spontaneous repetitive contractions) occur caused by a supersensitivity of the muscle to ACh as nACh receptors spread out over the entire cell membrane of the muscle fiber.

XI **Summation of Muscle Contractions.** A single contractile event (a muscle twitch) is initiated by a single action potential. If a second action potential is generated before the muscle fibers have relaxed, the second contractile event builds on the first contractile event and the two contractile events are said to summate. The summation of muscle contractions occurs when the action potentials reach ≈10 action potentials/second. As the frequency of action potentials increases, the muscle contractions continue to summate until a maximum is reached called **tetany.**

XII **Isometric Contractions (Figure 2-4A).** A good example of an isometric contraction is to imagine trying to curl (i.e., flexion at the elbow) a 500 lb dumbbell with one arm, which is literally impossible. In this example, muscle tension would be great but no muscle shortening would occur. In the laboratory, isometric contractions are measured when **muscle length (preload) is held constant,** the muscle is stimulated to contract, and the muscle tension is measured, thereby, generating a **muscle length-muscle tension relationship.** There are three types of muscle tension that can be described as indicated below.

A. **Total Tension.** The total tension is the muscle tension that develops when a muscle is stimulated to contract at different lengths (or preloads). Total tension = active tension + passive tension.

B. **Active Tension.** The active tension is the muscle tension that develops solely from the contraction of the muscle. The active tension is proportional to the number of crossbridges formed, which depends on the degree of overlap of the thin and thick filaments. When the muscle length is shortened, the overlap of thin and thick filament is reduced (i.e., the number of crossbridges is reduced because thin filaments collide) and the active tension is reduced. When the muscle length is optimal, the overlap of thin and thick filaments is maximal (i.e., the number of crossbridges is maximal) and the active tension is maximal. When the muscle length is stretched, the overlap of thin and thick filaments is reduced (i.e., the number of crossbridges is reduced) and the active tension is reduced. Active tension = total tension − passive tension.

C. **Passive Tension.** The passive tension is the muscle tension that develops solely from stretching the muscle to different lengths.

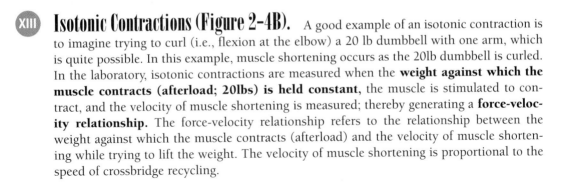

XIII **Isotonic Contractions (Figure 2-4B).** A good example of an isotonic contraction is to imagine trying to curl (i.e., flexion at the elbow) a 20 lb dumbbell with one arm, which is quite possible. In this example, muscle shortening occurs as the 20lb dumbbell is curled. In the laboratory, isotonic contractions are measured when the **weight against which the muscle contracts (afterload; 20lbs) is held constant,** the muscle is stimulated to contract, and the velocity of muscle shortening is measured; thereby generating a **force-velocity relationship.** The force-velocity relationship refers to the relationship between the weight against which the muscle contracts (afterload) and the velocity of muscle shortening while trying to lift the weight. The velocity of muscle shortening is proportional to the speed of crossbridge recycling.

XIV **Clinical Considerations.**

A. **Duchenne muscular dystrophy (DMD).** DMD is an **X-linked recessive disorder** caused by a mutation in the gene for **dystrophin** on the short arm of chromosome X (Xp21). X-linked recessive inheritance means that males who inherit only one defective copy of the DMD gene from the mother have the disease. Dystrophin anchors the cytoskeleton (actin) of skeletal muscle cells to the extracellular matrix through a transmembrane protein (α-dystroglycan and β-dystroglycan) and stablizes the cell membrane. A mutation of the DMD gene destroys the ability of dystrophin to anchor actin to the extracellular matrix. The characteristic dysfunction in DMD is **progressive muscle weakness and wasting.** Death occurs as a result of cardiac or respiratory failure, usually in late teens or twenties.

B. **Myasthenia gravis** is an autoimmune disease characterized by circulating antibodies against the nACh receptor (anti-nAChR) and decreased number of nACh receptors. The diagnosis of myasthenia gravis is made by the **edrophonium test** in which the patient is given edrophonium (an anticholinesterase). If improvement in muscle strength is observed after edrophonium administration, then myasthenia gravis is suggested. Myasthenia gravis is characterized by muscle weakness that fluctuates daily or even within hours. The extraocular muscles are generally involved, with ptosis and diplopia being the first disability.

C. **Tubocurarine, Pancuronium, Vecuronium, and Atracurium** are non-depolarizing drugs, which competitively block nACh receptors (i.e., a **nACh receptor antagonist**). These drugs decrease the size of EPPs. A maximal dose produces paralysis of respiratory muscles and death.

D. **Succinylcholine (Anectine, Quelicin, Sucostrin)** is a depolarizing drug that competes with acetylcholine for nACh receptor (i.e., a **nACh receptor agonist**). Succinylcholine maintains an open Na^+ channel, eventually causing skeletal muscle relaxation and paralysis. Succinylcholine may cause **malignant hyperthermia,** which is a major cause of anesthesia related deaths. Malignant hyperthermia results from an excessive release of Ca^{2+} from the sarcoplasmic reticulum and presents as hyperthermia, metabolic acidosis, tachycardia, and accelerated muscle contractions. Treatment includes: rapid cooling, 100% oxygen, control of acidosis, and administration of dantrolene, which blocks release of Ca^{2+} from the sarcoplasmic reticulum.

E. **Dantrolene** interferes with the release of Ca^{2+} and thereby reduces skeletal muscle contractions. Dantrolene is used in cerebral palsy, multiple sclerosis, and malignant hyperthermia.

F. **Botulinus Toxin** is a potent toxin produced by *Clostridium botulinus* bacteria that inhibits the release of acetylcholine [the latest beauty fad for facial skin wrinkles (BoTox injections)].

G. **Neostigmine** (an AChE inhibitor) inhibits the degradation of ACh, which prolongs its action at the neuromuscular junction.

H. **Hemicholinium** blocks the uptake of choline from the synaptic cleft into the synaptic terminal and thereby depletes ACh stores.

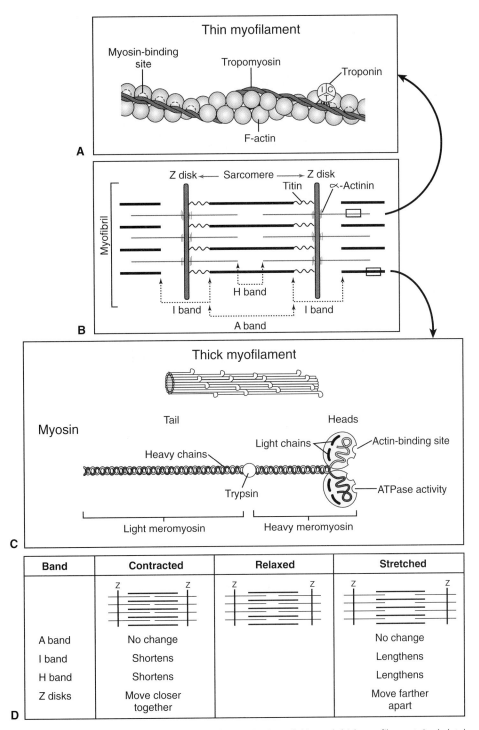

● **Figure 2-1: Myofilaments.** (A) Thin Myofilament. (B) Organization of thin and thick myofilaments in skeletal muscle. (C) Thick Myofilament. (D) Changes in contracted and stretched muscle compared to relaxed muscle.

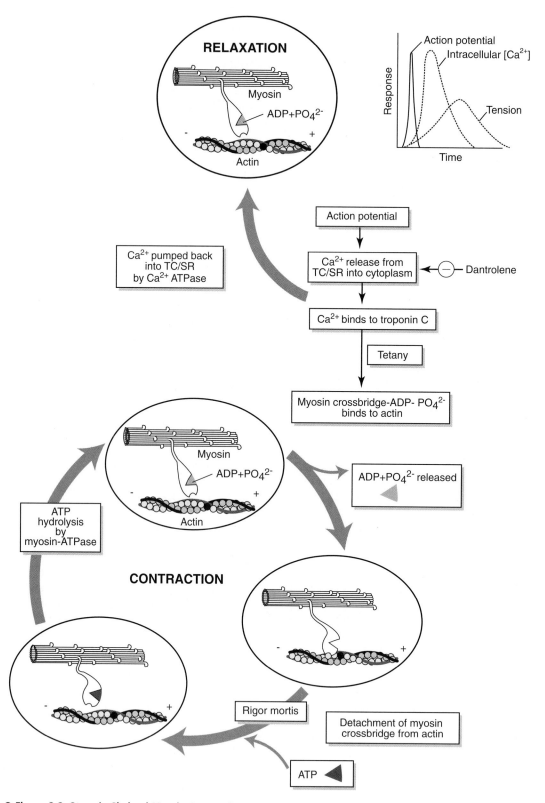

● Figure 2-2: Steps in Skeletal Muscle Contraction.

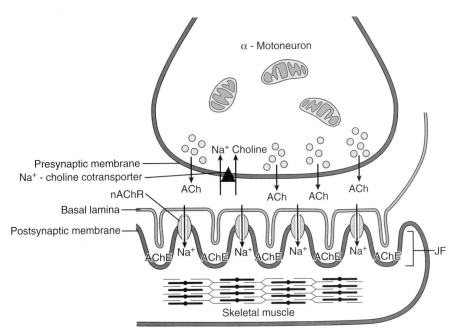

● **Figure 2-3: Diagram of the neuromuscular junction.** A collection of synaptic vesicles that contain acetylcholine (ACh) is indicated along with the presynaptic membrane where ACh is released. The postsynaptic membrane that contains nACh receptors (nAChR) is shown. The bracket indicates the postsynaptic membrane of the skeletal muscle fiber thrown into junctional folds (JF). The synaptic cleft containing the basal lamina and acetylcholinesterase (AChE) is shown.

Isometric contraction

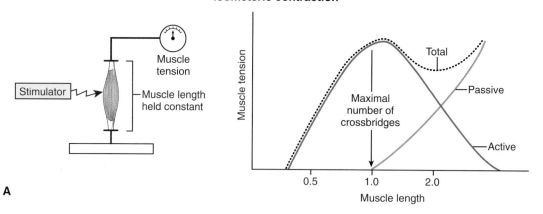

A

Isotonic contraction

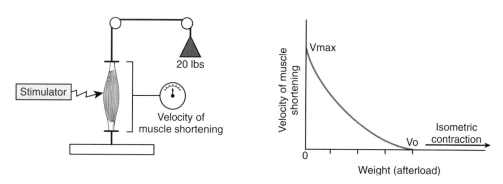

B

● **Figure 2-4: Muscle Contraction. (A) Isometric Contraction.** The muscle length-muscle tension relationship shows that maximal active tension occurs at a muscle length (1.0) where the number of crossbridges is maximal. When the muscle length is shortened (0.5) and held constant, the active tension is reduced because the number of crossbridges is reduced. When the muscle length is stretched (2.0) and held constant, the active tension is again reduced because the number of crossbridges is reduced. Note that passive tension begins only when the muscle is significantly stretched. Total tension = active tension + passive tension. The dip in total tension occurs because the active tension decreases but the total tension rises again because the passive tension increases. **(B) Isotonic Contraction.** The force-velocity relationship shows that maximal velocity of muscle shortening (V_{max}) occurs when the weight (afterload) on the muscle is zero. As the weight (afterload) increases, the velocity of muscle shortening steadily decreases until it reaches zero (V_0) such that any further effort to lift the weight will be an isometric contraction.

3

Smooth Muscle

I Single-unit (SU) Smooth Muscle (Figure 3-1A). SU muscle is found in the respiratory system, gastrointestinal tract, and genitourinary tract. SU smooth muscle demonstrates spontaneous rhythmic cycles of depolarization and repolarization called **slow waves.** Slow waves are not action potentials but do determine the pattern of action potentials. Action potentials that produce smooth muscle contraction occur at the crest of the depolarization phase of the slow wave. SU smooth muscle cells are connected by **gap junctions** that permit coordinated smooth muscle contraction. SU smooth muscle activity is modulated by a number of factors, which include:

A. **Post-ganglionic parasympathetic neurons** that release ACh, which binds to M_3 muscarinic ACh receptors (mAChR).

B. **Post-ganglionic sympathetic neurons** that release NE, which binds to α_1 and β_2 adrenergic receptors.

C. **Hormones (e.g., oxytocin, epinephrine, cholecystokinin).** For example, oxytocin stimulates smooth muscle cells of the uterine myometrium to contract thereby causing uterine contractions during childbirth. Oxytocin binds to the oxytocin receptor, which is a G-protein-linked receptor that generates IP_3. IP_3 opens IP_3-gated Ca^{2+} channels in the sarcoplasmic reticulum.

II Multi-unit (MU) Smooth Muscle (Figure 3-1A). MU smooth muscle is found in the **dilator and sphincter pupillae muscles of the iris, ciliary muscle of the lens,** and **arrector pili muscles.** MU smooth muscle behaves as individual motor units and is highly innervated. MU smooth muscle has no gap junctions. MU smooth muscle activity is modulated by a number of factors, which include:

A. **Post-ganglionic parasympathetic neurons** that release ACh, which binds to M_3 muscarinic ACh receptors (mAChR).

B. **Post-ganglionic sympathetic neurons** that release NE, which binds to α_1 and β_2 adrenergic receptors.

III SU/MU Smooth Muscle. has properties of both SU and MU smooth muscle and is found in the **tunica media of blood vessels.**

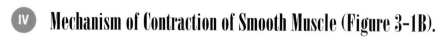

IV   **Mechanism of Contraction of Smooth Muscle (Figure 3-1B).**

V   **Comparison and Contrast of Skeletal, Cardiac, and Smooth Muscle (Table 3-1).**

TABLE 3-1		
Skeletal Muscle	**Cardiac Muscle**	**Smooth Muscle**
Types: Red Fibers (Type I) White fibers (Type II) Intermediate fibers	Types: Cardiac myocytes Purkinje myocytes Myocardial endocrine cells	Types: Single-unit Multi-unit Single/Multi-unit
Long parallel cylinders with multiple peripheral nuclei	Short branching cylinders with single central nucleus	Spindle-shaped, tapering ends with single central nucleus
A band, I band, H band, and Z disks are present	A band, I band, H band, and Z disks are present	Dense bodies and dense plaques connected by intermediate filaments; actin and myosin filaments
T tubules present at A-I junction and form triads with terminal cisternae	T tubules present at Z disks and form diads with a terminal cisterna	Caveolae present
Extensive sarcoplasmic reticulum	Intermediate sarcoplasmic reticulum	Limited sarcoplasmic reticulum
Cell junctions absent	Intercalated disks present (fascia adherens, desmosomes, gap junctions)	Gap junctions present in single unit Gap junctions absent in multi-unit
Muscle spindles present	Muscle spindles absent	Muscle spindles absent
Neuromuscular junction	Synapse en passant	Synapse en passant
Voluntary regulation of "all-or-none" contraction by α-motoneurons	Involuntary regulation of pacemaker-generated heart beat by autonomic nervous system	Involuntary regulation of contraction by autonomic nervous system and hormonal control
α-motoneuron releases ACh at neuromuscular junction, which binds to nicotinic ACh receptor (nAChR)	Post-ganglionic parasympathetic neuron releases ACh, which binds to M_2 muscarinic ACh receptor (mAChR)	Post-ganglionic parasympathetic neuron releases ACh, which binds to M_3 muscarinic ACh receptor (mAChR)
	Post-ganglionic sympathetic neuron releases NE, which binds to β_1 adrenergic receptor	Post-ganglionic sympathetic neuron releases NE, which binds to α_1 and β_2 adrenergic receptors
		Hormonal control: Oxytocin, Epinephrine, CCK
Troponin C is the Ca^{2+} binding protein	Troponin C is the Ca^{2+} binding protein	Calmodulin is the Ca^{2+} binding protein

TABLE 3-1	*(continued)*	
Intracellular Ca^{2+} stored in the TC/SR is released for contraction	Extracellular Ca^{2+} enters ("trigger Ca^{2+}") and induces more Ca^{2+} release from TC/SR	Extracellular Ca^{2+} enters ("trigger Ca^{2+}") and induces more Ca^{2+} release from SR (neural control) or Intracellular Ca^{2+} stored in the SR is released (hormone control)
Upstroke of action potential due to inward Na^+ current	Upstroke of action potential due to inward Ca^{2+} current	Upstroke of action potential due to inward Ca^{2+} current in the SA node Upstroke of action potential due to inward Na^+ current in the atria, ventricles, and Purkinje fibers
No action potential plateau	No action potential plateau	No action potential plateau in SA node Action potential plateau due to inward Ca^{2+} current in atria, ventricles, and Purkinje fibers
Action potential lasts $\approx$1msec	Action potential lasts $\approx$10msec	—————
Growth by hypertrophy	Growth by hypertrophy	Growth by hypertrophy and hyperplasia
Regeneration limited Satellite cells give rise to myoblasts	No Regeneration	Regeneration High Pericytes give rise to new cells
No mitosis	No mitosis	Mitosis

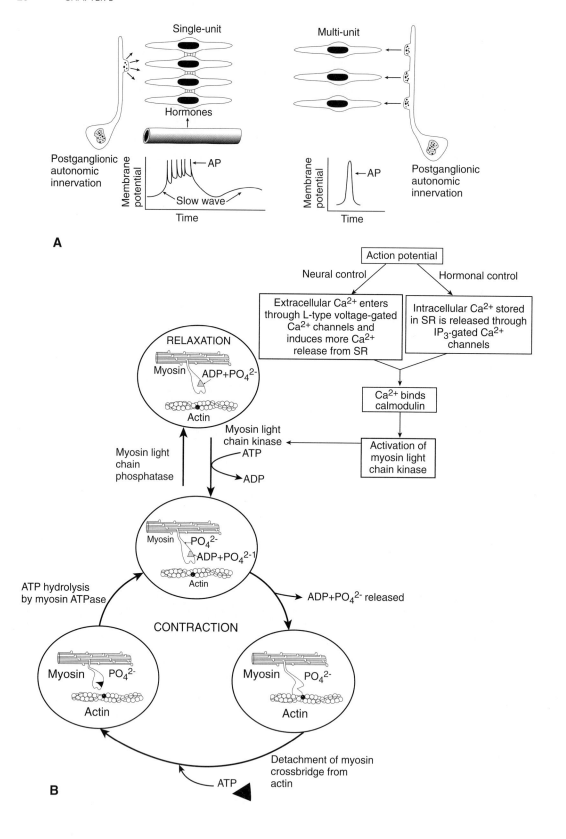

● **Figure 3-1: (A)** Characteristics of single-unit and multi-unit types of smooth muscle. Single-unit smooth muscle has characteristics that include: gap junctions, post-ganglionic autonomic nerves synapse en passant and diffuse neurotransmitter to numerous cells, hormonal control, and action potentials (AP) superimposed on slow waves. Multi-unit smooth muscle has characteristics, which include: no gap junctions, postganglionic autonomic nerves synapse en passant and diffuse neurotransmitter to an individual cell, and the action potential (AP) is spiked. **(B)** Events in smooth muscle contraction. An action potential is generated, which either: a) causes extracellular Ca^{2+} to enter through L-type voltage-gated Ca^{2+} channel proteins (L=long-lasting) and induces more Ca^{2+} release from SR (neural control) or b) intracellular Ca^{2+} stored in the SR is released through IP_3-gated Ca^{2+} channels (hormonal control). Ca^{2+} binds to calmodulin, which activates **myosin light chain kinase**. Myosin light chain kinase phosphorylates the myosin crossbridge-ADP-PO_4^{2-} complex. ADP+ PO_4^{2-} is released, leaving the phosphorylated myosin crossbridge bound to actin. Thin and thick filaments slide past each other (i.e., power stroke). The phosphorylated myosin crossbridge detaches from actin due to ATP binding. ATP hydrolysis by myosin ATPase occurs and the products (ADP + PO_4^{2-}) remain bound to the phosphorylated myosin crossbridge. **Myosin light chain phosphatase** dephosphorylates the myosin crossbridge causing relaxation. In the dephosphorylated state, myosin can still interact with actin but the attachments are called **latch-bridges.** The latch-bridges do not detach or detach very slowly, thereby maintaining a tonic level of tension in the smooth muscle.

4
Cardiac Muscle

I **Myogenic Heartbeat.** Cardiac myocytes contract through intrinsically generated action potentials, which are then passed on to neighboring myocytes by gap junctions; that is, the heartbeat is myogenic. The spontaneous, intrinsically generated action potentials are due to the expression of genes that code for various ion channel proteins and carrier (or transporter) proteins that get inserted into the myocyte cell membrane and begin the flux of ions. This flux of ions generates the action potential. There are two types of action potentials as indicated below.

II **Slow-Response Action Potentials (Figure 4-1A).** Slow-response action potentials are observed in the sinoatrial node (SA node) and atrioventricular node (AV node). Slow action potentials are due to the presence of **slow (funny) Na$^+$ channels** and are divided into three phases.

  A. Phase 0: is due to the **Ca^{2+} influx** into nodal cells through **L-type Ca^{2+} channels** (long-lasting voltage-gated channel).

  B. Phase 3: is due to the **K$^+$ efflux** through **K$^+$ channels** out of nodal cells.

  C. Phase 4: is due to the **Ca^{2+} influx** into nodal cells through **T-type Ca^{2+} channels** (transient voltage-gated channel) and **Na$^+$ influx** into nodal cells through **slow (funny) Na$^+$ channels.** Note that phase 4 is a gradual depolarization.

III **Fast-Response Action Potentials (Figure 4-1B).** Fast-response action potentials are observed in the atrial myocytes, Bundle of His, Purkinje myocytes, and ventricular myocytes. Fast action potentials are due to the presence of **fast Na$^+$ channels** and are divided into five phases.

  A. Phase 0: is due to **Na$^+$ influx into cardiac myocytes through fast Na$^+$ channels.**

  B. Phase 1: is due to **inactivation of fast Na$^+$ channels** and **K$^+$ efflux** out of cardiac myocytes through **K$^+$ channels.**

  C. Phase 2: is due to **Ca^{2+} influx** into cardiac myocytes through **L-type Ca^{2+} channels.** This Ca^{2+} influx (called trigger Ca^{2+}) is involved in the contraction of cardiac myocytes.

D. **Phase 3:** is due to **inactivation of Ca^{2+} channels** and **K^+ efflux** out of cardiac myocytes through K^+ channels.

E. **Phase 4:** is due to **high K^+ efflux**, **removal of the excess Na^+** that entered in Phase 0 by **Na^+-K^+ ATPase**, and **removal of the excess Ca^{2+}** that entered in Phase 2 by the **Na^+-Ca^{2+} exchanger.**

IV **Refractory Periods (Figure 4-1C).** Compared with action potentials in neurons or skeletal muscle, the fast-response action potential in cardiac muscle is much longer in duration, which results in a prolonged refractory period. A refractory period (about 250 msec) is the time at which a cardiac myocyte cell cannot be re-stimulated. A prolonged refractory period is necessary in cardiac myocytes to permit the ventricles sufficient time to empty their blood volume and refill with blood prior to the next contraction. The degree of refraction reflects the number of fast Na^+ ion channels that have recovered and are capable of re-opening during phase 3. The **absolute refractory period (ARP)** refers to the time during which a cardiac myocyte is **completely unexcitable** in response to a new stimulation. The **effective refractory period (ERP)** refers to a short time past the ARP during which a cardiac myocyte cell produces a **localized action potential that does not propagate** in response to a new stimulation. The **relative refractory period (RRP)** refers to the time interval during which a cardiac myocyte produces an action potential that is propagated but because the cardiac myocyte is stimulated at a voltage less negative than the resting potential, the upstroke of the action potential (phase 0) is less steep and of lower amplitude. During the RRP, a larger than normal stimulus is needed to cause an action potential.

V **Conduction System (Figure 4-2).**

A. **Sinoatrial (SA) Node** is the **pacemaker** of the heart and is located at the junction of the superior vena cava and right atrium just beneath the epicardium. From the SA node, the impulse spreads throughout the right atrium and to the AV node via the **anterior, middle, posterior internodal tracts** and to the left atrium via the **Bachmann bundle.** If all SA node activity is destroyed, the AV node will assume the pacemaker role.

B. **Atrioventricular (AV) Node** is located on the right side of the interatrial septum near the ostium of the coronary sinus in the subendocardial space.

C. **Bundle of His, Bundle Branches, Purkinje Myocytes.** The **bundle of His** travels in the subendocardial space on the right side of the interventricular septum and divides into the **right and left bundle branches.** The left bundle branch is thicker than the right bundle branch. The left bundle branch further divides into an **anterior segment** and **posterior segment.** The right and left bundle branches both terminate in a complex network of the intramural **Purkinje myocytes.**

VI **Parasympathetic Regulation of Heart Rate (Figure 4-2).**

A. **Decreases heart rate** ("vagal arrest") by decreasing $Na+$ influx associated with phase 4 depolarization in nodal tissue. This is also called a **negative chronotropism.**

B. **Decreases conduction velocity through the AV node (i.e., increases PR interval)** by decreasing Ca^{2+} influx associated with phase 0 depolarization in nodal tissue. This is also called a **negative dromotropism.**

C. **Decreases contractility of atrial myocytes** by decreasing Ca^{2+} influx associated with phase 2 in atrial myocytes. This is also called a **negative inotropism.**

VII. Sympathetic Regulation of Heart Rate (Figure 4-2).

A. **Increases heat rate** by increasing $Na+$ influx associated with phase 4 depolarization in nodal tissue. This is also called **positive chronotropism.**

B. **Increases conduction velocity through the AV node (i.e., increases PR interval)** by increasing Ca^{2+} influx associated with phase 0 in nodal tissue. This is also called a **positive dromotropism.**

C. **Increases contractility of atrial and ventricular myocytes** by increasing the Ca^{2+} influx associated with phase 2 of the action potential in atrial and ventricular myocytes and increases the activity of the **Ca^{2+}ATPase pump** by **phosphorylation of phospholamban** so that more Ca^{2+} re-accumulates during relaxation and therefore is available for release during later heartbeats. This is also called **positive inotropism.**

● **Figure 4-1: (A)** Slow-response action potential and associated ion fluxes observed in the SA node and AV node. **Class IV Ca^{2+} ion channel antagonists** (Diltiazem and Verapamil) block L-type Ca^{2+} ion channels. **Adenosine** binds to adenosine receptors, which results in the activation of K^+ ion channels and inhibits T-type Ca^{2+} ion channels. **Note that phase 0 is due to Ca^{2+} ion influx. (B)** Fast-response action potential and associated ion fluxes observed in atrial myocytes, Bundle of His, Purkinje myocytes, and ventricular myocytes. Various **antiarrhythmic drugs** are indicated along with their specific effect on ion channels. **Class I Na^+ ion channel antagonists** include Class IA, IB, and IC. **Class IA** (Quinidine, Procainamide, Disopyramide) blocks open Na^+ ion channels. **Class IB** (Lidocaine, Tocainide, Mexiletine, Phenytoin) blocks open and closed Na^+ ion channels. **Class IC** (Flecainide, Propafenone, Moricizine) blocks Na^+ ion channels. **Class III K^+ ion channel antagonists** (Amiodarone and Bretylium) block K^+ ion channels. **Cardiac glycosides** (Digoxin and Digitoxin) are Na^+-K^+ ATPase antagonists that elevate intracellular Na^+ ions. The elevated Na^+ ions overwhelm the Na^+-Ca^{2+}exchanger so that more Ca^{2+} ions can be re-accumulated by terminal cisternae (TC). During the next contraction, more Ca^{2+} ions are released from TC increasing the force of contraction. Cardiac glycosides are used in congestive heart failure (CHF) to increase the strength of contraction. The antiarrhythmic effect of cardiac glycosides is due to their indirect effect on the autonomic nervous system (increase parasympathetic activity and decrease sympathetic activity). Note that phase 0 is due to Na^+ ion influx and the long plateau (phase 1 and phase 2) of about 300 msec. **(C) Refractory Periods.** ARP=absolute refractory period; ERP = effective refractory period; RRP = relative refractory period.

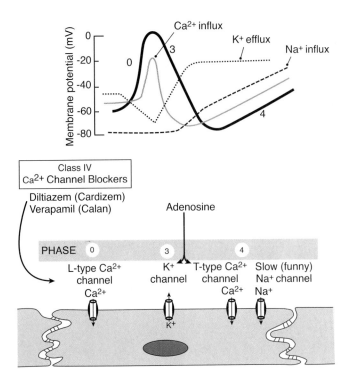

A Slow

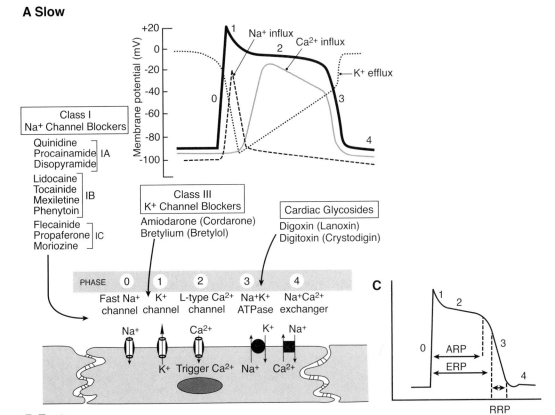

B Fast

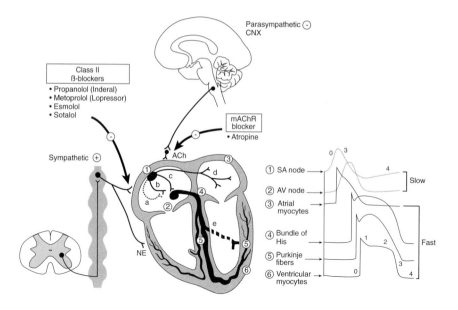

ECG	Heart Action
P wave	Represents atrial depolarization (0.08-0.1 sec)
PR interval	Is the interval from start of atrial depolarization to the start of ventricle depolarization (0.12-0.20 sec)
	Gets shorter as the heart rate increases
	Gets longer as conduction velocity through AV node is slowed (e.g., heart block)
QRS complex	Represents ventricle depolarization (0.06-0.10 sec)
QT interval	Represents the entire period of ventricle depolarization and ventricle repolarization (0.32 sec)
ST segment	Represents the period when the entire ventricle is depolarized
T wave	Represents ventricle repolarization (0.1-0.25 sec)

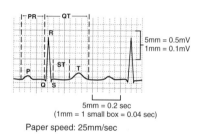

5mm = 0.5mV
1mm = 0.1mV

5mm = 0.2 sec
(1mm = 1 small box = 0.04 sec)
Paper speed: 25mm/sec

● **Figure 4-2: Diagram of the conduction system of the heart.** Action potentials from various areas of the heart are shown. The electrocardiogram (ECG) is a record of the electrical activation of the heart and is the body surface manifestation of all these action potentials (1-6). As a wave of depolarization progresses through the heart, the area (outside the depolarized cardiac muscle cell) becomes electrically negative relative to areas not yet depolarized. This makes the heart a dipole or an electrical source consisting of asymmetrically distributed electrical charge. Due to the ions present in body fluids and other body structures, the body acts as a conductor that conducts electrical activity generated by the heart to the body surface, which can be recorded by body surface electrodes. The various components of the ECG are indicated along with their associated heart function. Parasympathetic regulation of heart rate is solely a negative effect. **Atropine** is the classic cholinergic antagonist ("mACHR blocker"; muscarinic blocker; antimuscarinic). Sympathetic regulation of heart rate is solely a positive effect. **Class II β-blockers** (Propanolol, Metoprolol, Esmolol, Sotalol) block β-adrenergic receptors. The antiarrhythmic effect of β-blockers is due to a decrease in phase 4 depolarization in nodal tissue resulting in decreased SA node activity and AV nodal conduction. The antianginal effect of β-blockers is due to a decrease in heart rate (chronotropism) and decrease in contractility (inotropism), which decreases myocardial oxygen demand. a = posterior internodal tract; b = middle internodal tract; c = anterior internodal tract; d = Brachmann bundle; e = posterior segment of the left bundle branch; CN X = cranial nerve X (vagus nerve).

5
Cardiac Muscle Mechanics

① **Contraction of Cardiac Myocytes.** Cardiac muscle differs from skeletal muscle in that cardiac myocytes branch and are connected by intercalated disks to form a **syncytium.** The syncytium provides easy movement of an action potential so that when one cardiac myocyte becomes excited, the action potential spreads to all adjoining cells. The atrial syncytium is separated from the ventricular syncytium by the **annulus fibrosis** so that action potentials are conducted from the atria→ventricles only through the Purkinje system.

A. Cardiac myocytes demonstrate a **diad** that consists of a **T tubule** located at the Z disk and flanked by one **terminal cisterna (TC).** A T tubule is an invagination of the cell membrane. A TC is a dilated sac of sarcoplasmic reticulum (SR), which stores, releases, and reaccumulates Ca^{2+}.

B. The Ca^{2+} influx that occurs at the cell membrane and T tubule in **Phase 2** of the action potential through L-type Ca^{2+} channels is <u>not</u> sufficient to cause contraction but acts as **trigger Ca^{2+}** that stimulates release of a large pool of Ca^{2+} stored in TC **(i.e., intracellular Ca^{2+} increases).**

C. Ca^{2+} binds to **troponin C,** which allows the **myosin head-ADP-PO_4^{2-}** complex to bind actin. From this point on, cardiac myocyte contraction resembles skeletal muscle contraction.

D. ADP+PO_4^{2-} is released leaving the myosin head bound to actin, forming a **crossbridge.** Thick and thin filaments slide past each other **(i.e., power stroke).** The magnitude of the force of contraction is proportional to the intracellular Ca^{2+}.

E. The myosin head binds ATP, which detaches the myosin crossbridge from actin.

F. ATP hydrolysis by **myosin ATPase** occurs and the products (ADP + PO_4^{2-}) remain bound to the myosin head, thereby reforming the myosin head-ADP-PO_4^{2-} complex so that myosin can bind to a new site on actin toward the + end.

G. As Ca^{2+} influx begins to decrease at the end of Phase 2, Ca^{2+} is pumped from the cytoplasm back into the TC/SR by **Ca^{2+} ATPase** that is regulated by an intramembranous SR protein called **phospholamban (i.e, relaxation).**

H. Troponin C is freed of Ca^{2+}.

I.   The phases of contraction of the entire heart are called **systole** (period during which cardiac contraction occurs)and **diastole** (period during which cardiac relaxation and filling occurs.

II **Preload.** Preload is the load on ventricular myocytes at the end of diastole. Therefore, preload is the load on the heart prior to contraction. The preload of the right ventricle and left ventricle are equal. The best index of preload is **end-diastolic volume,** which is the volume of blood contained in the left ventricle at the end of diastole or just before contraction. **Pulmonary artery wedge pressure (PAWP)** measured by a Swan-Ganz catheter is another index used clinically because of ease of measurement.

A. **Factors that increase preload.**
   1. **Overinfusion of saline**
   2. **Edema**
   3. **Exercise**

B. **Factor that decreases preload. Venous dilation [e.g., Nitroglycerin, Isosorbide dinitrate (Isordil), Amyl nitrite (Aspirols)].** These drugs relax predominately **venous** smooth muscle leading to peripheral venous dilation via the active metabolite **nitric oxide (NO),** which activates guanylate cyclase and **increases cGMP.** The increase in cGMP cause dephosphorylation of myosin light chains.

III **Afterload.** Afterload is the load on ventricular myocytes during contraction. Therefore, afterload is the magnitude of load the heart must overcome to eject blood. The best index of afterload is **aortic pressure** (for left ventricle) and **pulmonary artery pressure** (for right ventricle).

A. **Factor that increases afterload. Arteriolar constriction (e.g., hypertension).**

B. **Factors that decrease afterload.**
   1. **Vasodilators [e.g., Hydralazine (Apresoline), Minoxidil (Loniten)].** These drugs relax predominately **arteriolar** smooth muscle, leading to a decrease in peripheral vascular resistance (PVR). The action of hydralazine is uncertain but may involve NO. Minoxidil is a K^+ channel agonist that causes an increased K^+ efflux, hyperpolarization, and relaxation of smooth muscle.
   2. **Angiotensin Converting Enzyme (ACE) Inhibitors [e.g., Captopril (Capoten), Enalapril (Vasotec), Lisinopril (Zestril).** These drugs reversibly inhibit ACE, thereby preventing the conversion of angiotensin I to angiotensin II (a potent vasoconstrictor).
   3. **Angiotensin II Receptor Antagonist [e.g., Losartan (Cozaar)].** This drug blocks the angiotensin II receptor.

IV **Contractility (Inotropism) and Frank-Starling Law (Figure 5-1A).** Contractility is the force of contraction of ventricular myocytes at a given muscle length (preload), which is classically describe by the **Frank-Starling curve (or cardiac function curve).** Therefore, contractility is an index that measures the ability of the heart to pump blood. The Frank-Starling Law indicates that as cardiac muscle is stretched, its ability to contract is augmented. This means that when an additional amount of blood returns to the ventricles, the ventricles are stretched, which results in an augmented contraction that propels the additional blood out of the ventricles. This ensures that both ventricles pump the same volume of blood within one heartbeat, thereby preventing any overfilling of the pulmonary or systemic circulations. The best clinical index of contractility is **ejection fraction,** which is the percentage of blood pumped by the heart on each beat. The ejection fraction = stroke volume/end-diastolic volume, which is normally **55%.**

A. **Factors that increase contractility (positive inotropism).**
1. **Increased heart rate (Bowditch Staircase)** strengthens the force of contraction in a stepwise fashion as intracellular Ca^{2+} is elevated cumulatively over several heartbeats.
2. **Sympathetic stimulation [e.g., catecholamines via β_1 adrenergic receptor, Dobutamine (Dobutrex)].** Dobutamine is a β_1 adrenergic agonist.
3. **Cardiac glycosides [e.g. Digoxin (Lanoxin) and Digitoxin (Crystodigin).** These drugs are Na^+-K^+ ATPase blockers that elevate intracellular Na^+. The elevated Na^+ overwhelms the Na^+-Ca^{2+} exchanger so that more Ca^{2+} can be reaccumulated by terminal cisternae (TC). During the next contraction, more Ca^{2+} is released from TC, increasing the force of contraction.

B. **Factors that decrease contractility (negative inotropism).**
1. **Heart failure**
2. **Acidosis**
3. **Hypoxia/hypercapnia**
4. **Parasympathetic stimulation (e.g., ACh via M_2 muscarinic ACh receptor).** See Chapter 4IV
5. **β_1 adrenergic antagonist [e.g., Metoprolol (Lopressor)]**

V **Swan-Ganz Catheter** is a relatively soft, flexible right heart catheter with an inflatable balloon at its tip. The balloon allows the catheter to float through the right heart chambers and into the pulmonary artery before "wedging" in a distal branch of the pulmonary artery. The information gained from a Swan-Ganz catheter is as follows:

A. **Cardiac Output (CO)** is measured by the thermodilution technique.

B. **Pulmonary Artery Wedge Pressure (PAWP)** is obtained by inflating the balloon while the catheter is positioned in a distal branch of the pulmonary artery. This shields the catheter tip from the proximal pressure in the pulmonary artery proximally, so that the distal pressure in the pulomonary arterioles can be measured (or PAWP). The PAWP approximates the pressure in the left atrium. Assuming no obstruction between the left atrium and left ventricle, the PAWP approximates the end-diastolic <u>pressure</u> in the left ventricle (LVEDP). The LVEDP is the clinical measure of **LV preload.** Technically, LV end-diastolic <u>volume</u> determines LV preload (not pressure), but LV end-diastolic <u>volume</u> is very difficult to measure.

C. **CO and PAWP** are important physiologic parameters to measure with the Swan-Ganz catheter because CO and PAWP allow the physician to apply the Frank-Starling Law, which states that an increase in preload (PAWP) produces an increase in CO at any given level of myocardial contractility.

D. **Pulmonary Artery Pressure** is measured when the balloon is deflated.

E. **Right Atrium Pressure** is measured using a port 15cm proximal to the catheter tip. This port is also used to infuse drugs or fluids into the central circulation.

F. **Mixed Venous Oxyhemoglobin Saturation (SvO₂)** is measured using fiberoptics.

VI   Left Ventricle Pressure-Volume Curves (Figure 5-1 B-F).

The events of the cardiac cycle can be summarized by the relationship between left ventricular pressure and left ventricular volume. The effects of preload, afterload, and contractility can also be graphically depicted using the pressure-volume curve.

VII   Cardiac Calculations (Figure 5-2A).

A. **Stroke Volume (SV)** is the volume of blood ejected from the ventricle on each heartbeat.

B. **Cardiac output (CO)** is the stroke volume multiplied by the heart rate.

C. **Ejection Fraction (EF)** is the fraction of the end-diastolic volume ejected in each stroke volume.

VIII   Pressures Within Heart Chambers and Great Vessels (Figure 5-2B).

A. **Right Atrium (0–6mm Hg; 4mm Hg).** The right atrium is a very compliant chamber that holds blood as it moves from the systemic circulation to return to the heart. Due to its high degree of compliance and weak contraction, the pressure within the right atrium undergoes little change. As the right atrium fills with blood, the pressure rises from **0–6mm Hg** with a mean pressure of about **4mm Hg.**

B. **Right Ventricle (25/0mm Hg).** The right ventricle pumps blood into the pulmonary artery and has pressures ranging from **25 mm Hg systolic to 0mm Hg diastolic.**

C. **Pulmonary Artery (28/4mm Hg).** The pressure within the pulmonary artery ranges from **28mm Hg systolic to 4mm Hg diastolic.**

D. **Left Atrium (0–10mm Hg; 8mm Hg).** The left atrium receives blood returning from the pulmonary circulation and has pressure ranging from **0–10mm Hg** with a mean pressure of about **8mm Hg.**

E. **Left Ventricle (125/8mm Hg).** The left ventricle pumps blood into the aorta and has pressures ranging from **125mm Hg systolic to 8mm Hg diastolic.**

F. **Aorta (120/80mm Hg).** The pressure within the **aorta** ranges from **120mm Hg systolic to 80mm Hg diastolic.**

IX   The Cardiac Cycle (Figure 5-3).

The cardiac cycle includes both **electrical events** of the heart (measured by ECG) and **mechanical events** associated with the contraction and relaxation of the heart. A cardiac cycle refers to the period from the start of one heart beat through the start of the next heart beat. A cardiac cycle is divided into seven phases and key points in each phase are indicated below.

A. **Atrial Systole.** The **P wave** initiates atrial systole and ejects more blood into the ventricles. Atrial systole generates the **a wave,** which is reflected back into the large veins and may be recorded from the jugular vein. The appearance of **distended jugular veins** in a patient indicates excessive pressure in the right atrium which may be caused by congestive heart failure (CHF) or tricuspid valve dysfunction. Atrial systole contributes to (but is not essential for) ventricle filling and causes the **S4 heart sound,** which is not audible in normal adults.

B. **Isovolumetric Ventricular Contraction.** After the onset of the **QRS complex,** the ventricles begin to contract and the ventricular pressure begins to rise. As the ventricular pressure exceeds atrial pressure, the AV valves (mitral and tricuspid) close. Closure of the AV valves causes the **S1 heart sound.** The mitral valve closes before tricuspid valve so that the S1 heart may be split (**S1 splitting**). Note that during this phase even though the ventricles contract there is no change in blood volume (i.e., isovolumetric) because **all the valves are closed** (mitral, tricuspid, aortic, and pulmonic).

C. **Rapid Ventricular Ejection.** When ventricular pressure exceeds the pressure within the aorta and pulmonary artery, the **aortic valve and pulmonic valve open,** respectively. Right ventricular ejection occurs before left ventricular ejection because the pressure is lower in the pulmonary artery than the aorta. A **majority of the stroke volume is ejected** during this phase. The **T wave** marks the end of the rapid ventricular ejection phase. Note that **atrial filling** begins during this phase.

D. **Reduced Ventricular Ejection.** During this phase, ventricular pressure begins to decrease while ejection of blood from the ventricles continues but is slower. The pressure within the aorta and pulmonary artery decreases as blood flows from the large arteries into smaller arteries. Atrial filling continues.

E. **Isovolumetric Ventricular Relaxation.** As the **T wave** has already been completed, the ventricles are now repolarized. The aortic valve and pulmonic valve close, which produces the **S2 heart sound.** Normally, the aortic valve closes first, producing the aortic component of S2 called A_2. Then, the pulmonic valve closes, producing the pulmonic component of S2 called P_2. During this phase, ventricular pressure decreases rapidly. Note also that during this phase there is no change in blood volume (i.e, isovolumetric) because **all the valves are closed** (mitral, tricuspid, aortic, and pulmonic). However, when the ventricular pressure falls below the atrial pressure, the **AV valves open.** A "blip" in aortic pressure (called the **dicrotic notch**) occurs after closure of the aortic valve.

F. **Rapid Ventricular Filling.** Rapid ventricular filling begins as the AV valves open. The flow of blood from the atria to the ventricles produces the **S3 heart sound.** Pressure within the aorta and pulmonary artery continues to decrease as blood continues to flow from the large arteries into smaller arteries.

G. **Reduced Ventricular Filling (diastasis).** Filling of the ventricles continues although at a slower rate. This is the longest phase of the cardiac cycle. Note that the time required for rapid ventricular filling and diastasis depends on the heart rate. The faster the heart rate the shorter time available for ventricle filling.

X **Clinical Considerations.**

A. Right Ventricle (RV) Failure

1. **General Features.** The RV is susceptible to failure in situations that cause an increase in afterload on the RV. Pure RV failure most often occurs with **cor pulmonale,** which can be induced by intrinsic diseases of the lung or **pulmonary arterial hypertension (PAH). Acute cor pulmonale** is RV dilation caused by a large **thrombopulmonary embolism. Chronic cor pulmonale** is RV hypertrophy followed by RV enlargement and RV failure caused by PAH. PAH is defined as pulmonary artery pressures above the normal systolic value of 30mm Hg. There are numerous causes of PAH, which include: **v**asculitis, **i**diopathic ("primary PAH), **c**hronic pulmonary emboli, **c**hronic lung disease, **e**mphysema, **E**isenmenger syndrome (mnemonic: "VICE")

2. **Clinical findings include:** right hypogastric quadrant discomfort due to hepatomegaly, a cut section of the liver demonstrates a "nutmeg" pattern of chronic passive congestion, peripheral edema (e.g., hallmark of RV failure is ankle swelling), pulmonary edema absent, jugular vein and portal vein distention, enlarged spleen, peritoneal cavity ascites, pleural effusion, palpable parasternal "heave", presence of S4 heart sound ("atrial gallop"), tricuspid valve murmur, ascent to high altitudes is contraindicated due to hypoxic pulmonary vasoconstriction, which will exacerbate the condition.

B. Left Ventricle (LV) Failure (Myocardial Infarction)

1. **General Features.** LV failure most often occurs due to impaired left ventricle function caused by myocardial infarction (MI). The left ventricle is usually hypertrophied and quite massively dilated. In LV failure, there is progressive damming of blood within the pulmonary circulation such that pulmonary vein pressure mounts and pulmonary edema with wet, heavy lungs is apparent. Coughing is a common feature of LV failure. Transferrin and hemoglobin that leak from the congested capillaries are phagocytosed by macrophages in the alveoli (called heart failure cells). In LV failure, the decreased cardiac output causes a reduction in kidney perfusion, which may lead to acute tubular necrosis and also activates the renin-angiotensinogen system.

2. **Clinical findings include:** patient is overweight, has a poor diet, and has occasional episodes of angina; crushing pressure on the chest with pain radiating down the left arm ("referred pain"), nausea, profuse sweating and cold, clammy skin due to stress-induced release of catecholamines (epinephrine and norepinephrine) from adrenal medulla that stimulate sweat glands and cause peripheral vasoconstriction, dyspnea, orthopnea, auscultation of pulmonary rales due to "popping open" of small airways that were closed off due to pulmonary edema, noisy breathing ("cardiac asthma"), pulmonary wedge pressure (indicator of left atrial pressure) increased versus normal (30 vs. 5mm Hg, respectively), ejection fraction decreased versus normal (0.35 vs. 0.55, respectively).

3. **Treatment includes:** sublingual nitroglycerin; β-adrenergic antagonist (e.g., propranolol "β-blocker") to relieve tachycardia and hypertension, although there is a risk because β-blockers will further decrease an already compromised cardiac output; streptokinase IV or tissue plasminogen activator (TPA) reduces amount of infarcted tissue if administered within 6 hours of MI; atropine to relieve bradycardia; heparinization and warfarin therapy to prevent ventricular aneurysms; thrombopulmonary embolisms; and deep vein thrombosis.

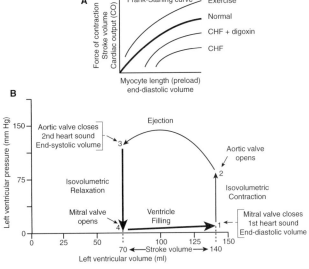

	Increase	Decrease
Preload	• Overinfusion of saline • Edema • Exercise	• Venous dilation (nitroglycerin, isosorbide, dinitrate, amyl nitrate)
Afterload	• Arteriolar constriction (hypertension)	• Vasodilators (hydralazine, minoxidil) • ACE Inhibitors (captopril, enalapril, lisinopril) • Angiotensin II receptor antagonists (losartan)
Contractility	• Increased heart rate (Bowditch staircase) • Sympathetic stimulation (catecholamines, dobutamine) • Cardiac glycosides (digoxin, digitoxin)	• Heart failure • Acidosis • Hypoxia/Hypercapnea • Parasympathetic stimulation (ACh) • β_1-adrenergic antagonist (metoprolol)

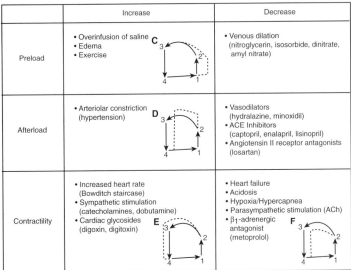

● **Figure 5-1: (A) The Frank-Starling Curve or Cardiac Function Curve.** Note the relationship of the force of contraction to myocyte length (preload). In the ventricle, stroke volume is a good indicator of force of contraction and end-diastolic volume is a good indicator of myocyte length. Note that as the end-diastolic volume (or venous return) increases, the stroke volume increases. Note the changes in the curve due to congestive heart failure (CHF), CHF plus treatment with digoxin, and exercise. **(B)** Left ventricular pressure-volume curve through one cardiac cycle. Thin lines (1→2 and 2→3) indicate the **systolic portion** of the curve. Thick lines (3→4 and 4→1) indicate the **diastolic portion** of the curve. Note the events at points 1, 2, 3, and 4 as indicated by the arrows. Beginning at point 1, the left ventricle begins to contract, which leads to mitral valve closure. However, the aortic valve has not yet opened so that the **period 1→2 is the isovolumetric ventricular contraction phase**. At point 2, the aortic valve opens when sufficient pressure has been generated to overcome aortic pressure and blood is pumped from the ventricle into the aorta. The **period 2→3 is the rapid and reduced ventricular ejection phase**. The amount of blood ejected during period 2→3 is called the **stroke volume** 140mLs −70mLs = 70mLs. At point 3, the left ventricle begins to relax and the pressure falls rapidly, resulting in closure of the aortic valve. The mitral valve remains closed until point 4. The **period 3→4 is the isovolumetric ventricular relaxation phase.** At point 4, the mitral valve opens to permit ventricular filling when left atrial pressure exceeds left ventricular pressure. The **period 4→1 is the rapid and reduced ventricular filling phase. (C)** Left ventricular pressure-volume curve depicting an increase in preload (dotted line). Note the **shift to the right** of the curve and the **increase in stroke volume. (D)** Left ventricular pressure-volume curve depicting an increase in afterload (dotted line). Note the increase in **left ventricle pressure** and **decrease in stroke volume. (E)** Left ventricular pressure-volume curve depicting an increase in contractility (dotted line). Note the **increase in stroke volume** and **no change in end-diastolic volume. (F)** Left ventricular pressure-volume curve depicting a decrease in contractility (dotted line). Note the **decrease in stroke volume** and **increase in end-systolic volume.**

A

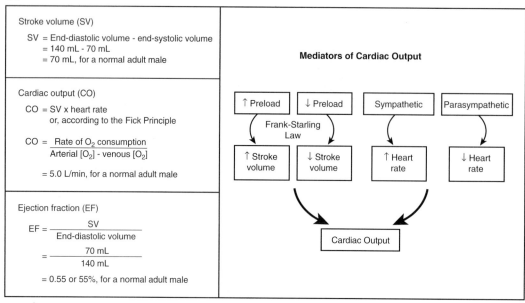

Stroke volume (SV)	
SV = End-diastolic volume - end-systolic volume	
= 140 mL - 70 mL	
= 70 mL, for a normal adult male	

Cardiac output (CO)

CO = SV x heart rate
  or, according to the Fick Principle

$$CO = \frac{\text{Rate of } O_2 \text{ consumption}}{\text{Arterial } [O_2] - \text{venous } [O_2]}$$

= 5.0 L/min, for a normal adult male

Ejection fraction (EF)

$$EF = \frac{SV}{\text{End-diastolic volume}}$$

$$= \frac{70 \text{ mL}}{140 \text{ mL}}$$

= 0.55 or 55%, for a normal adult male

Mediators of Cardiac Output

↑ Preload | ↓ Preload | Sympathetic | Parasympathetic

Frank-Starling Law

↑ Stroke volume | ↓ Stroke volume | ↑ Heart rate | ↓ Heart rate

Cardiac Output

B

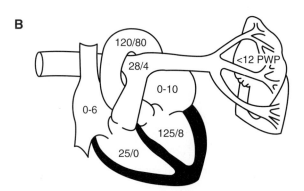

120/80
28/4
<12 PWP
0-10
0-6
125/8
25/0

● **Figure 5-2: (A) Calculations of Stroke volume (SV), cardiac output (CO), and ejection fraction (EF).** A flow chart of the key mediators of cardiac output is shown. Note that cardiac output is effected by both stroke volume and heart rate (i.e., CO = SV × heart rate). This indicates that an increase (or decrease) in either stroke volume or heart rate will increase (or decrease) cardiac output. What causes an increase (or decrease) in stroke volume? The stroke volume is determined primarily by the preload as defined by the Frank-Starling Law, which indicates that as preload increases the stroke volume increases until the stroke volume reaches a plateau. And, as the preload decreases the stroke volume decreases. What causes an increase (or decrease) in heart rate? The heart rate is determined primarily by the sympathetic innervation (increases heart rate) and the parasympathetic innervation (decreases heart rate). If heart rate increases, then cardiac output increases. If heart rate decreases, then cardiac output decreases. However, when the heart rate increases to >150 beats/min, cardiac output decreases because the stroke volume decreases significantly. At >150 beats/min, the stroke volume decreases because the heart spends less time in diastole and therefore the time available for the rapid and reduced ventricular filling phase of the cardiac cycle is decreased. If the heart fills with less blood, the preload is reduced, which affects the stroke volume. **(B) Diagram of normal blood pressures (mm Hg; systole/diastole) within heart chambers and great vessels.** Note that pulmonary wedge pressure (PWP) measured with a Swan-Ganz catheter is a good estimate of left atrial pressure (<12mm Hg).

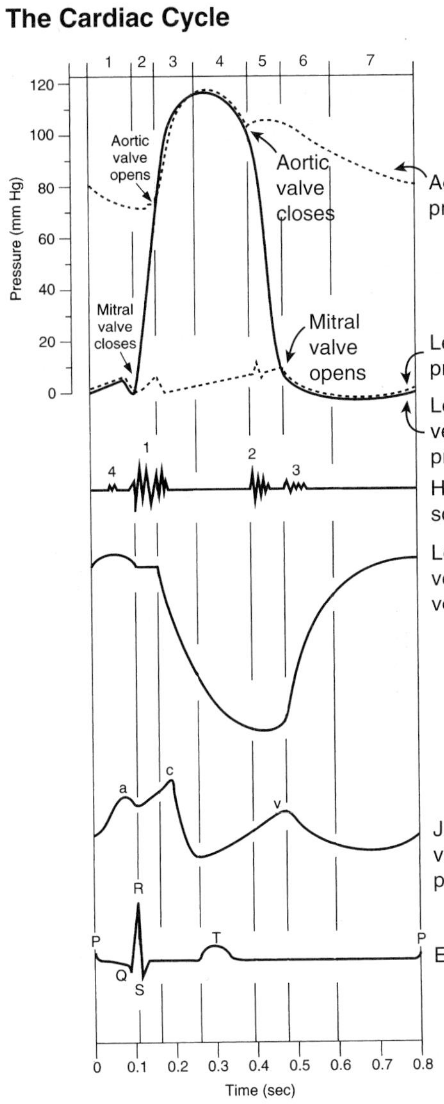

The Cardiac Cycle

● **Figure 5-3: The Cardiac Cycle**. The events in the cardiac cycle are summarized for the left side of the heart. Similar events occur for the right side of the heart although the pressures are reduced. The seven phases (1-7) of the cardiac cycle are separated by the vertical lines. 1: atrial systole 2: isovolumetric ventricular contraction 3: rapid ventricular ejection 4: reduced ventricular ejection 5: isovolumetric ventricular relaxation 6: rapid ventricular filling 7: reduced ventricular filling. Use the ECG (electrocardiogram) as an event marker and note how the jugular venous pressure, left ventricle volume, heart sounds, left ventricle pressure, left atrium pressure, and aortic pressure change during the ECG. **ECG:** P = P wave; QRS = QRS complex; T = T wave.

Jugular venous pressure: The **a wave** is produced by right atrial systole. The a wave increases in amplitude as the vigor of atrial systole increases. A giant a wave (called a **cannon wave**) is observed when the right atrium contracts against a closed tricuspid valve. The **c wave** is produced by right ventricle systole (i.e, the tricuspid valve bulging into atrium). The **v wave** is produced by an increase in right atrial pressure due to filling against the closed tricuspid valve. The v wave terminates when the tricuspid valve opens.

6

General Principles of Cardiovascular System

① Types of Blood Vessels.

A. Elastic (Conducting) Arteries (e.g., pulmonary artery, aorta) have a tunica media with a prominent elastic fiber component that responds to the high systolic pressure generated by the heart.

B. Muscular (Distributing) Arteries have a tunica intima with a prominent internal elastic lamina and a tunica media with a prominent smooth muscle cell component. These vessels are under high pressure and deliver oxygenated blood to tissues.

C. Arterioles have a tunica media that consists of only 1–2 layers of smooth muscle cells and play a major role in regulation of blood pressure. **Metarterioles** are the smallest (or terminal) branches of the arterial system and play a role in regulation of blood flow to capillary beds. Arterioles are the **site of highest resistance** in the cardiovascular system, which is regulated by many of the factors listed above (see IB1-5). At any point in time the blood volume within the arterial circulation is $\cong$ **1L or $\cong$ 25% of total blood volume.**

D. Arteriovenous Anastomoses (AVA) allow arteriolar blood to bypass the capillary bed and empty directly into venules. AVA is found primarily in the skin to regulate body temperature. Constriction of the arteriolar component directs blood to the capillary bed, causing depletion of body heat. Dilation of the arteriolar component directs blood to the venules causing conservation of body heat.

E. Capillaries consist of a single layer of endothelial cells surrounded by a basal lamina. Capillaries have the **largest total cross-sectional and surface area** in the cardiovascular system, are the **site of exchange** of CO_2, O_2, H_2O, nutrients, etc. between blood and cells, and have the **slowest blood velocity.** Although the total cross-sectional and surface area is large, the individual volume of capillaries is small so that at any point in time the blood volume within capillaries is only $\cong$ **200mL or $\cong$ 5% of total blood volume.** Microvasculature damage associated with Type 1 and Type 2 diabetes is due to **nonenzymatic glycosylation** of various proteins, which causes the release of harmful cytokines.

F. Venules are the **most permeable** component of the microcirculation.

G. Veins are thin-walled vessels that are under **low pressure.** The largest blood volume at any point in time is present within the venous circulation ($\cong$ **2L or $\cong$ 70% of total blood volume).**

II **Pumps.** The cardiovascular system consists of two pumps: the **right ventricle** whose output produces the **pulmonary blood flow,** and the **left ventricle** whose output produces the **systemic blood flow.**

III **Factors (Figure 6-1B, C).** The general factors involved in cardiovascular physiology include:

A. **Arterial Pressure**
   1. **Systolic pressure (SP)** is measured after the heart contracts and blood is ejected into the arterial system. SP is the highest arterial pressure during the cardiac cycle.
   2. **Diastolic pressure (DP)** is measured when the heart is relaxed and blood is returning to the heart via the veins. DP is the lowest arterial pressure during the cardiac cycle.
   3. **Pulse pressure (PP)** is the difference between the systolic pressure and diastolic pressure. **Stroke volume** is the most important determinant of PP. SP, DP, and PP increase with **aging** due to a decreased compliance of blood vessels.

$$PP = SP - DP$$
$$= 125 - 85 \text{ mmHg}$$
$$= 40 \text{ mmHg}$$

   4. **Mean arterial pressure (MAP)** is the average arterial pressure over time, is the driving force for blood flow, and decreases as blood moves farther out along the arterial tree. MAP is calculated as indicated below.

$$MAP = DP + 1/3 \ PP$$
$$= DP + 1/3 \ (SP - DP)$$
$$= 85 + 1/3 \ (125 - 85)$$
$$= 85 + 13$$
$$= 98 \text{ mmHg}$$

B. **Venous Pressures**
   1. The pressure within veins is very low ($\cong 15$ mm Hg).
   2. The pressure within the atria is even lower than that within the veins (right atrium: 4 mm Hg vs 15 mm Hg; left atrium: 8 mm Hg vs 15 mm Hg).

C. **Velocity of blood flow** refers to the movement of blood within blood vessels with respect to time (i.e., distance/time or cm/sec) and is expressed by the equation below.

$$V = \frac{Q}{A}$$

where,

V = velocity (cm/sec)
Q = blood flow (cm^3/sec)
A = cross-sectional area of vessel (cm^2)

Note that velocity of blood flow (V) is directly proportional to blood flow (Q). Also, note that velocity of blood flow is indirectly proportional to the cross-sectional area (A) at any level of the cardiovascular system. For example, $A_{aorta} \cong 3cm^2$ and the $A_{capillaries} \cong 1350cm^2$. This means that the velocity of blood flow in the aorta is high whereas the velocity of blood flow in capillaries is low.

D. **Blood Flow** refers to the movement of a volume of blood with respect to time (i.e., volume/time or cm³/sec or ml/min)and is expressed by the equation below.

$$Q = \frac{\Delta P}{R}$$

where,

Q = blood flow (ml/min)
ΔP = pressure gradient (mm Hg)
R = resistance (mmHg/ml/min)

Note that blood flow (Q) is directly proportional to the pressure gradient (ΔP) and therefore blood flow is driven by ΔP such that blood flows from a high pressure to a low pressure. Also, note that blood flow (Q) is indirectly proportional to the resistance (R) of blood vessels.

Or, Cardiac Ouput (CO) = $\dfrac{\text{mean arterial pressure} - \text{right atrial pressure}}{\text{total peripheral resistance (TPR)}}$

E. **Compliance** refers to the distensibility of a blood vessel and is expressed by the equation below.

$$C = \frac{\Delta V}{\Delta P}$$

where,

C = compliance
ΔV = change in volume
ΔP = change in pressure

Note that compliance is the slope relationship between a change in volume and a change in pressure. The compliance of veins is much greater (about 20-fold) than the compliance of arteries, since arteries have much more elastic fibers. Consequently, the largest blood volume at any point in time is present within the venous circulation (≅2L or ≅70% of total blood volume).

 Venous Return and Cardiac Output (Figure 6-2). The relationship between venous return and cardiac output indicates that **venous return must equal cardiac output** over any significant period of time.

A. **Vascular function curve** describes the relationship between **venous return** and **right atrial pressure** (i.e., venous pressure).

B. **Cardiac Function Curve (or Frank Starling curve)** describes the relationship between **cardiac output** and **end-diastolic volume** (see Chapter 5IV).

C. **Cardiovascular Function Curve.** Because both venous return and cardiac output depend upon venous pressure, these two curves are typically combined. The point at which these two curves intersect (called the **steady-state point** or **operating point**) is the only point where the cardiovascular system can operate because venous return must equal cardiac output. Although physiological changes may cause the steady-state point to shift, venous return will always equal cardiac output. These changes are indicated below.

1. **Blood volume changes** shift the only vascular function curve.
2. **Positive and Negative Inotropic factors** shift the only cardiac function curve.
3. **Total peripheral resistance (TPR) changes** shift both the vascular function curve and cardiac output curve. TPR is the resistance of all vessels in the systemic circulation, with by far the largest component being the resistance in the arterioles.

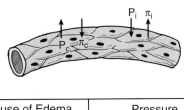

Cause of Edema	Pressure
Heart failure Mitral valve stenosis	Increase in pulmonary P_c
Nephrotic syndrome Liver failure Protein malnutrition	Decrease in π_c
Lymphatic blockage	Increase in π_i
Toxins Infections Burns	Increase in K_f Increase in π_i
Prolonged standing	Increase in P_c

A

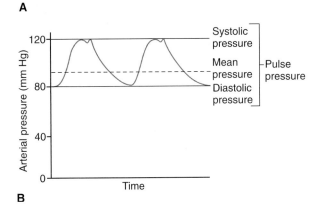

B

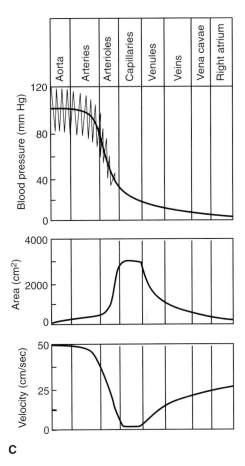

C

● **Figure 6-1: (A)** Fluid exchange across a capillary. There are two pressures associated with the lumen of the capillary. P_c (capillary hydrostatic pressure) favors fluid movement <u>out of</u> the capillary and π_c (capillary oncotic pressure) favors fluid movement <u>into</u> the capillary. There are two pressures associated with the interstitium. P_i (interstitial hydrostatic pressure) favors fluid movement <u>into</u> the capillary and π_i (interstitial oncotic pressure) favors fluid movement <u>out of</u> capillary. K_f is a filtration coefficient that estimates capillary permeability. Edema is a condition whereby excess fluid flows into the interstitium. In left ventricular heart failure or mitral valve stenosis, pulmonary capillary hydrostatic pressure (P_c) will increase and cause pulmonary edema. In nephrotic syndrome, liver failure, or protein malnutrition (starvation), capillary oncotic pressure (π_c) will decrease due to a decrease in plasma protein levels and cause accumulation of fluid in the interstitial space. In lymphatic blockage (e.g., pregnancy, filariasis, or worm infection), interstitial oncotic pressure (π_i) will increase and cause accumulation of fluid in the interstitial space. In toxin exposure, infections, or severe burns, capillary permeability (K_f) will increase and significant amounts of protein and fluid leaks out of the capillaries into the interstitial space. The escaped protein increases interstitial oncotic pressure (π_i), which leads to additional fluid loss. In prolonged standing, capillary hydrostatic pressure (P_c) will increase due to venous pooling of blood and increase local venous pressure and cause accumulation of fluid in the interstitial space. If the lymphatics cannot return the fluid to the circulation, edema will result.Note the various clinical conditions and the causative pressure that lead to edema. **(B)** Diagram of arterial pressures during the cardiac cycle. **(C)** Diagram of the blood pressure, cross-sectional area, and velocity in the aorta → right atrium. As blood flows through the peripheral circulation, the pressure progressively decreases from the aorta → right atrium. The spikes represent the systolic and diastolic pressures during the cardiac cycle. Spikes are not normally observed beyond the arterioles. Note that the largest drop in blood pressure occurs across the arterioles. The largest collective cross-sectional area is the capillaries. The largest velocity is found within the aorta, whereas the slowest velocity is found within the capillaries.

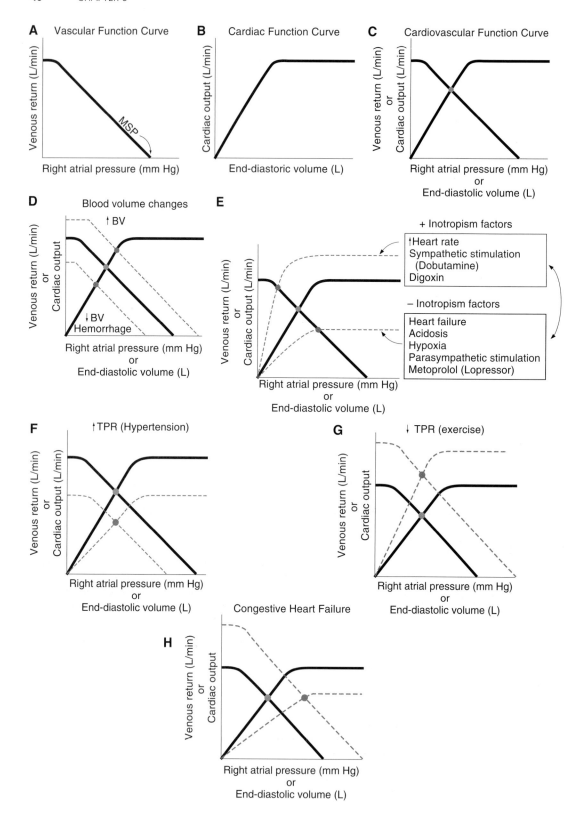

A Vascular Function Curve

Venous return (L/min)

Right atrial pressure (mm Hg)

MSP

B Cardiac Function Curve

Cardiac output (L/min)

End-diastoric volume (L)

C Cardiovascular Function Curve

Venous return (L/min) or Cardiac output (L/min)

Right atrial pressure (mm Hg) or End-diastolic volume (L)

D Blood volume changes

↑BV

↓BV Hemorrhage

Venous return (L/min) or Cardiac output

Right atrial pressure (mm Hg) or End-diastolic volume (L)

E

Venous return (L/min) or Cardiac output (L/min)

Right atrial pressure (mm Hg) or End-diastolic volume (L)

+ Inotropism factors

↑Heart rate
Sympathetic stimulation (Dobutamine)
Digoxin

− Inotropism factors

Heart failure
Acidosis
Hypoxia
Parasympathetic stimulation
Metoprolol (Lopressor)

F ↑TPR (Hypertension)

Venous return (L/min) or Cardiac output (L/min)

Right atrial pressure (mm Hg) or End-diastolic volume (L)

G ↓ TPR (exercise)

Venous return (L/min) or Cardiac output

Right atrial pressure (mm Hg) or End-diastolic volume (L)

H Congestive Heart Failure

Venous return (L/min) or Cardiac output

Right atrial pressure (mm Hg) or End-diastolic volume (L)

● **Figure 6-2: (A) Vascular Function Curve.** Note that as the right atrial pressure (i.e., venous pressure) increases, the venous return decreases. When the right atrial pressure is maximal [called the **mean systemic pressure (MSP)**] the venous return is zero. The MSP is the point at which the vascular function curve intersects the X-axis and is measured when the heart is stopped experimentally. **(B) Cardiac Function Curve.** See Chapter 5IV and Figure 5-2A. **(C) Cardiovascular Curve.** The vascular function curve and cardiac function curve are combined. Note the point at which the two curves intersect (steady-state point or operating point) where venous return and cardiac output are equal. **(D) Blood Volume Changes.** An increased blood volume (BV) shifts the vascular function curve upward. This causes an increased MSP. A new steady-state point is established whereby the cardiac output and right atrial pressure are increased. A decreased blood volume (e.g., hemorrhage) shifts the vascular function curve downward. This causes a decreased MSP. A new steady-state point is established whereby the cardiac output and right atrial pressure are decreased. **(E) Positive and Negative Inotropic Factors.** A positive inotropic factor shifts the cardiac function curve upward. A new steady-state point is established whereby the cardiac output is increased at a correspondingly lower right atrial pressure. The right atrial pressure is lower because more blood is ejected during each heartbeat (i.e., increased stroke volume). A negative inotropic factor shifts the cardiac function curve downward. A new steady-state point is established whereby the cardiac output is decreased at a correspondingly higher right atrial pressure. The right atrial pressure is higher because less blood is ejected during each heartbeat (i.e., decreased stroke volume). **(F) Total Peripheral Resistance (TPR) Changes.** An increased TPR (e.g., hypertension) shifts the vascular function curve downward and the cardiac function curve downward. A new steady-state point is established whereby venous return and cardiac output are decreased, but right atrial pressure is unchanged. A decreased TPR (e.g., exercise) shifts the vascular function curve upward and the cardiac function curve upward. A new steady-state point is established whereby venous return and cardiac output are increased, but right atrial pressure is unchanged. **(G) Congestive Heart Failure.** The primary defect in congestive heart failure is decreased contractility of the heart. This causes the cardiac function curve to shift downward thereby decreasing cardiac output. The renin-angiotensin-aldosterone system causes the kidneys to retain fluids. This causes the vascular function curve to shift upward thereby raising the right atrial pressure. A new steady-state point is established whereby cardiac output tends toward normal, but right atrial pressure is increased.

7
Regulation of Blood Flow

I   **Resistance.** The factors that affect the resistance in blood vessels are derived from the **Poiseuille equation** as indicated below:

$$R = \frac{8nl}{\pi r^4}$$

where,

     R = resistance
     n = viscosity of blood
     l = length of blood vessel
     r = radius of blood vessel

A. **Viscosity of blood.** Resistance is directly proportional to the viscosity of blood. The viscosity of blood is measured by the **hematocrit,** which is the percent volume of blood occupied by the red blood cells (RBCs). A normal hematocrit is **45%.**
   1. **Hematocrit <45%** (e.g., anemia) will decrease resistance in blood vessels and therefore increase blood flow.
   2. **Hematocrit >45%** (e.g., polycythemia, hyperproteinemia caused by multiple myeloma, hereditary spherocytosis) will increase resistance in blood vessels and therefore decrease blood flow.

B. **Length of blood vessel.** Resistance is directly proportional to the length of a blood vessel.

C. **Radius of blood vessel.** Resistance is inversely proportional to r^4. This powerful relationship indicates that if blood vessel radius is decreased by a factor of 2, then resistance increases by a factor of 16 (2^4). For example, **coronary artery atherosclerosis** will increase resistance in blood vessels and therefore decrease blood flow leading to myocardial infarction (MI) or angina.

II   **Resistance in Series and Parallel Circulations (Figure 7-1A,B).**

A. **Series Circulation.** A circulation arranged in series may be illustrated by the arrangement of blood vessels within an individual organ (e.g., kidney). The kidneys are supplied by a large renal artery, smaller arteries, arterioles, capillaries, venules, and large renal vein arranged in series. Under steady-state conditions for a series circulation, blood flow (Q) through all the vascular elements is equal (i.e., Q through the renal artery = 1.1 L/min and Q through the renal capillaries = 1.1 L/min, etc.). The total resistance of a series circulation is the sum of the individual resistances as indicated below.

$$R_T = R_{arteries} + R_{arterioles} + R_{capillaries} + R_{venules} + R_{veins}$$

where,

R_T = total resistance

B. Parallel Circulations. A circulation arranged in parallel may be illustrated by the numerous arteries that branch off the aorta to supply particular areas of the body (e.g., coronary, skin, brain, splanchnic, renal, and muscle). Under steady-state conditions for a parallel circulation, blood flow (Q) to particular areas of the body is not equal (i.e., Q to the brain = 0.8L/min, whereas Q to the muscle = 1.1 L/min, etc.). The total resistance of a parallel circulation is the sum of the reciprocals of the individual resistances as indicated below.

$$R_T = \frac{1}{R_{coronary}} + \frac{1}{R_{skin}} + \frac{1}{R_{brain}} + \frac{1}{R_{other}} + \frac{1}{R_{splanchnic}} + \frac{1}{R_{renal}} + \frac{1}{R_{muscle}}$$

where,

R_T = total resistance

III Laminar versus Turbulent Blood Flow (Figure 7-10).

A. Laminar Flow is flow in layers where the highest velocity is in the center of the blood vessel. Laminar flow occurs throughout the normal cardiovascular system, except the heart. Laminar flow does not generate an audible sound. A **Reynold number <2000** indicates laminar flow.

B. Turbulent Flow is non-layered flow. A **Reynold number >2000** and audible vibration called **bruits** indicate turbulent flow.

C. Measurement of Blood Pressure. Blood pressure is commonly measured by the **Korotkoff auscultatory method** that indirectly measures brachial artery pressure.

IV Methods of Regulation. Regulation of blood flow to an organ is explained by the **metabolic hypothesis,** which states that vasodilator metabolites are released upon an increase in tissue activity, or the **myogenic hypothesis,** which states that vascular smooth muscle contracts upon stretching. Regulation of blood flow to an organ is modified in a number of ways, which include:

A. Autoregulation: is the phenomenon whereby blood flow to an organ remains constant over a wide range of pressures.

B. Active Hyperemia: is the phenomenon whereby blood flow to an organ is proportional to its metabolic activity.

C. Reactive Hyperemia: is the phenomenon whereby blood flow to an organ is increased after a period of occlusion.

Types of Circulation.

TABLE 7-1		TYPES OF CIRCULATION		
Circulation	% of cardiac output	Blood Flow Demonstrates	Control
Coronary	5%	Autoregulation Active hyperemia Reactive hyperemia	**Hypoxia, adenosine, and NO** cause vasodilation Increased O2 demand is met by increased coronary blood flow
Cerebral	15%	Autoregulation Active hyperemia Reactive hyperemia	**Increased P_{aCO2} or decreased pH** cause vasodilation
Skeletal Muscle	20%	Autoregulation Active hyperemia Reactive hyperemia	**During exercise:** **Lactate, adenosine,** and **K**+ cause vasodilation **At rest:** Sympathetic innervation through NE* release stimulates α_1**-adrenergic receptors,** causing vasoconstriction Sympathetic innervation through NE release stimulates β_2**-adrenergic receptors,** causing vasodilation
Kidney	25%	Autoregulation	Renal blood flow remains constant from 100–200 mm of Hg arterial pressure Highest blood flow per gram of tissue
Respiratory	100%	**Hypoxic vasoconstriction**	Hypoxia causes vasoconstriction so that blood is directed away from poorly ventilated areas to well-ventilated areas of the lung; it is the only circulation that responds to hypoxia by vasoconstriction
Skin	5%	Temperature regulation	Increase in temperature: Sympathetic innervation causes vasodilation directing blood to the surface

NE = norepinephrine; NO = nitric oxide

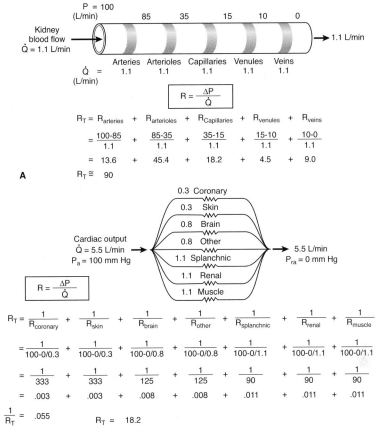

A

$$P = 100 \quad 85 \quad 35 \quad 15 \quad 10 \quad 0$$
(L/min)

Kidney blood flow $\dot{Q} = 1.1$ L/min → → 1.1 L/min

$$\begin{array}{cccccc} & \text{Arteries} & \text{Arterioles} & \text{Capillaries} & \text{Venules} & \text{Veins} \\ \dot{Q} = & 1.1 & 1.1 & 1.1 & 1.1 & 1.1 \\ \text{(L/min)} \end{array}$$

$$R = \frac{\Delta P}{\dot{Q}}$$

$$R_T = R_{arteries} + R_{arterioles} + R_{Capillaries} + R_{venules} + R_{veins}$$

$$= \frac{100\text{-}85}{1.1} + \frac{85\text{-}35}{1.1} + \frac{35\text{-}15}{1.1} + \frac{15\text{-}10}{1.1} + \frac{10\text{-}0}{1.1}$$

$$= 13.6 + 45.4 + 18.2 + 4.5 + 9.0$$

$$R_T \cong 90$$

B

0.3 Coronary
0.3 Skin
0.8 Brain
0.8 Other
1.1 Splanchnic
1.1 Renal
1.1 Muscle

Cardiac output $\dot{Q} = 5.5$ L/min $P_a = 100$ mm Hg → → 5.5 L/min $P_{ra} = 0$ mm Hg

$$R = \frac{\Delta P}{\dot{Q}}$$

$$R_T = \frac{1}{R_{coronary}} + \frac{1}{R_{skin}} + \frac{1}{R_{brain}} + \frac{1}{R_{other}} + \frac{1}{R_{splanchnic}} + \frac{1}{R_{renal}} + \frac{1}{R_{muscle}}$$

$$= \frac{1}{100\text{-}0/0.3} + \frac{1}{100\text{-}0/0.3} + \frac{1}{100\text{-}0/0.8} + \frac{1}{100\text{-}0/0.8} + \frac{1}{100\text{-}0/1.1} + \frac{1}{100\text{-}0/1.1} + \frac{1}{100\text{-}0/1.1}$$

$$= \frac{1}{333} + \frac{1}{333} + \frac{1}{125} + \frac{1}{125} + \frac{1}{90} + \frac{1}{90} + \frac{1}{90}$$

$$= .003 + .003 + .008 + .008 + .011 + .011 + .011$$

$$\frac{1}{R_T} = .055 \qquad R_T = 18.2$$

C Korotkoff sounds

None	Repetitive crisp sounds	Muffled	None
Cuff pressure >120 mm Hg	Cuff pressure 120-60 mm Hg	Cuff pressure 60-50 mm Hg	Cuff pressure <50 mm Hg
Blood flow Occluded	Turbulent	Turbulent	Laminar

Korotkoff sounds	Systolic	Diastolic
Normal	<120	<80
Pre-hypertension	120-139	80-89
Stage 1 hypertension	140-159	90-99
Stage 2 hypertension	160-179	100-109
Stage 3 hypertension	>180	>110

● **Figure 7-1: (A) Series Circulation.** Note that under steady-state conditions for a series circulation, blood flow (Q) through all the vascular elements is equal. Blood flow (Q) into the kidney = 1.1 L/min, Q through the renal arteries, arterioles, capillaries, venules, and veins = 1.1 L/min, and Q out of the kidney = 1.1. L/min. Note also that the pressure (P) decreases (from 100 → 0 mm Hg) as blood flows through a series circulation like the kidney; and, therefore the ΔP varies across the various vascular elements. **(B) Parallel Circulations.** Note that under steady-state conditions for a parallel circulation, blood flow (Q) to particular areas of the body is not equal. Q varies from 0.3 L/min to 1.1 L/min. Note also that the pressure (P) is the same in each parallel circulation, and therefore the ΔP does not vary with each parallel circulation (100 − 0 = 100 mm Hg). The total resistance (18.2) is less than the resistance in each parallel circulation (e.g., $R_{coronary}$ = 333, R_{brain} = 125, R_{renal} = 90). When an artery is added in parallel, the total resistance decreases. P_a = arterial pressure; P_{ra} = pressure in right atrium. **(C) Measurement of Blood Pressure.** An inflatable cuff is wrapped around the arm at the level of the heart. The cuff is inflated to a pressure higher than the systolic pressure (e.g., >120 mm Hg) which completely occludes blood flow in the brachial artery and no Korotkoff sounds are heard. As the cuff pressure is lowered below systolic pressure (e.g., 120 → 60 mm Hg), blood flow through the brachial artery becomes turbulent and repetitive, faint, crisp sounds (Korotkoff sounds) are heard with a stethoscope. As cuff pressure is further reduced (e.g., 60 → 50 mm Hg), blood flow through the brachial artery becomes continuous but is still relatively turbulent such that muffled Korotkoff sounds are heard. Muffled Korotkoff sounds are heard when the blood pressure is 5–10 mm Hg greater than diastolic pressure. As cuff pressure is further reduced below diastolic pressure (e.g., <50 mm Hg), blood flow through the brachial artery becomes continuous and laminar such that no Korotkoff sounds are heard. The latest guidelines for normal blood pressure, pre-hypertensive stage, Stage 1, Stage 2, and Stage 3 hypertension are indicated.

8
Regulation of Arterial Blood Pressure

General Features. In most people, the daily average mean arterial blood pressure is strictly regulated at about **100 mm Hg** with fluctuations of $\pm$**20 mm Hg.** This strict regulation provides organs with a blood flow at a constant perfusion pressure and minimizes cardiac, vascular, and renal damage. There are two main mechanisms that regulate arterial blood pressure as indicated below.

A. **Baroreceptor Mechanism** involves the **autonomic nervous system** and regulates blood pressure in a **fast, moment-to-moment, neurotransmitter fashion.** The baroreceptors are stretch receptors that monitor **changes in blood pressure** and are located in the walls of the common carotid arteries (i.e., **carotid sinus**), great veins, atria, and aortic arch. **CN IX** (also called **Hering nerve** or **carotid sinus nerve**) innervates the carotid sinus and relays information to the central nervous system (CNS). **CN X** innervates the baroceptors in the great veins, atria, and aortic arch and relays information to the CNS. The CNS elicits control of the parasympathetic and sympathetic nervous system as indicated below.

1. **Parasympathetic Control.** The parasympathetic innervation elicits the following actions in the heart.
   a. Decreases heart rate (negative chronotropism)
   b. Decreases conduction velocity (negative dromotropism)
   c. Decreases contractility (negative inotropism).
2. **Sympathetic Control.** The sympathetic innervation elicits the following actions in the heart, arterioles, and veins.
   a. Increases heart rate (positive chronotropism)
   b. Increases conduction velocity (positive dromotropism)
   c. Increases contractility (positive inotropism).
   d. Increases vasoconstriction of arterioles and veins

B. **Renin-Angiotensin II Mechanism** involves the **juxtaglomerular (JG) complex** of the kidney and regulates blood pressure in a **slow, long-term, hormonal fashion.** The JG complex regulates blood pressure in three different ways, all of which effect **renin** release from JG cells (modified smooth muscle cells of the afferent arteriole).

1. The JG complex contains **macula densa (MD) cells** that monitor **changes in Na^+** within the fluid of the distal straight tubule (DST) and effect **renin** release.
2. The JG complex contains **JG cells** (which act as intrarenal baroreceptors) that monitor **changes in blood pressure** and effect **renin** release.

3. JG cells are innervated by sympathetic nerves under the control of peripheral baroreceptors (e.g., carotid sinus) that monitor **changes in blood pressure** and effect **renin** release.

4. **Renin** is an enzyme that converts **angiotensinogen** (produced by the liver) to **angiotensin I**. Angiotensin I is converted to **angiotensin II** (primarily by endothelium of lung capillaries) by **angiotensin converting enzyme (ACE).** Angiotensin II has widespread actions as indicated below.

   a. Affects vascular smooth muscle
   b. Affects CNS and PNS to modulate sympathetic activity
   c. Affects the adrenal cortex to modulate aldosterone
   d. Affects the kidneys to modulate Na^+ reabsorption and glomerular filtration rate (GFR)
   e. Affects the CNS to modulate anti-diuretic hormone (ADH)
   f. Affects the CNS to modulate thirst.

Ⅱ Clinical Considerations.

A. **Hemorrhagic or Hypovolemic Shock: Response to Decreased Blood Pressure. (Figure 8-1).** The physiological response to hemorrhage involves both the baroreceptor mechanism and the renin-angiotensin II mechanism.

1. **Baroreceptor Mechanism.**

   a. A decreased stretch on the baroreceptors is relayed via CN IX and CN X to the CNS, which in turn inhibits the parasympathetic nervous system. This elicits the following actions: increases heart rate (positive chronotropism), increases conduction velocity (positive dromotropism), increases contractility (positive inotropism). These actions will increase arterial blood pressure.

   b. A decreased stretch on the baroreceptors is relayed via CN IX and CN X to the CNS, which in turn stimulates the sympathetic nervous system. This elicits the following actions: increases heart rate (positive chronotropism), increases conduction velocity (positive dromotropism), increases contractility (positive inotropism) and increases vasoconstriction of arterioles and veins. These actions will increase arterial blood pressure.

2. **Renin-Angiotensin II Mechanism.** The MD cells sense a decreased Na^+ in the DST fluid while the JG cells and sympathetic nerves sense a decreased blood pressure. This causes an increased renin release and increased angiotensin II. Increased angiotensin II elicits the following actions:

   a. Affects vascular smooth muscle to contract, which increases arteriolar and venous constriction and leads to increased peripheral resistance.

   b. Affects the CNS and PNS to increase sympathetic activity which increases arteriolar and venous constriction and leads to increased peripheral resistance and to increased cardiac output.

   c. Affects the adrenal cortex to increase aldosterone (ALD) secretion, which increases Na^+ reabsorption and leads to decreased Na^+ and H_2O excretion in the urine.

   d. Affects the kidneys to increase Na^+ reabsorption by the proximal convoluted tubule (PCT) and decrease glomerular filtration rate (GFR) by vasoconstriction of the afferent and efferent arterioles, both of which lead to decreased Na^+ and H_2O excretion in the urine.

   e. Affects the CNS (i.e., neurohypophysis) to increase anti-diuretic hormone (ADH) secretion, which works synergistically with ALD and increases H_2O reabsorption, both of which lead to decreased Na^+ and H_2O excretion in the urine.

f.   Affects the CNS to increase the sensation of thirst, which increases H_2O ingestion and leads to decreased Na^+ and H_2O excretion in the urine.

g.   The increased peripheral resistance, increased cardiac output, and decreased Na^+ and H_2O excretion in the urine are physiological actions that increase arterial blood pressure.

B. **Hypertension (HTN): Response to Increased Blood Pressure. (Figure 8-2).** Stage 1 HTN is defined as blood pressure $\geq$140/90 measured on three separate days. Almost all cases of HTN (95%) are **idiopathic** and called **essential or primary HTN.** The remainder of the cases (5%) are called **secondary HTN.** The causes of secondary HTN are aortic regurgitation, patent ductus arteriosus, coarctation of the aorta, glomerular disease, renal artery stenosis, Cushing syndrome, Conn syndrome, pheochromocytoma, hyperthyroidism, and iatrogenic causes ("white coat HTN"). The physiological response to HTN involves both the baroreceptor mechanism and the renin-angiotensin II mechanism.

1. **Baroreceptor Mechanism.**

a.   An increased stretch on the baroreceptors is relayed via CN IX and CN X to the CNS, which in turn stimulates the parasympathetic nervous system. This elicits the following actions: decreases heart rate (negative chronotropism), decreases conduction velocity (negative dromotropism), decreases contractility (negative inotropism). These actions will decrease arterial blood pressure.

b.   An increased stretch on the baroreceptors is relayed via CN IX and CN X to the CNS, which in turn inhibits the sympathetic nervous system. This elicits the following actions: decreases heart rate (negative chronotropism), decreases conduction velocity (negative dromotropism), decreases contractility (negative inotropism) and decreases vasoconstriction of arterioles and veins. These actions will decrease arterial blood pressure.

2. **Renin-Angiotensin II Mechanism.** The MD cells sense a increased Na^+ in the DST fluid while the JG cells and sympathetic nerves sense an increased blood pressure. This causes an decreased renin release and decreased angiotensin II. Decreased angiotensin II elicits the following actions:

a.   Affects vascular smooth muscle to relax, which decreases arteriolar and venous constriction and leads to decreased peripheral resistance.

b.   Affects the CNS and PNS to decrease sympathetic activity, which decreases arteriolar and venous constriction and leads to decreased peripheral resistance and to decreased cardiac output.

c.   Affects the adrenal cortex to decrease aldosterone (ALD) secretion, which decreases Na^+ reabsorption and leads to increased Na^+ and H_2O excretion in the urine.

d.   Affects the kidneys to decrease Na^+ reabsorption by the proximal convoluted tubule (PCT) and increase glomerular filtration rate (GFR) because the vasoconstriction effect by angiotensin II on the afferent and efferent arterioles is not present; both of which lead to increased Na^+ and H_2O excretion in the urine.

e.   Affects the CNS (i.e., neurohypophysis) to decrease anti-diuretic hormone (ADH) secretion, which works synergistically with ALD and decreases H_2O reabsorption, both of which lead to increased Na^+ and H_2O excretion in the urine.

f.   Affects the CNS to decrease the sensation of thirst, which decreases H_2O ingestion and leads to increased Na^+ and H_2O excretion in the urine.

g.   The decreased peripheral resistance, decreased cardiac output, and increased Na^+ and H_2O excretion in the urine are physiological actions that decrease arterial blood pressure.

Ⅲ **Pressure Natriuresis and Pressure Diuresis Theory.** This theory indicates that the ability of the kidneys to excrete Na^+ and H_2O in the urine is directly dependent on arterial blood pressure. Consequently, as arterial blood pressure rises, excretion of Na^+ and H_2O in the urine increases, which results in a decrease of blood volume. The consequence of this theory is that long-term blood pressure control is dependent on kidney excretory ability, whereas, short-term blood pressure control is dependent of peripheral vascular resistance.

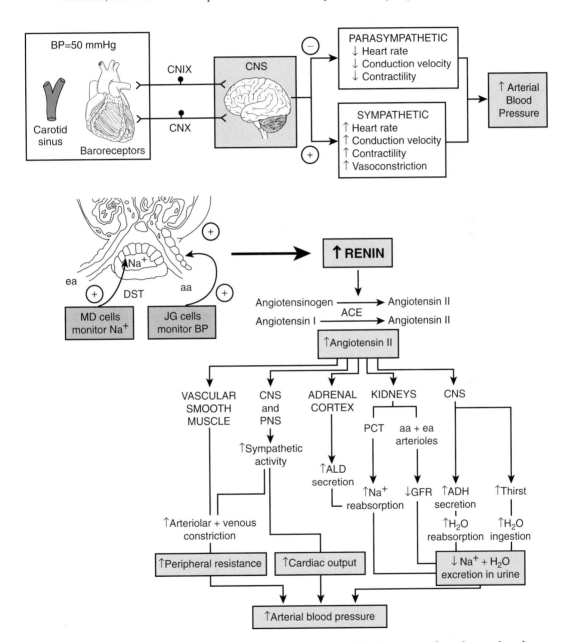

● **Figure 8-1: Flow chart of physiological responses to decreased blood pressure (e.g., hemorrhage).** + = stimulation; − = inhibition; ↑ = increases; ↓ = decreases; DST = distal straight tubule; ea = efferent arteriole; aa = afferent arteriole; JG = juxtaglomerular; ACE = angiotensin converting enzyme; PCT = proximal convoluted tubule; ALD = aldosterone; ADH = anti-diuretic hormone; GFR = glomerular filtration rate; BP = blood pressure; CNS = central nervous system; PNS = peripheral nervous system; MD = macula densa cells; CN X = cranial nerve X (vagus nerve); CN IX = cranial nerve IX (glossopharyngeal nerve).

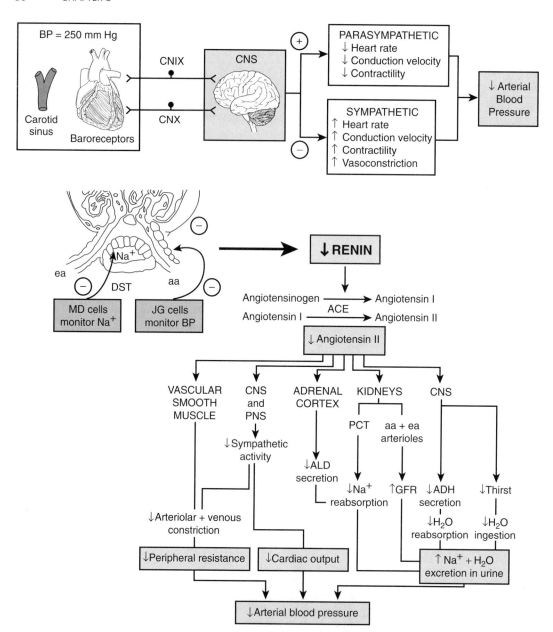

● **Figure 8-2: Flow chart of physiological responses to increased blood pressure (e.g., hypertension).** The efferent arteriole is more sensitive to angiotensin II than the afferent arteriole. Therefore, constriction of the efferent arteriole predominates at low angiotensin II levels, and constriction of both the efferent and afferent arteriole occurs at high angiotensin II levels. + = stimulation; − = inhibition; ↑ = increases; ↓ = decreases; DST = distal straight tubule; ea = efferent arteriole; aa = afferent arteriole; JG = juxtaglomerular; ACE = angiotensin converting enzyme; PCT = proximal convoluted tubule; ALD = aldosterone; ADH = anti-diuretic hormone; GFR = glomerular filtration rate; BP = blood pressure; CNS = central nervous system; PNS = peripheral nervous system; MD = macula densa cells; CN X = cranial nerve X (vagus nerve); CN IX = cranial nerve IX (glossopharyngeal nerve).

9
Cardiovascular Responses to Gravity

I ## Effect of Gravity in the Upright Position.

A. **Above the level of the heart,** venous pressure quickly becomes subatmospheric (or negative) and arterial pressure progressively decreases towards subatmospheric (or negative). Superficial veins above the heart cannot maintain a subatmospheric pressure. Consequently, if a superficial vein is severed or punctured, air may be introduced into the circulatory system (air embolus).

B. **At the level of the heart,** venous pressure equals **2 mm Hg** and arterial pressure equals **100 mm Hg.** The pressure difference is **98 mm Hg** (100 − 2 = 98).

C. **Below the level of the heart,** venous pressure and arterial pressure increase equally (by ~80 mm Hg) assuming no muscular action, so that venous pressure equals **82 mm Hg** and arterial pressure equals **180 mm Hg.** The pressure difference is still **98 mm Hg** (180 − 82 = 98). Note that the pressure difference at the level of the heart and the level of the ankles is the same (i.e., 98 mm Hg). Because veins are very compliant, the higher venous pressure in veins below the level of the heart indicates a significant **venous pooling** of blood (this pool of blood does not contribute to the cardiac output).

II ## Movement From Supine to Upright Position (Figure 9-1).

A. **In the supine position,** the legs are at the same level as the heart so that the gravitational forces that come into play in the upright position are diminished. Therefore, venous pressure and venous pooling of blood in the legs is decreased in the supine position.

B. **When a person stands,** gravitational forces come into play. Therefore, venous pressure and venous pooling of blood in the legs is increased. This decreases blood volume and venous return to the heart. As a result of the decreased venous return, **stroke volume** and **cardiac output decrease.**

C. The decrease in cardiac output causes a **decrease in arterial blood pressure.** If cerebral blood pressure decreases low enough, **fainting or lightheadedness when a person stands (i.e., orthrostatic hypotension)** may occur.

D. The physiological response to the decrease in arterial blood pressure that occurs when a person stands involves the **baroreceptor mechanism** which results in a **compensatory increase in arterial blood pressure** (see Chapter 8IIA and Figure 8-1)

E. In patients being treated with sympatholytic drugs (e.g., α_1-blockers, β-blockers) for hypertension, the sympathetic response necessary for the compensatory increase in arterial blood pressure when a person stands is impaired. These patients generally experience orthostatic hypotension.

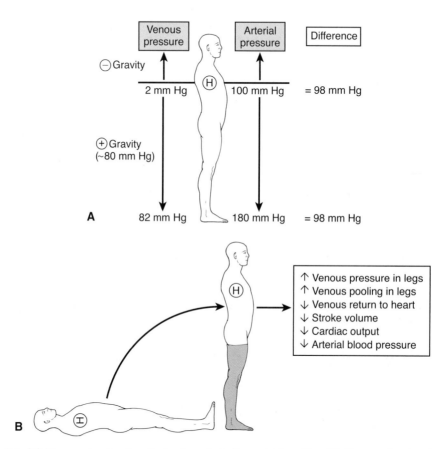

● **Figure 9-1: (A)** Diagram showing the effects of gravity in the upright position. **(B)** Diagram showing the effects of movement from the supine to upright position. Note the physiological changes that occur due to the movement from the supine to upright position (boxed area). The decrease in arterial blood pressure is quickly corrected by a compensatory increase in arterial blood pressure using the baroreceptor mechanism and the autonomic nervous system. Note also that sympatholytic drugs may block the compensatory increase in arterial blood pressure leading to orthostatic hypotension. H = heart

10

Lung Mechanics

I Lung Volumes and Capacities (Figure 10-1).

A. Static pulmonary mechanics refers to the mechanical forces acting on the lung and chest wall that determine lung volume. **Lung volumes** are compartments of the lung that contain air and are measured by various techniques (lung volumes are not visible on radiographs). **Lung capacities** are two or more volumes that are added together. The lung increases in size from birth to late teens, plateaus, the declines with aging. Age-related changes in the lung volumes include: decrease in vital capacity (VC), total lung capacity (TLC), and expiratory reserve volume (ERV); increase in residual volume (RV); no change in functional residual capacity (FRC).

B. The Physiologic Role of FRC. Breathing is a cyclical process, whereas blood flow through the lung capillary bed is continuous process. During the respiratory cycle, short periods of apnea occur, at which times there is no ventilation but blood flow continues. The FRC acts as a reservoir for continued gas exchange during the apneic periods. Without FRC, high levels of deoxygenated blood from the pulmonary capillaries would empty into pulmonary veins and consequently lower the partial pressure of arterial oxygen (P_{aO2}). This would in effect constitute an intrapulmonary shunt.

II Breathing.

A. The Breathing Cycle (Figure 10-2A). In order to understand the breathing cycle, three parameters are considered:
1. **Lung volumes,** particularly the **functional residual capacity (FRC)** and **tidal volume (TV).**
2. **Alveolar pressure (P_A)** is expressed relative to atmospheric pressure (P_{atm}; 760 mm Hg at sea level). When P_A equals P_{atm}, the P_A is said to be **zero.** When P_A is greater than P_{atm}, the P_A is said to be **positive.** When P_A is less than P_{atm}, the P_A is said to be **negative.**
3. **Intrapleural pressure (P_{IP})** is the pressure within the pleural cavity lying between the chest wall and lung. At rest, there is an outward expanding force on the chest wall and an inward collapsing force on the lung. As a result of these two opposing forces, P_{IP} is **negative (-4 mm Hg or -5 cm H_2O).**

B. Clinical consideration. Open Pneumothorax occurs when the parietal pleura is pierced and the pleural cavity is opened to the outside atmosphere. This causes a loss of the negative P_{IP} because P_{IP} now equals P_{atm} (P_{IP} changes from -4 mm Hg $\rightarrow$ $+760$ mm Hg). This results in the **expanded chest wall** (its natural tendency) and a **collapsed lung** (its natural tendency).

III **Elastance** of the lung is the collapsing force that develops in the lung as the lung expands. Elastance always acts to collapse the lung. One can think of elastance as the collapsing force that builds up in a balloon completely inflated with air. The components that contribute to elastance are:

A. Collagen and **elastic fibers** within the lung (minor component)

B. Surface tension of the alveoli (major component)
   1. Surface tension is created at the air/surfactant interface. The relationship between elastance and surface tension is describe by the **Laplace law** below:

$$E = \frac{2T}{r}$$

where,

   E = collapsing force (elastance)
   T = surface tension
   r = radius of alveolus

The Laplace law indicates that:
   a. **Large alveoli ($\uparrow r$)** have a low collapsing force (elastance) and are easy to keep open.
   b. **Small alveoli ($\downarrow r$)** have a high collapsing force (elastance) and are difficult to keep open.

   2. Surfactant is a surface-active detergent that consists of **phosphatidylcholine** (mainly **dipalmitoyl lecithin**) and **surfactant proteins A, B, and C** produced by **Type II pneumocytes.** Surfactant lines alveoli and reduces surface tension and therefore prevents collapse of small alveoli (atelectasis).

   3. Clinical consideration. Neonatal Respiratory Distress Syndrome (NRDS) is caused by a deficiency of surfactant, which may occur due to prolonged intrauterine asphyxia, in premature infants, or in infants of diabetic mothers. Lung maturation is assessed by the **lecithin:sphingomyelin ratio** in amniotic fluid (a ratio $>$ 2:1 = maturity). **Thyroxine** and **cortisol** treatment can increase surfactant production. Pathologically, the lung shows hemorrhagic edema, atelectasis, and **hyaline membrane disease** characterized by eosinophilic material consisting of proteinaceous fluid (fibrin, plasma) and necrotic cells.

IV **Compliance of the lung (Figure 10-2B)** is the change in lung volume (ΔLV) divided by the change in intrapleural pressure (ΔP_{IP}) given by the equation below. Or, compliance of the lung is the slope of the line between any two points on a **pressure-volume curve.** One can think of compliance as describing the **distensibility** of the lung (or the ease with which a balloon can be inflated with air). Compliance of the lung is **increased** in obstructive lung diseases (e.g. emphysema) and compliance is **decreased** in restrictive lung diseases (e.g., idiopathic pulmonary fibrosis)

$$C = \frac{\Delta LV}{\Delta P_{IP}}$$

where,

    C = compliance
    ΔLV = change in lung volume
    ΔP_{IP} = change in intrapleural pressure

V Flow-Volume Curves (Figure 10-2C).

A flow-volume curve is generated by having an individual inspire maximally to total lung capacity (TLC) and then exhale to residual volume (RV) forcibly, rapidly, and as completely as possible.

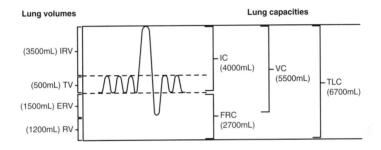

Volume/Capacity	Normal Value	Description
Inspiratory Reserve Volume (IRV)	3500mL	Volume inspired above the tidal volume
Tidal Volume (TV)	500mL	Volume of a normal breath
Expiratory Reserve Volume (ERV)	1500mL	Volume expired after expiration of tidal volume Decreases with age
Residual Volume (RV)	1200mL	Volume that remains after maximal expiration Increases with age Cannot be measured by spirometry RV = FRC − ERV
Inspiratory Capacity (IC)	4000mL	IC = IRV + TV
Functional Residual Capacity (FRC)	2700mL	Volume remaining after TV is expired No change with age FRC = ERV − RV
Vital Capacity (VC)	5500mL	Volume expired after maximal inspiration Decreases with age VC = TLC − RV
Total Lung Capacity (TLC)	6700mL	Volume that lung can maximally hold Decreases with age TLC = IRV + TV + ERV + RV
Dead Space (DS)	Anatomic DS = 150mL	**Anatomic DS:** Portion of the breath that remains in the conducting airways **Alveolar DS:** Portion of the breath entering alveoli that receive no or reduced blood flow **Physiologic DS:** Portion of breath that does not participate in gas exchange **Physiologic DS = Anatomic DS + Alveolar DS**
Forced Vital Capacity (FVC)	5500mL	Volume forcibly expired after maximal inspiration Pulmonary function tests measure FVC
Forced Expiratory Volume (FEV$_1$)	4400mL (80% of FVC) FEV$_1$/FVC=0.8	Volume expired in 1 second during an FVC maneuver

* Physiologic DS = TV x $\dfrac{P_{aco_2} - P_{Eco_2}}{P_{aco_2}}$ where TV = tidal volume, $P_{aco_2} = P_{co_2}$ of arterial blood, $P_{Eco_2} = P_{co_2}$ of expired air

● **Figure 10-1:** Spirometry diagram of lung volumes and capacities.

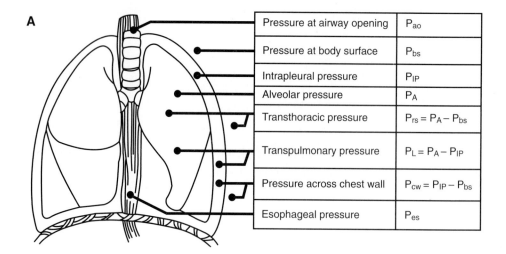

Pressure at airway opening	P_{ao}
Pressure at body surface	P_{bs}
Intrapleural pressure	P_{IP}
Alveolar pressure	P_A
Transthoracic pressure	$P_{rs} = P_A - P_{bs}$
Transpulmonary pressure	$P_L = P_A - P_{IP}$
Pressure across chest wall	$P_{cw} = P_{IP} - P_{bs}$
Esophageal pressure	P_{es}

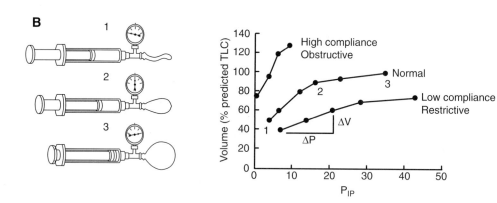

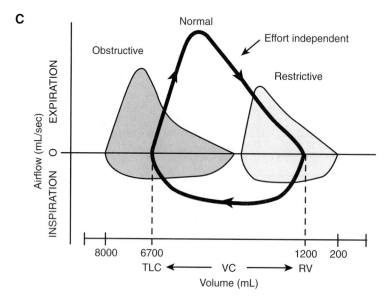

● **Figure 10-2: (A)** Diagram of the various pressures involved in breathing. The transthoracic pressure (P_{rs}) is the pressure across the entire respiratory system. The transpulmonary pressure (P_L) is the pressure across the lung. **(B)** A simple way to visualize compliance is inflating a balloon and measuring the pressure. For each change in pressure (1, 2, 3; note change in syringe and manometer), the balloon inflates to a new volume, so that compliance can be defined as the slope of the line ($\Delta V/\Delta P$) between any two points on a pressure-volume curve. In a lung with normal compliance, for a given change in intrapleural pressure, a certain amount of air will enter the lung. In a lung with low compliance (as seen in restrictive lung diseases), for a given change in intrapleural pressure, less air will flow into the lung. In a lung with high compliance (as seen in obstructive lung diseases), for a given change in intrapleural pressure, more air will flow into the lung. **(C)** Flow-volume curve. A normal maximal flow-volume curve is shown (thick line). Note that the air flow rises rapidly at the beginning of expiration near the total lung capacity (TLC = 6700mL). Then air flow decreases linearly as lung volume decreases to residual volume (RV = 1200mL), which is called the effort independent phase. During the effort independent phase, no matter how hard the individual tries (i.e., effort), they will be unable to change this part of the curve. This occurs because during forced expiration high intrathoracic pressures (5–10 times above resting) place airways under considerable pressure. If the airways are histologically normal, the airways will become somewhat compressed (but remain patent) during forced expiration and thereby limit airflow. Vital capacity (VC) equals TLC minus RV. In obstructive lung diseases, the flow-volume curve is shifted to the left as the TLC and RV are both increased. If airways are histologically abnormal due to a disease process (e.g., emphysema), during a forced expiration the high intrathoracic pressures will significantly compress the airways and significantly reduced the airway diameter. In severe cases, the airways may completely collapse during forced expiration and cause air trapping. In restrictive lung diseases, the flow-volume curve is shifted to the right as the TLC and RV are both decreased.

11

Alveolar-Blood Gas Exchange

I **Partial Pressure (P) (Table 11-1)** of a gas in air is described by the **Dalton Law** as given below:

$$P = P_{atm} \times F_{gas}$$

where,

P	=	partial pressure
P_{atm}	=	atmospheric pressure (760 mm Hg)
P_{water}	=	partial pressure of water (47 mm Hg)
F_{gas}	=	fractional gas concentration; the composition of air is: $N_2 = 78\%$, $O_2 = 21\%$, $CO_2 = \approx 0\%$

TABLE 11-1	PARTIAL PRESSURES OF O_2 AND CO_2	
Dry air	$P_{O2} = 160$ mm Hg $P_{CO2} = 0$	$P_{O2} = 760$ mm Hg $\times$ 0.21 = 160 $P_{CO2} = 760$ mm Hg $\times$ 0.0 = 0
Inspired humidified air	$P_{IO2} = 150$ mm Hg $P_{ICO2} = 0$	$P_{O2} = (760 - 47$ mm Hg$) \times 0.21 = 150$ $P_{CO2} = 760$ mm Hg $\times$ 0.0 = 0
Alveolar air	$P_{AO2} = 100$ mm Hg $P_{ACO2} = 40$ mm Hg	O_2 diffuses from alveoli $\rightarrow$ capillary blood CO_2 diffuses from capillary blood $\rightarrow$ alveoli
Systemic arterial blood	$P_{aO2} = 95$ mm Hg $P_{aCO2} = 40$ mm Hg	Blood has equilibrated with alveolar air P_{O2} is <100 mm Hg because of the physiologic shunt*
Mixed venous blood	$P_{vO2} = 40$ mm Hg $P_{vCO2} = 46$ mm Hg	O_2 has diffused from arterial blood $\rightarrow$ tissues CO_2 has diffused from tissues $\rightarrow$ venous blood

II **Air flow** through the lung from the bronchi to alveoli is inversely proportional to airway resistance.

A. Airway resistance is described by the **Poiseuille Law** as shown below:

$$R = \frac{8n\,l}{\pi\,r^4}$$

where,

    R = resistance
    n = viscosity of inspired gas
    l = length of airway
    r = radius of airway

Note the strong relationship of r to R. If airway radius (r) is reduced by a factor of 2, then airway resistance (R) is increased by a factor of 16 (2^4). Therefore, air flow will be dramatically reduced.

    B. The **medium-sized bronchi** are the **main site of airway resistance** through the contraction or relaxation of bronchial smooth muscle.

III **Blood-Air Barrier.** The components of the blood-air barrier are the: **surfactant layer, Type I pneumocyte, basement membrane,** and **capillary endothelial cell.**

IV **Rate of Diffusion (RD) of O_2 and CO_2** across the blood-air barrier is governed by the **Fick Law** indicated below:

$$RD = \frac{A}{T} \times D \times (P_1 - P_2)$$

where,

    A = surface area of alveoli
    T = thickness of blood–air barrier
    D = solubility of the gas
    $P_1 - P_2$ = pressure difference across blood–air barrier

Note that increases in the surface area of alveoli, solubility of gas, and pressure difference will increase the rate of diffusion of O_2 and CO_2 across the blood–air barrier. However, increases in the thickness of the blood–air barrier will decrease the rate of diffusion of O_2 and CO_2 across the blood–air barrier.

V **Alveolar-arterial (A-a) Gradient** is the difference between the alveolar P_{O2} (P_{AO2} = A) and arterial P_{O2} (P_{aO2} = a). The A-a gradient indicates how well O_2 is equilibrating across the blood–air barrier.

    A. Normal Condition. In a normal lung, P_{AO2} = 100 mm Hg and P_{aO2} = 95 mm Hg (see Table 12-1) such that the **A-a gradient =100 − 95 = 5.** This is due to the fact that normally **2% of cardiac output** bypasses alveolar ventilation caused almost exclusively by the **bronchial circulation** (i.e, deoxygenated bronchial venous blood drains into oxygenated pulmonary venous blood; called **venous admixture**). This is referred to as a right-to-left **physiologic shunt.**

    B. Tetralogy of Fallot is a congenital heart condition such that there is skewed development of the aorticopulmonary (AP) septum. This results in a condition characterized by: **pulmonary stenosis, overriding aorta, interventricular (IV) septal defect,** and **right ventricular hypertrophy.** The resultant right-to-left shunt of blood leads to a decrease in P_{aO2} (P_{aO2} = 40 mm Hg) and cyanosis. The **A-a gradient = 100 − 40 = 60.** The dramatic increase in the A-a gradient (60 versus 5) is because about 50% of the cardiac output bypasses alveolar ventilation in Tetralogy of Fallot.

VI Ventilation.

A. **Total (or Minute) Ventilation (V_{total})** is the total volume of air moved in or out of the respiratory system per minute.

Normally,

$$
\begin{aligned}
V_{total} &= \text{Tidal volume} \times \text{breaths/min} \\
&= 500 \text{ mL} \times 15 \text{ breaths/min} \\
&= 7500 \text{ mL/min}
\end{aligned}
$$

B. **Alveolar Ventilation (V_A)** is the volume of air moved in or out of the alveoli per minute.

Normally,

$$
\begin{aligned}
V_A &= (\text{Tidal volume} - \text{Dead space}) \times \text{breaths/min} \\
&= (500 \text{ mL} - 150 \text{ mL}) \times 15 \text{ breaths/min} \\
&= 350 \text{ mL} \times 15 \text{ breaths/min} \\
&= 5250 \text{ mL/min}
\end{aligned}
$$

C. **Alveolar Ventilation Equation.** This equation describes the most important relationship in pulmonary physiology, which is the **inverse relationship between alveolar ventilation (V_A) and P_{ACO2}** and by inference P_{aCO2} since $P_{ACO2} = P_{aCO2}$ in a normal lung. This equation indicates that **CO_2 is the controlled variable for the regulation of ventilation.**

$$
V_A = \frac{V_{CO2} \times K}{P_{ACO2} \text{ or } P_{aCO2}}
$$

where,

V_A = alveolar ventilation
V_{CO2} = rate of CO_2 production
K = constant (0.863)
P_{ACO2} = alveolar P_{CO2}
P_{aCO2} = arterial P_{CO2}

D. **Alveolar Gas Equation.** This equation allows one to calculate the alveolar P_{O2} (P_{AO2}) as long as the alveolar P_{CO2} (P_{ACO2}) is known.

$$
P_{AO2} = P_{IO2} - P_{ACO2} \left(F_{IO2} + \frac{1 - F_{IO2}}{R} \right)
$$

where,

P_{IO2} = P_{O2} in inspired gas
F_{IO2} = fractional concentration of O_2 in inspired gas

For a healthy individual who is breathing room air, has a measured $P_{aO2} = 40$ mm Hg (which closely approximates the P_{ACO2}), at barometric pressure of 760mm Hg, and water vapor pressure of 47 mm Hg. Hence,

$$P_{AO2} = [(760-47) \times 0.21] - 40[0.21 + (1 - 0.21)/0.8]$$
$$= 149 - 48$$
$$= 101 \text{ mm Hg}$$

E. Relationship between V_A, P_{ACO2}, and P_{AO2} (Table 11-2). The alveolar ventilation equation and alveolar gas equation are important in assessing hyperventilation and hypoventilation states as indicated below. **Hyperventilation** is ventilation in excess of metabolic needs and may be caused by: infections, drugs, hormones (e.g., progesterone), anxiety, and exercise. **Hypoventilation** is ventilation less than metabolic needs and may be caused by: depression of central nervous system (e.g., anesthesia, head trauma), respiratory muscle disease, thoracic cage deformities, scleroderma, and obstructive or restrictive pulmonary disease. Note that the alveolar ventilation equation demonstrates the inverse relationship between alveolar ventilation (V_A) and P_{ACO2}. Note that the alveolar gas equation demonstrates the direct relationship between alveolar ventilation (V_A) and P_{AO2}.

TABLE 11-2	RELATIONSHIP BETWEEN V_A, P_{ACO2}, P_{AO2}		
	Alveolar Ventilation Equation	**Alveolar Gas Equation**	**pH**
Hyperventilation ($\uparrow V_A$)	$P_{ACO2} = 20$ mm Hg $P_{aCO2} = 20$ mm Hg	$P_{AO2} = 126$ mm Hg $P_{aO2} = 126$ mm Hg	>7.45 alkalosis
Normal V_A	$P_{ACO2} = 40$ mm Hg* $P_{aCO2} = 40$ mm Hg*	$P_{AO2} = 101$ mm Hg $P_{aO2} = 101$ mm Hg	7.3–7.4
Hypoventilation ($\downarrow V_A$)	$P_{ACO2} = 80$ mm Hg $P_{aCO2} = 80$ mm Hg	$P_{AO2} = 54$ mm Hg $P_{aO2} = 54$ mm Hg	<7.35 acidosis

* See Table 11-1

VII Pulmonary Perfusion (Q) is the blood flow through the lung. Pulmonary arterial blood pressure is much lower than systemic arterial blood pressure (15 mm Hg versus 100 mm Hg, respectively). **Hypoxic vasoconstriction** is a clinically important phenomenon that is unique to pulmonary circulation. If a local decrease in P_{AO2} occurs, a local vasoconstriction is produced that diverts blood flow away from the hypoxic region toward well-ventilated regions of the lung.

VIII Ventilation/Perfusion Ratio (V_A/Q) (Figure 11-1A). In the normal condition, the V_A/Q ratio equals 0.8, assuming that alveolar ventilation $V_A = 4$ L/min and pulmonary blood flow Q = 5 L/min. There are two important clinical conditions that involve the V_A/Q ratio as indicated below:

A. Airway Blockage (e.g., child swallows a small toy). If V_A is blocked and blood flow is normal, then the **V_A/Q ratio equals 0 (no gas exchange).** As a result, P_{aO2} and P_{aCO2} values will approach P_{vO2} and P_{vCO2} values (see Table 12-1).

B. **Blood Flow Blockage** (e.g., pulmonary embolism). If V_A is normal and blood flow is blocked, then the **V_A/Q ratio equals infinity (no gas exchange).** As a result, P_{AO2} and P_{ACO2} values will approach P_{IO2} and P_{ICO2} (see Table 11-1).

IX Apex versus Base of the Lung (Figure 11–1B). There are regional lung differences in both V_A and Q that are both **gravity-dependent.**

A. **V_A Differences.** In an upright individual, the lung does <u>not</u> hang from the trachea or sit on the diaphragm. Instead, each level of lung is suspended by the lung level above it. As the mass of lung that must be suspended increases, the weight of the lung pulling down or away from the chest wall will increase, thereby creating a gradient in intrapleural pressure (P_{IP}).
   1. At the lung apex, P_{IP} is decreased (more negative; **−10 cm H_2O**). Recall that transpulmonary pressure $P_L = P_A - P_{IP}$. It follows then that the P_L at the apex will be increased. This results in **larger diameter alveoli at the apex.**
   2. At the lung base, P_{IP} is increased (more positive; **−4 cm H_2O**). Recall that transpulmonary pressure $P_L = P_A - P_{IP}$. It follows then that the P_L at the base will be decreased. This results in **smaller diameter alveoli at the base.**

B. **Q Differences.** In an upright individual, there are regional differences in blood flow through the lung caused by gravity.
   1. At the lung apex, pulmonary arterial pressure is decreased. This results in **smaller diameter blood vessels at the apex.**
   2. At the lung base, pulmonary arterial pressure is increased. This results in **larger diameter blood vessels at the base.**

X Five Causes of Hypoxemia.

A. **Hypoventilation (↑P_{ACO2})** causes hypercapnia and hypoxemia. Hypoxemia due to hypoventilation can be corrected by oxygen therapy. Causes of hypoventilation include:
   1. **Primary hypoventilation** is due to **CNS dysfunction** [e.g., narcotics, myxedema, brain damage, trauma, or central hypoventilation (Ondine curse); often seen in obese patients; sometimes called Obesity Hypoventilation Sydrome].
   2. **Secondary hypoventilation** is due to **PNS** or **neuromuscular dysfunction** (e.g., polio, Guillain-Barre, myasthenia gravis, Duchenne muscular dystrophy, kyphoscoliosis, or sleep apnea).
   3. **Obstructive or Restrictive lung disease.**

B. **V/Q Mismatch. This is a common cause of hypoxemia. V/Q mismatch** causes hypoxemia but not necessarily hypercapnia because of a reflexive increased ventilation. Hypoxemia due to V/Q mismatch can be corrected by oxygen therapy. Causes of V/Q mismatch include:
   1. **Airway blockage (increased alveolar shunt)**
   2. **Blood flow blockage (increased alveolar dead space)**

C. **Diffusion Impairment.** This is the rarest of the five causes of hypoxemia, whereby O_2 cannot diffuse from the alveoli to the capillary blood. Hypoxemia due to diffusion impairment can be corrected by oxygen therapy. Causes of diffusion impairment include:
   1. **Increased diffusion path** (e.g., idiopathic pulmonary fibrosis).
   2. **Decreased transit time** (e.g., ↑cardiac output, anemia).

D. Right→Left Blood Shunt. Hypoxemia caused by a right–left shunt **cannot** be overcome by oxygen therapy. Causes of a right–left shunt include:
1. **Pulmonary edema**
2. **Pneumonia**
3. **Heart septal defects**
4. **Chronic liver disease**

E. Low Inspired P_{O2}. This occurs due to ascent to a **high altitude.** Hypoxemia due to low inspired P_{O2} can be corrected by oxygen therapy.

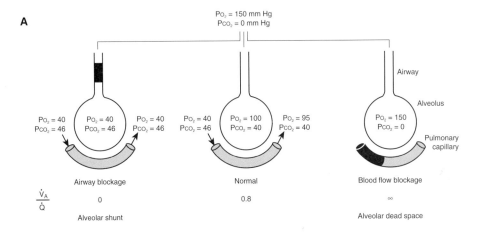

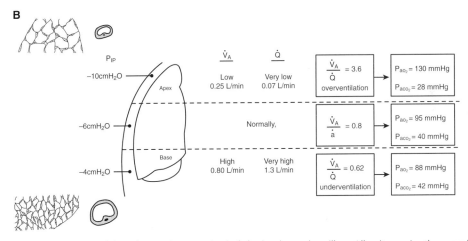

● **Figure 11-1:** (A) Diagram of three lung units comprised of an alveolus and capillary. All units receive the same inspired gas and mixed venous blood. The blackened areas indicate blockage sites in the airway and capillary. In the airway blockage, the respiratory unit receives no ventilation ($V_A = 0$), so that the $V_A/Q = 0$, which is also called an alveolar shunt. An alveolar shunt occurs when a portion of the cardiac output goes through the pulmonary capillaries but does not contact alveolar air. In the blood flow blockage, the respiratory unit receives no blood flow ($Q = 0$) so that the $V_A/Q = \infty$, which is also called an alveolar dead space. (B) Apex versus Base of Lung. Apex: V_A and Q are lower at the apex of the lung than at the base. Even though V_A is low, it is still too high for the very low Q. Hence, $V_A/Q = 3$ (overventilation or wasted ventilation) and gas exchange is more efficient. Organisms that thrive in a high O_2 environment (e.g., *Mycobacterium tuberculosis*) will flourish in the apex of the lung. During inspiration at the apex, the P_{IP} decreases from -10 to -13 cm H_2O. But because the alveoli at the apex have a large diameter (i.e., almost completely inflated before inspiration begins), very little room air flows into these alveoli. Hence, V_A is low (0.25 L/min). Base: V_A and Q are higher at the base of the lung than at the apex. Even though V_A is high, it is not high enough for the very high Q. Hence, $V_A/Q = 0.6$ (underventilation or wasted perfusion) and gas exchange is less efficient. During inspiration at the base, the P_{IP} decreases from -2 to -5 cm H_2O. Since the alveoli at the base have a small diameter (i.e., almost completely deflated before inspiration begins), a large amount of room air flows into these alveoli. Hence, V_A is high (0.80 L/min).

12

Transport of Oxygen and Carbon Dioxide

I **Transport of Oxygen (O_2).** O_2 **is transported in blood in two forms:**

  A. **O_2 dissolved in blood.** The amount of O_2 dissolved in blood is **0.3 mL O_2/dL blood** (at a P_{O2} of 100 mm Hg; arterial blood). Hence, O_2 is not very soluble in blood.

  B. **O_2 bound to Hemoglobin (Hb).** The amount of O_2 bound to Hb is **19.7 mL O_2/dL blood** (at a P_{O2} of 100 mm Hg; arterial blood).

II **Total O_2 Content of Arterial Blood.**

$$\text{Total } O_2 \text{ content} = \text{dissolved } O_2 + O_2 \text{ bound to Hb}$$
$$= 0.3 \text{ mL } O_2/\text{dL blood} + 19.7 \text{ mL } O_2/\text{dL blood}$$
$$= 20.0 \text{ mL } O_2/\text{dL blood}$$

III **Hemoglobin (Hb).**

  A. Is a globular protein consisting of four subunits.
   1. **Adult Hb (HbA)** consists of two alpha-globin subunits and two beta-globin subunits designated **Hb $\alpha_2\beta_2$.**
   2. **Fetal Hb (HbF)** consists of two alpha-globin subunits and two gamma-globin subunits designated **Hb $\alpha_2\gamma_2$.** HbF is the major form of Hb during **fetal development** since the O_2 affinity of HbF is higher than the O_2 affinity of HbA and thereby "pulls" O_2 from the maternal blood into fetal blood. The higher O_2 affinity of HbF is explained by **2,3 bisphosphoglycerate (BPG).** When 2,3 BPG binds HbA, the O_2 affinity of HbA is lowered. However, 2,3 BPG does not bind HbF and therefore O_2 affinity of HbF is higher.

  B. Contains a **heme** moiety, which is an **iron (Fe)-containing porphyrin.** Fe^{+2} (ferrous state) binds O_2, forming **oxyhemoglobin.** Fe^{+3} (ferric state) does not bind O_2, forming **deoxyhemoglobin.** The heme moiety is synthesized partially in mitochondria and partially in cytoplasm.

  C. In males, the normal blood concentration of Hb is **13.5–17.5 g/dL.** In females, the normal blood concentration of Hb is **12.0–16.0 g/dL.**

D. **Clinical Consideration.**
1. **Thalassemia Syndromes** are a heterogeneous group of genetic defects character-ized by the lack of or decreased synthesis of either α-globin (**α-thalassemia**) or β-globin (**β-thalassemia**) of Hb $\alpha_2\beta_2$.
   a. **Hydrops fetalis** is the most severe form of α-thalassemia. It causes severe pal-lor, generalized edema, and massive hepatosplenomegaly, and invariably leads to intrauterine fetal death.
   b. **β-Thalassemia Major** is the most severe form of β-thalassemia. It causes a severe, transfusion-dependent anemia. It is most common in Mediterranean countries and parts of Africa and southeast Asia.
2. **Type 1 and 2 Diabetes.** The amount of **glycosylated Hb (HbA_{1C})** is an indicator of blood glucose normalization over the previous three months (since the half-life of RBCs is three months) in Type 1 and Type 2 diabetes. Long periods of elevated blood glucose levels will result in a glycosylated Hb of 12–20%, whereas normal levels are about 5%.

IV **Hemoglobin-O_2 Dissociation Curve (Figure 12-1A).** Each Hb molecule can carry up to **four O_2 molecules.** A Hb-O_2 dissociation curve is **sigmoid-shaped** because each successive O_2 that binds to Hb increases the affinity for the next O_2 (called **positive cooperativity**). Hence, the affinity for the fourth O_2 is the highest. There are three impor-tant points on the curve as follows:

A. **P_{O2} = 25 mm Hg.** At this point, Hb is **50% saturated** (called the **P_{50}**). This means that Hb is bound to two O_2 molecules.

B. **P_{O2} = 75 mm Hg (venous blood).** At this point, Hb is **75% saturated.** This means that Hb is bound to three O_2 molecules.

C. **P_{O2} = 100 mm Hg (arterial blood).** At this point, Hb is almost **100% saturated.** This means that Hb is bound to four O_2 molecules.

V **Shifts in the Hemoglobin-O_2 Dissociation Curve (Figure 12-1B,C).**

A. **A shift to the left** occurs when the **affinity of Hb for O_2 is increased.** This makes the unloading of O_2 from arterial blood to tissues more difficult. A shift to the left is caused by a number of different factors:
1. **Decreased P_{aCO2}, increased arterial pH** (e.g., alkalosis)
2. **Decreased body temperature**
3. **Decreased 2,3-BPG** (e.g., stored blood, HbF). Stored blood loses 2,3BPG. HbF does not bind 2,3-BPG.

B. **A shift to the right** occurs when the **affinity of Hb for O_2 is decreased.** This makes the unloading of O_2 from arterial blood to tissues easier. A shift to the right is caused by a number of different factors:
1. **Increased P_{aCO2}, decreased arterial pH** (e.g., acidosis)
2. **Increased body temperature** (e.g., exercise)
3. **Increased 2,3 BPG** (e.g., living at high altitude)

VI **Clinical Considerations (Figure 12-1D).**

A. **Polycythemia vera** is a myeloproliferative disorder whereby the RBC precursors dominate and result in an increased RBC mass.

B. **Anemias. Iron-deficiency anemia** (the most common type of anemia) reduces **heme synthesis. Vitamin B$_{12}$ (pernicious anemia) and Folate Deficiency** reduce **DNA synthesis** in hematopoietic stem cells, thereby hindering erythropoiesis.

C. **Carbon Monoxide (CO) Poisoning.** CO binds to Hb with an affinity 200-fold greater than that of O$_2$, forming **carboxyhemoglobin (HbCO)**, that gives blood a characteristic **cherry-red color.** CO poisoning **decreases the O$_2$ content** of the blood and causes a **shift to the left** of the hemoglobin-O$_2$ dissociation curve. Patients with CO poisoning are given 100% O$_2$ to breathe in order to competitively displace CO from Hb and to increase the amount of dissolved O$_2$ content in the blood.

VII **Transport of Carbon Dioxide (CO$_2$).** CO$_2$ is transported in blood in three forms:

A. **CO$_2$ dissolved in blood.** 5% of the total CO$_2$ is transported in this form.

B. **CO$_2$ bound to Hb (HbCO$_2$; carbaminohemoglobin).** 5% of the total CO$_2$ is transported in this form.

C. **HCO$_3^-$.** 90% of the total CO$_2$ is transported in this form.

VIII **Control of Breathing.** The rate and depth of breathing are regulated so that arterial P$_{CO2}$ = 40 mm Hg. Under normal circumstances, the P$_{aCO2}$ is the major determinant of breathing and is held to within +/− 3 mm Hg. A 1–2 mm Hg increase in P$_{aCO2}$ evokes a 30–40% increase in ventilation.

A. **Receptors**
   1. **Medulla receptors** are indirectly stimulated by an **increased P$_{aCO2}$.** CO$_2$ freely crosses the blood–brain barrier to enter the cerebrospinal fluid (CSF). In the CSF, CO$_2$ combines with H$_2$O to form H$_2$CO$_3$ (carbonic acid), which dissociates to H+ and HCO$_3^-$. The medulla receptors sense high levels of [H+] in CSF and therefore respond to a **decrease in CSF pH (normal CSF pH = 7.32).** Note that the medulla receptors do NOT respond to O$_2$ at all.
   2. **Carotid Body and Aortic Bodies** are peripheral **chemoreceptors** that are primarily stimulated by a **decreased P$_{aO2}$ (<60 mm Hg) and a decreased arterial pH (acidosis).** The carotid body (innervated by CN IX) and aortic bodies (innervated by CN X) are the **only sites that detect changes in P$_{aO2}$.** In **diabetic ketoacidosis,** there is a decreased arterial pH (acidosis), which leads to an increased tidal volume (TV) and minute ventilation (amount of air inspired or expired each minute). This is called **Kussmaul breathing.**

B. **CNS Respiratory Centers.** CNS respiratory centers include the cerebral cortex, pneumotaxic center in the upper pons, apneustic center in the lower pons, and medulla. Breathing is normally a smooth, cyclic process. However, in some CNS diseases and congestive heart failure, **Cheyne-Stokes breathing** is observed. Cheyne-Stokes breathing is rapid breathing of increasing (↑TV) and decreasing (↓TV) depth followed by apnea lasting 10–20 seconds. **Apneustic breathing** is characterized by prolonged inspirations followed by brief periods of expiration.

IX **Physiology of High Altitude (Figure 12-2).** When a person ascends from sea level (P_{atm} = 760 mm Hg) to a high altitude (P_{atm} = 400 mm Hg), the P_{O2} of humidified air decreases from 150 mm Hg to 80 mm Hg, respectively. This decreases P_{AO2} and as a result **decreases P_{aO2} (< 60 mm Hg)**, that is, **hypoxemia.** Hypoxemia stimulates a number of processes as indicated in Figure 13-4.

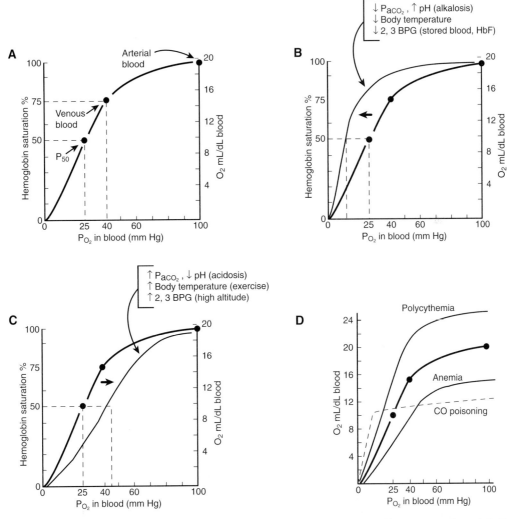

● **Figure 12-1: (A)** Hemoglobin-O_2 dissociation curve. P_{O2} in the blood is usually measured by an oxygen electrode in blood taken by a puncture of the radial artery (i.e., arterial P_{O2}). Generally, arterial P_{CO2} and arterial pH are measured at the same time. Normal ranges are: arterial P_{O2} = 75–105 mm Hg, arterial P_{CO2} = 33–45 mm Hg, arterial pH = 7.35–7.45, serum HCO_3^- = 22–28 mEq/L. Whenever you read a report of arterial P_{O2}, you should recall the hemoglobin-O_2 dissociation curve. Remember the three anchor points on the curve: P_{O2} = 25 mm Hg (the P_{50}), P_{O2} = 40 mm Hg (venous blood), and P_{O2} = 100 mm Hg (arterial blood) as indicated. Also note that the curve is flat between P_{O2} = 60–100 mm Hg, which means that humans can tolerate relatively large changes in P_{O2} without changing the oxygen-carrying capacity of Hb. **(B)** A shift to the left of the hemoglobin-O_2 dissociation curve. Note the various factors that cause a shift to the left and that the P_{50} is decreased. **(C)** A shift to the right of the hemoglobin-O_2 dissociation curve. Note the various factors that cause a shift to the right and that the P_{50} is increased. **(D)** O_2 content of the blood is shown in polycythemia, anemia, and carbon monoxide (CO) poisoning. In polycythemia, the O_2 content of the blood is above normal (24 versus 20 mL of O_2/dL blood) because of the increased Hb concentration. In anemia, the O_2 content of the blood is below normal (14 versus 20 mL of O_2/dL blood) because of the decreased Hb concentration. In CO poisoning, the O_2 content of the blood is below normal (12 versus 20 mL of O_2/dL blood) because CO binds to Hb with a high affinity taking up O_2 sites. In addition, CO poisoning causes a shift to the left of the curve. Note that the main change in these curves compared to normal is at the plateau or the total O_2 carrying capacity of the blood.

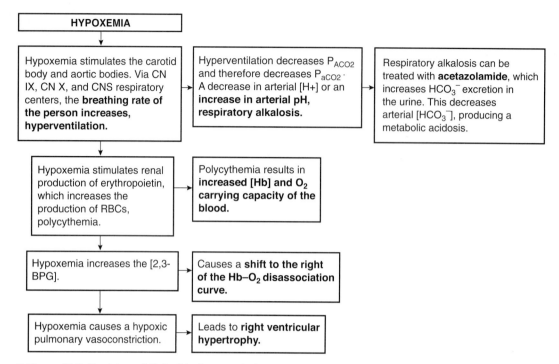

● **Figure 12-2:** Physiology of High Altitude. Note the biological processes stimulated by hypoxemia.

13

Pathophysiology of the Lung

① **Obstructive Lung Diseases** are characterized by an **increase in airway resistance (particularly expiratory airflow)**. **Obstructive ventilatory impairment** is the impairment of airflow during expiration with concomitant air trapping and hyperinflation. The increase in airway resistance (due to narrowing of the airway lumen) can be caused by conditions: **in the wall of the airway** where smooth muscle hypertrophy may cause airway narrowing (e.g., asthma), **outside the airway** where destruction of lung parenchyma may cause airway narrowing upon expiration due to loss of radial traction (e.g., emphysema), and **in the lumen of the airway** where increased mucus production may cause airway narrowing (e.g., chronic bronchitis).

A. **Asthma.** Asthma is associated with **smooth muscle hyperactivity within bronchi and bronchioles, increased mucus production, and edema of the bronchial wall.** Patients with asthma have the following characteristics: a decreased P_{aO2} (hypoxemia) leads to stimulation of the carotid and aortic bodies and hyperventilation, a decreased P_{aCO2} (hypocapnia), and respiratory alkalosis. As the asthma attack worsens, hypoventilation occurs and leads to a further decreased P_{aO2}, a severely increased P_{aCO2} (hypercapnia), respiratory acidosis, and death.

B. **Emphysema** is a type of chronic obstructive pulmonary disease (COPD). Emphysematous patients have much less difficulty inhaling air into the lung (↑compliance) than a normal individual. However, emphysematous patients have much more difficulty exhaling air out of the lung, which increases the work of breathing (i.e, respiratory muscles), which is manifested by shortness of breath (dyspnea). Emphysematous patients breathe slower with large tidal volumes. Patients are referred to as **"pink puffers"** with the following characteristics: a thin, barrel-shaped chest, increased breathing rate (tachypnea), a mildly decreased P_{aO2} (mild hypoxemia), and a mildly decreased or normal P_{aCO2} (hypocapnia or normocapnia), decreased diffusion-limited carbon monoxide (DLCO).

C. **Chronic Bronchitis** is a type of COPD that is related to **smoking.** Patients are referred to as **"blue bloaters"** with the following characteristics: a muscular, barrel-shaped chest, severely decreased P_{aO2} (severe hypoxemia with cyanosis), increased P_{aCO2} (hypercapnia) leads to chronic respiratory acidosis, increased HCO_3^- reabsorption by kidneys to buffer the acidemia, right ventricular failure, and systemic edema.

II **Restrictive Lung Diseases** are characterized by a **decrease in compliance** (i.e., the distensibility of the lung is restricted). The lungs are said to be "**stiff**". **Restrictive ventilatory impairment** is the inability to fully expand the lung, which results in a decrease in total lung capacity (TLC).

   A. **Idiopathic Pulmonary Fibrosis.** Patients with idiopathic pulmonary fibrosis have the following characteristics: a decreased P_{aO2} (hypoxemia) and a mildly decreased or normal P_{aCO2} (hypocapnia or normocapnia). **During exercise, the hypoxemia worsens without hypercapnia.** As the condition worsens, hypoventilation leads to a further decreased P_{aO2}, a severely increased P_{aCO2} (hypercapnia), respiratory acidosis, decreased diffusion limited carbon monoxide (DLCO), and death.

   B. **Others.** Other types of restrictive lung diseases include: coal workers' pneumoconiosis ("black lung disease"), silicosis, asbestosis, byssinosis (reaction to cotton or hemp fibers), farmer lung (reaction to mold in hay dust), silo-filler lung (reaction to nitrous oxides found in corn silos), bagassosis (reaction to moldy sugar cane), and sarcoidosis.

III **Obstructive Versus Restrictive (Figure 13-1).** Obstructive lung diseases (e.g. asthma, emphysema, chronic bronchitis) and restrictive lung diseases (e.g., idiopathic pulmonary fibrosis) demonstrate distinct differences in various lung parameters.

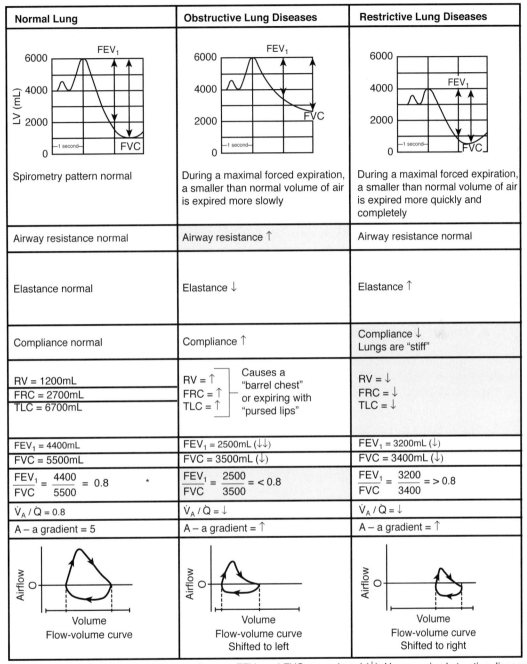

Normal Lung	Obstructive Lung Diseases	Restrictive Lung Diseases
Spirometry pattern normal	During a maximal forced expiration, a smaller than normal volume of air is expired more slowly	During a maximal forced expiration, a smaller than normal volume of air is expired more quickly and completely
Airway resistance normal	Airway resistance ↑	Airway resistance normal
Elastance normal	Elastance ↓	Elastance ↑
Compliance normal	Compliance ↑	Compliance ↓ Lungs are "stiff"
RV = 1200mL FRC = 2700mL TLC = 6700mL	RV = ↑ FRC = ↑ Causes a "barrel chest" or expiring with "pursed lips" TLC = ↑	RV = ↓ FRC = ↓ TLC = ↓
FEV_1 = 4400mL	FEV_1 = 2500mL (↓↓)	FEV_1 = 3200mL (↓)
FVC = 5500mL	FVC = 3500mL (↓)	FVC = 3400mL (↓)
$\dfrac{FEV_1}{FVC} = \dfrac{4400}{5500} = 0.8$ *	$\dfrac{FEV_1}{FVC} = \dfrac{2500}{3500} = <0.8$	$\dfrac{FEV_1}{FVC} = \dfrac{3200}{3400} = >0.8$
$\dot{V}_A / \dot{Q} = 0.8$	$\dot{V}_A / \dot{Q} = ↓$	$\dot{V}_A / \dot{Q} = ↓$
A – a gradient = 5	A – a gradient = ↑	A – a gradient = ↑
Flow-volume curve	Flow-volume curve Shifted to left	Flow-volume curve Shifted to right

* In both obstructive and restrictive lung disease, FEV_1 and FVC are reduced (↓). However, in obstructive disease, FEV_1 is more dramatically reduced (↓↓), resulting in a $\dfrac{FEV_1}{FVC}$ ratio < 0.8.

● **Figure 13-1:** Comparison of various lung parameters in normal lung, obstructive lung disease (asthma, emphysema, chronic bronchitis), and restrictive lung disease (idiopathic pulmonary fibrosis). Shaded blocks indicate the hallmark signs of obstructive versus restrictive lung disease. LV = lung volume.

14

Physiological Responses to Exercise

I   **At the start of exercise,** muscle spindle and joint receptors are stimulated by muscle activity, which carries information to the CNS centers via the dorsal column-medial lemniscal pathway.

II   ## Cardiovascular Responses to Exercise.

     A. During exercise, CNS centers inhibit the parasympathetic nervous system. This elicits the following actions: increases heart rate (positive chronotropism), increases conduction velocity (positive dromotropism), increases contractility (positive inotropism).

     B. During exercise, CNS centers stimulate the sympathetic nervous system. This elicits the following actions: increases heart rate (positive chronotropism), increases conduction velocity (positive dromotropism), increases contractility (positive inotropism) and increases vasoconstriction in the skin, gut, and inactive muscles. This results in an increased cardiac output and decreased blood flow to the skin initially (later, skin blood vessels dilate for heat dissipation), gut, and inactive skeletal muscles.

     C. There is **increased blood flow to the heart.**

     D. There is **no change in blood flow to the brain or kidney.**

III   ## Skeletal Muscle Responses to Exercise.

     A. During exercise, the increased metabolism of active skeletal muscle produces vasodilator metabolites (i.e., **lactate, adenosine, and K^+**). These metabolites cause vasodilation in active skeletal muscle. This results in **increased blood flow (i.e., active hyperemia)** and **increased O_2 delivery to active skeletal muscle.**

     B. The vasodilation within active skeletal muscle also accounts for the **overall decrease in total peripheral resistance (TPR)** that occurs during exercise. Even though sympathetics cause vasoconstriction (see above), the vasodilation within active skeletal muscle is the overwhelming factor.

IV **Blood Values Response to Exercise.**   During exercise:

A. **Arterial P_{O2} (P_{aO_2})** remains unchanged.

B. **Arterial P_{CO2} (Pa_{CO2})** remains unchanged.

C. **Arterial pH** remains unchanged during moderate exercise. During strenuous exercise, a **decreased arterial pH** occurs because of **lactic acidosis.**

D. **Venous P_{CO2} (P_{vCO2}) increases** because the excess CO_2 produced by the active skeletal muscle is transported to the lungs via venous blood.

V **Respiratory Responses to Exercise.**

A. During exercise, CNS centers stimulate lower motor neurons of cranial nerve XI, cervical spinal nerves (C5-C8), phrenic nerve, and intercostal nerves that innervate the breathing muscles. This causes an **increased breathing rate.**

B. The increased breathing rate causes a **greatly increased alveolar ventilation (V_A).** Note that V_A = (Tidal volume − Dead space) × breaths/min. Resting $V_A \cong$ 5L/min, whereas exercise $V_A \cong$ 100 L/min. The increased V_A matches the increased O_2 consumption and CO_2 production by the body during exercise. In a normal subject, **exercise is limited by the capacity of the heart.** A normal subject (trained or untrained) will reach maximal heart rate long before maximal V_A is reached.

C. Due to the increased cardiac output, **increased pulmonary blood flow (Q)** occurs.

D. During exercise, the **V_A/Q > 0.8** (i.e., V_A increases much more than Q) and the **V_A/Q ratios are more evenly distributed** in lung.

15

Body Fluids

① **Total Body Water (TBW) Figure 15-1A,B.** TBW for the average person is about **60% of body weight. Adult males, lean/muscular persons, and newborns** have the highest percentage of TBW, whereas **adult females and obese individuals** have the lowest percentage of TBW. TBW is divided into two main compartments.

A. Intracellular Fluid (ICF). ICF represents the fluid contained within cells. The ICF is about **40% of body weight or 66% of TBW (2/3 of TBW).** The major cations of ICF are **K^+ and Mg^{2+}.** The major anions of ICF are **proteins and organic phosphates (e.g, AMP, ADP, ATP).**

B. Extracellular Fluid (ECF). ECF represents the fluid outside the cells. The ECF is about **20% of body weight or 33% of TBW (1/3 of TBW).** The major cation of ECF is **Na^+.** The major anions of ECF are **Cl^- and HCO_3^-.** The ECF is divided into two main compartments (ISF and Plasma) and a third minor compartment (TCF) as indicated below.

   1. Interstitial Fluid (ISF). ISF represents the fluid that surrounds all cells (except blood cells) and includes **lymph.** The ISF is about **25% of TBW or 75% of ECF. Edema** is the palpable swelling caused by an increase in the ISF.

   2. Plasma. Plasma represents the fluid portion of blood. Plasma is about **7% of TBW or 20% of ECF.**

   3. Transcellular Fluid (TCF). TCF represents the following fluids: digestive fluid with the gut, cerebrospinal (CSF), pleural, pericardial, peritoneal, synovial, and bile). The TCF is **about 1% of TBW or 5% of ECF.**

② **Measurement of Body Fluid Compartments** is based on the **indicator dilution principle** described by the equation below:

$$V = \frac{A}{C}$$

where,

     V = volume of compartment (L)
     A = amount of marker injected (mCi, g, or cpm)
     C = concentration of marker (mCi/L, g/L, or cpm/L)

A. **Measurement of TBW** is accomplished using the markers **tritiated water (^3H_2O)** or **deuterium oxide (D_2O)** as shown in the example below.

A 60 kg patient is infused intravenously with 1 mCi of ^3H_2O. After 2 hours of equilibration, a plasma sample is measured and has a concentration of 0.025 mCi/L. Because the concentration of ^3H_2O throughout the body fluids should be same, as in plasma after equilibration, the TBW is calculated as given below.

$$V_{TBW} = \frac{1\ mCi}{0.025\ mCi/L}$$
$$= 40.0\ L$$

B. **Calculation of ICF.** The ICF cannot be measured directly by the indicator dilution principle because no marker is confined exclusively to the ICF compartment. Instead, the volume of ICF is calculated as given below.

$$V_{ICF} = V_{TBW} - V_{ECF}$$
$$= 40\ L - 12.5\ L$$
$$= 27.5\ L$$

C. **Measurement of ECF** is accomplished using the markers **mannitol, sodium (^{22}Na), ^{125}I-iothalamate,** or ^3H**-inulin** as shown in the example below.

A 60 kg patient is infused intravenously with 0.5 g of mannitol. After 2 hours of equilibration, a plasma sample is measured and has a concentration of 0.04 g/L. The ECF is calculated as given below.

$$V_{ECF} = \frac{0.5\ g}{0.04\ g/L}$$
$$= 12.5\ L$$

D. **Calculation of ISF.** The ISF cannot be measured directly by the indicator dilution principle because no marker is confined exclusively to the ISF compartment. Instead, the volume of ISF is calculated as given below.

$$V_{ISF} = V_{ECF} - V_{PLASMA}$$
$$= 12.5\ L - 3.5\ L$$
$$= 9.0\ L$$

E. **Measurement of Plasma** is accomplished using the markers **Evans blue dye** or ^{125}I**-albumin (RISA)** as shown in the example below.

A 60 kg patient is infused intravenously with 300,000 cpm of RISA. After 2 hours of equilibration, a plasma sample is measured and has a concentration of 100,000 cpm/L. The plasma volume is calculated as given below.

$$V_{PLASMA} = \frac{300,000\ cpm}{100,000\ cpm/L}$$
$$= 3.0\ L$$

F. **Calculation of TCF.** The TCF cannot be measured directly by the indicator dilution principle because no marker is confined exclusively to the TCF compartment. Instead, the volume of TCF is calculated as given below.

$$V_{TCF} = V_{ECF} - V_{ISF} - V_{PLASMA}$$
$$= 12.5\ L - 9.0\ L - 3.0\ L$$
$$= 0.5\ L$$

G. **Calculation of Blood Volume** is given below.

$$V_{BLOOD} = \frac{V_{PLASMA}}{1-hematocrit}$$
$$= \frac{3.0\ L}{1 - 0.40}$$
$$\cong 5.0\ L$$

III Water Consumption and Elimination.

A. **Consumption.** The average water consumption by an individual through **food and drink** is about **2 L/day**. In addition, **metabolism** produces about **0.2 L/day**.

B. **Elimination.** Water elimination by an individual occurs in a number of different ways.
1. **Through the urine (0.5–1.5 L/day).** Water excretion by the **kidneys** is the main regulator of body water and electrolyte balance.
2. **Through the skin (≈0.3 L/day).** This water loss is not dependent on sweating and is minimized by the stratum corneum of the skin. When the stratum corneum is damaged by severe burns, water loss through the skin increases dramatically (≈3–5 L/day).
3. **Through respiration (≈0.3 L/day).** During breathing, dry atmospheric air becomes saturated with water as air passes through the conducting airway passages.
4. **Through the feces (≈0.2 L/day).** During diarrhea, water loss through the feces increases dramatically.
5. **Through sweating at rest (≈0.1 L/day).** During exercise, water loss due to sweating increases dramatically (1–2 L/hour).

IV Hormonal Regulation of Body Fluids.
The steroid hormone **aldosterone (ALD)** regulates the **volume of body fluids** (by increasing Na^+ reabsorption) through its action on the cortical collecting ducts of the kidney. The protein hormone **anti-diuretic hormone (ADH)** regulates the **concentration of body fluids** (by increasing H_2O reabsorption) through its action on both the cortical and medullary collecting ducts of the kidney.

V Dehydration States (Figure 15-10).

A. **Isosmotic Dehydration (hemorrhage, diarrhea, vomiting, and severe burns).** In isosmotic dehydration, the person loses a $H_2O + NaCl$ fluid out of the ECF.

B. **Hyperosmotic Dehydration (sweating in a desert, strenuous exercise, fever, lack of drinking water, alcoholism, and diabetes insipidus).** In hyperosmotic dehydration, the person loses a H_2O fluid (sweat excretes more H_2O than NaCl) out of the ECF.

C. **Hyposmotic Dehydration (adrenal gland insufficiency, lack of aldosterone, Addison disease).** In hyposmotic dehydration, the person loses a NaCl fluid (kidneys excrete more NaCl than H_2O) out of the ECF.

VI Overhydration States (Figure 15-10).

A. **Isosmotic Overhydration (parenteral administration of a large volume of isotonic NaCl solution).** In isosmotic overhydration, the person gains a $H_2O + NaCl$ fluid into the ECF.

B. **Hyperosmotic Overhydration (excessive NaCl intake).** In hyperosmotic overhydration, the person gains NaCl into the ECF.

C. **Hyposmotic Overhydration [syndrome of inappropriate antidiuretic hormone (SIADH; elevated ADH)].** In hyposmotic overhydration, the person gains a H_2O fluid into the ECF.

A

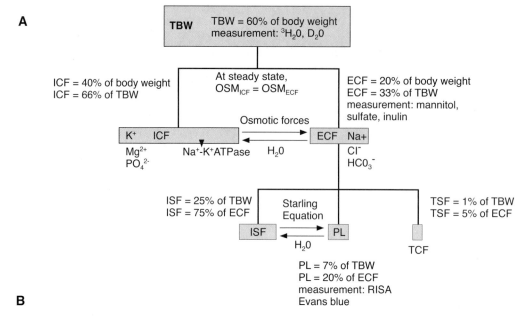

TBW = 60% of body weight
measurement: ^3H_2O, D_2O

ICF = 40% of body weight
ICF = 66% of TBW

At steady state,
$OSM_{ICF} = OSM_{ECF}$

Osmotic forces

ECF = 20% of body weight
ECF = 33% of TBW
measurement: mannitol,
sulfate, inulin

K^+ ICF
Mg^{2+}
PO_4^{2-}
Na^+-K^+ATPase H_2O

ECF Na^+
Cl^-
HCO_3^-

ISF = 25% of TBW
ISF = 75% of ECF

Starling
Equation

ISF H_2O PL

TSF = 1% of TBW
TSF = 5% of ECF

TCF

PL = 7% of TBW
PL = 20% of ECF
measurement: RISA
Evans blue

B

Bedside Estimates for a 60kg patient

TBW = 60% of body weight	60% X 60KG = 36L
ICF = 66% of TBW	66% X 36L = 24L
ECF = 33% of TBW	33% X 36L = 12L
Plasma = 20% of ECF	20% X 12L = 2.4L
Blood volume = Plasma volume / 1-hematocrit	2.4L ÷ (1-0.40) = 4L

C

Volume Status	ECF Volume	ECF Osmolarity	H20 Shift	IFC Volume	IFC Osmolarity	[PP]	Hmt	BP	P_{Na} mEq/L
Isosmotic Dehydration	↓	–	–	–	–	↑	↑	↓	145
Hyperosmotic Dehydration	↓	↑	ICF→ECF	↓	↑	↑	–	↓	>145
Hyposmotic Dehydration	↓	↓	ECF→ICF	↑	↓	↑	↑	↓	<145
Isosmotic Overhydration	↑	–	–	–	–	↓	↓	↑	145
Hyperosmotic Overhydration	↑	↑	ICF→ECF	↓	↑	↓	↓	↑	>145
Hyposmotic Overhydration	↑	↓	ECF→ICF	↑	↓	↓	–	↑	<145

[PP] = plasma protein concentration, Hmt = hematocrit

P_{Na} = plasma sodium concentration, BP = blood pressure

● **Figure 15-1: (A)** Flow chart of body fluid compartments. Note that only the total body water (TBW) extracellular fluid (ECF), and plasma (PL) can be directly measured. Note also that the ICF and ECF are in osmotic equilibrium such that at steady state the ICF osmolarity (OSM_{ICF}) equals the ECF osmolarity (OSM_{ECF}) i.e., 280–300 mOsm/L. To achieve this osmotic equality, water moves between the ICF and ECF compartments (i.e., NOT through the movement of osmotically active substances. The distribution of H_2O between the ICF and ECF is governed by osmotic forces. The distribution of K^+ in the ICF and Na^+ in the ECF is maintained by the enzyme Na^+-K^+ ATPase located on the cell membrane of various cells. Na^+-K^+ ATPase plays a critical role in actively pumping Na^+ out of cells (against the electrochemical gradient of Na^+) and pumping K^+ into cells. Although Na^+ diffuses into cells driven by its electrochemical gradient, the Na^+ that diffuses into cells is actively pumped out by Na^+-K^+ ATPase in order to maintain a low intracellular Na^+ concentration, whereas K^+ is actively pumped into cells. The distribution of H_2O between the ISF and plasma is governed by the Starling equation, which describes exchange of fluid across capillaries. In general, the forces favoring filtration prevail slightly, which leads to a net filtration out of plasma and into ISF, which is collected as lymph and returned to circulation. **(B)** Table of bedside estimates of body fluid compartments for a 60kg patient. **(C)** Table summarizing the various changes that occur in the six different volume states. The most commonly used clinical index of body fluid is plasma Na^+ (P_{Na}). Because Na^+ is the major cation of the ECF, P_{Na} is a good indicator of volume status. Under normal conditions, P_{Na} = 145mEq/L. **Hypernatremia** occurs when $P_{Na} > 145$mEq/L. **Hyponatremia** occurs when $P_{Na} < 145$mEq/L. Hyponatremia is the most common disorder of body fluid and electrolyte imbalance in hospitalized patients.

16

Basic Renal Processes

① Renal Blood Flow (RBF). The RBF in a typical normal adult is **~1.1 L/min or ~25% of the cardiac output (5L/min).** A majority of the RBF (90%) goes to the kidney cortex where the glomeruli are located. **RBF $= \Delta P/R$,** where ΔP = mean renal artery pressure minus renal vein pressure and R = total vascular resistance overwhelmingly determined by the **afferent arterioles.** The kidney vasculature is unique in that it contains **two types of arterioles** (i.e., afferent arteriole and efferent arteriole) and **two types of capillary beds** (i.e., glomerular and peritubular). The peritubular capillary bed is separated from the glomerular capillary bed by the efferent arteriole so that the hydrostatic pressure in the peritubular capillary bed is lower than the hydrostatic pressure in the glomerular capillary bed (20 mmHg vs 60 mmHg). RBF remains constant even when arterial pressure varies from 100–200mmHg by **autoregulation,** which occurs by two mechanisms: the **myogenic mechanism** whereby afferent arterioles constrict in response to stretch; and the **tubuloglomerular mechanism** whereby afferent arterioles constrict in response to **adenosine** secreted by the macular densa cells, which detect increased Na^+ and Cl^- ion concentrations.

A. Measurement of Renal Plasma Flow (RPF). RPF is measured by the **clearance of para-aminohippuric (PAH)** but underestimates true RPF by ~10%. PAH is excreted by glomerular filtration and tubular secretion (plasma → tubular fluid). The RPF in a typical normal adult is **0.605 L/min.**

$$RPF = C_{PAH} = \frac{[U]_{PAH}V}{[P]_{PAH}}$$

Where:

RPF = renal plasma flow (mL/min)
C_{PAH} = clearance of PAH (mL/min)
$[U]_{PAH}$ = urine concentration of PAH (mg/mL)
V = urine flow rate (mL/min)
$[P]_{PAH}$ = plasma concentration of PAH (mg/mL)

B. Measurement of RBF

$$RBF = \frac{RPF}{1 - hematocrit}$$

❚ **Glomerular Filtration Rate (GFR).** The formation of urine begins with the process of glomerular filtration, which is the bulk-flow of fluid from the glomerular capillaries → Bowman's space forming, a glomerular filtrate (or tubular fluid). The GFR = amount of glomerular filtrate formed per unit time. The GFR in a typical normal adult is **0.125 L/min** (or an incredible **180 L/day**).

A. **Measurement of GFR.** GFR is measured by the **clearance of inulin.** Inulin is excreted by glomerular filtration only (no tubular reabsorption or tubular secretion is involved).

$$GFR = \frac{[U]_{inulin} \, V}{[P]_{inulin}}$$

Where:

GFR = glomerular filtration rate (mL/min)
$[U]_{inulin}$ = urine concentration of inulin (mg/mL)
V = urine flow rate (mL/min)
$[P]_{inulin}$ = plasma concentration of inulin (mg/mL)

B. **Filtration Fraction (FF).** The FF in a typical normal adult is 0.20 or 20%. This means that 20% of the RPF is filtered into Bowman's space and the remaining 80% of the RPF enters the efferent arteriole → peritubular capillary bed → renal vein.

$$FF = \frac{GFR}{RPF}$$

Where:

FF = filtration fraction
GFR = glomerular filtration rate
RPF = renal plasma flow

C. **GFR-Starling Forces.** The filtration in any capillary in the body is determined by capillary permeability, capillary surface area, and net filtration pressure (NFP). The NFP always favors movement of fluid out of the glomerular capillaries. The GFR is described by the **Starling equation.**

$$GFR = KF[(PGC - PBS) - (\Pi GC - \Pi BS)]$$

Where:

K_F = filtration coefficient of the glomerular capillaries
P_{GC} = hydrostatic pressure exerted by the fluid in the glomerular capillaries. Afferent arteriole dilation and efferent arteriole constriction both increase P_{GC}.
P_{BS} = hydrostatic pressure exerted by the fluid in Bowman's space. Ureter blockage or constriction increase P_{BS}.
Π_{GC} = oncotic pressure of the glomerular capillary. Π_{GC} increases along the length of the glomerular capillary because the protein concentration in the glomerular capillary increases as H_2O is forced into Bowman's space.
Π_{BS} = oncotic pressure of Bowman's space. Π_{BS} is normally zero.

III **Physiological Regulation of RBF and GFR.** Despite autoregulation of RBF by the myogenic mechanism and tubuloglomerular mechanism, RBF and GFR (to a lesser extent) can be altered by the **sympathetic nervous system** and **angiotensin II,** both of which cause afferent and efferent arteriole constriction. This results in: **decrease in RBF** and a **small decrease in GFR.**

IV **Renal Clearance.** Renal clearance is the volume of plasma from which a substance is completely cleared by the kidneys per unit time. The clearance of inulin (C_{inulin}) is used as a benchmark because inulin is freely filterable at the glomerulus and does not undergo tubular secretion or tubular reabsorption. Note that $C_{inulin} = GFR = 0.125L/min$.

A. Renal clearance is described by the equation below.

$$C_X = \frac{[U]_X \, V}{[P]_X}$$

Where:

C_X = clearance of X (mL/min)
$[U]_X$ = urine concentration of X (mg/mL)
V = urine volume/time (mL/min)
$[P]_X$ = plasma concentration of X (mg/mL)

B. Physiological Implications.
   A.   If substance A is present in the plasma but is not excreted in the urine, then $C_A = 0.$
   B.   If substance B (like inulin) is freely filterable at the glomerulus and does not undergo tubular secretion or tubular reabsorption, then the clearance of inulin can be used to measure GFR. $C_{inulin} = GFR = 0.125 \, L/min.$
   C.   If substance C is freely filterable at the glomerulus and undergoes tubular secretion, then $C_C > C_{inulin} > 0.125 \, L/min$
   D.   If substance D is freely filterable at the glomerulus and undergoes tubular reabsorption, then $C_D < C_{inulin} < 0.125 \, L/min$

C. Clearance of Creatinine (C_{CR}). Creatinine is freely filterable at the glomerulus and undergoes a small amount of tubular secretion but no tubular reabsorption. If the small amount of tubular secretion is ignored, then $C_{CR} \approx C_{inulin} \approx GFR \approx 0.125 \, L/min$. In clinical practice, it is more common to measure plasma creatinine levels (P_{CR}) as an indicator of GFR because there is an excellent inverse relationship between P_{CR} and GFR.

V **Glomerular Filtration.** Urine formation begins with filtration that occurs where the glomerulus and Bowman's capsule interact to form a **glomerular filtration barrier (GFB).** The functions of the GFB include:

A. Prevents passage of red blood cells, leukocytes, and platelets

B. Restricts passage of proteins >70,000d (**"size filter"**) and negatively charged substances (**"charge filter"**). The GFB provides no hindrance to molecules <**7000d** and almost total hindrance to plasma albumin (**70,000d**). For molecules between **7000d** ⇔ **70,000d,** the amount filtered becomes progressively smaller as the molecule becomes larger.

C. Permits passage of water, ions (both + and −), and other small molecules.

D. Forms an ultrafiltrate of blood.

VI Tubular Reabsorption (tubular fluid → plasma).

A. Paracellular Route. Tubular reabsorption via the paracellular route occurs **between** renal tubular epithelial cells at the zonula occludens. Tubular reabsorption via the paracellular route occurs by **diffusion** ("downhill") or **solvent drag** (movement of water drags dissolved solutes with it).

B. Transcellular Route. Tubular reabsorption via the transcellular route occurs **across** renal tubular epithelial cells and therefore the substance must cross the luminal cell membrane → cytoplasm of the cell → basolateral cell membrane. Tubular reabsorption via the transcellular route occurs by **diffusion** ("downhill") for lipid-soluble substances or by **active transport** ("uphill") for lipid-insoluble substances.

C. Transport Maximum (T_m). Active reabsorption by renal tubules generally has a limit (called the T_m) to the amount of substance that can be reabsorbed per unit time. The T_m occurs because carrier proteins responsible for reabsorption become saturated. **The T_m for glucose equals 350 mg/dL.** For example, when plasma glucose concentration is <T_m, all the filtered glucose will be reabsorbed and the urine will be glucose free. When plasma glucose concentration is >T_m, all the filtered glucose will not be reabsorbed and glucose will appear in the urine as in the case of diabetes. However, in actuality, glucose appears in the urine before the T_m of 350 mg/dL is reached. The plasma concentration where glucose first appears in the urine is called the renal plasma threshold for glucose. **The renal plasma threshold for glucose equals 250 mg/dL. Splay** is a term used to describe the appearance of glucose in the urine before the T_m is reached and occurs between **250 mg/dL** → **350 mg/dL.** Splay is explained by the heterogeneity of nephrons i.e., not all nephrons have the same T_m for glucose.

VII Tubular Secretion (plasma → tubular fluid).

A. Paracellular Route. Tubular secretion via the paracellular route occurs **between** renal tubular epithelial cells at the zonula occludens. Tubular secretion via the paracellular route occurs by **diffusion** ("downhill").

B. Transcellular Route. Tubular secretion via the transcellular route occurs **across** renal tubular epithelial cells and therefore the substance must cross the basolateral cell membrane → cytoplasm of the cell → luminal cell membrane. Tubular secretion via the transcellular route occurs by **diffusion** ("downhill") for lipid-soluble substances or by **active transport** ("uphill") for lipid-insoluble substances.

Pump-Leak Systems involve active transport using carrier (or transporter) proteins (the "pump" component) that establish a diffusion gradient that opposes its own action by favoring back-diffusion (or a "leak"). The "leak" component is the paracellular route based on the permeability of the zonula occludens. Consequently, epithelia are classified as "leaky" if the zonula occludens has a high permeability and as "tight" if the zonula occludens has a low permeability.

Fluid Uptake by the Peritubular Capillary Bed. The major mechanism by which this occurs in the peritubular capillary bed is **bulk-flow of interstitial fluid** into peritubular capillaries. The bulk-flow of interstitial fluid always favors movement into the plasma of the peritubular capillary bed because the hydrostatic pressure in peritubular capillaries is low (20 mm Hg) and the oncotic pressure of the plasma entering the peritubular capillaries is high because the plasma proteins are concentrated due to the loss of protein-free filtrate during passage through the glomerular capillary bed.

17

Renal Handling of Organic Substances

I **Renal Handling of Organic Nutrients [Glucose, Amino acids, Water-soluble vitamins (B complex and C), Lactate, Acetate, Ketones (β-hydroxybutyrate and acetoacetate), and Krebs Cycle intermediates].** Organic nutrients are freely-filtered from the glomerular capillaries → Bowman's space and then are reabsorbed almost completely by the **proximal convoluted tubule.** In organic nutrient reabsorption, the key factor is that the reabsorption of all organic nutrients occurs by a transport mechanism very similar to that of glucose.

A. **Proximal Convoluted Tubule (PCT).** The PCT reabsorbs **100%** of the filtered organic nutrients. The carrier proteins involved include:
   1. **Na^+-K^+ATPase** transports Na^+ across the basolateral membrane into the interstitial fluid (i.e., "pumps" Na^+ out of the cell) keeping cytoplasmic $[Na^+]$ low.
   2. **Na^+-organic nutrient Cotransporters**
   3. **Organic nutrient Transporters**

B. No other portion of the nephron is involved in organic nutrient reabsorption.

II **Renal Handling of Proteins, Polypeptides, and Urea.**

A. **Proximal Convoluted Tubule (PCT).** The PCT reabsorbs **100%** of filtered proteins, **100%** of filtered polypeptides, and **50%** of filtered urea.
   1. **Proteins.** Proteins are NOT freely-filtered from the glomerular capillaries → Bowman's space. However, a small amount of protein is filtered from the glomerular capillaries → Bowman's space such that the Total Filtered Protein = GFR × concentration of protein in the tubular fluid = 170 L/day × 10mg/L = 1.8 g/day. **Close to 100%** of the **1.8 g of filtered protein** is reabsorbed by the proximal convoluted tubule so that only about **100 mg/day** is excreted in the urine. The cell membrane receptors involved are: **Specific Protein Receptors** located on the luminal cell membrane that bind filtered proteins within the tubular fluid and then undergo **endocytosis.** The endocytic vesicles fuse with endolysosomes where various lysosomal enzymes digest the protein to amino acids. The amino acids exit the basolateral cell membrane into the interstitial fluid.
   2. **Polypeptides.** Small polypeptides are freely-filtered from the glomerular capillaries → Bowman's space, then are reabsorbed almost completely by the

proximal convoluted tubule. The cell surface enzymes involved are: **Peptidases** located on the luminal cell membrane that digest polypeptides to amino acids within the tubular fluid. The amino acids (which are organic nutrients) are then handled as indicated above.

3. **Urea** (end product of protein catabolism). Urea is freely-filtered from the glomerular capillaries → Bowman's space and then 50% of the urea is reabsorbed by the PCT and an additional 10% is reabsorbed by the inner medullary collecting ducts. In the PCT, reabsorption of **50%** of the filtered urea occurs by **diffusion or passive transport ("downhill")** due to concentration gradients. As urea flows through the proximal convoluted tubule, reabsorption of H_2O occurs which increases the concentration of urea within the tubular fluid so that it is greater than the concentration of urea within the plasma. Consequently, the transport of urea across the luminal and basolateral membranes into the interstitial fluid occurs by diffusion.

B. **Collecting Duct (CD).** The inner medullary CD reabsorbs **10%** of filtered urea. In the inner medullary CD, reabsorption of **10%** of filtered urea occurs by **facilitated diffusion or passive transport ("downhill").** The carrier protein involved is the **urea transporter,** which transports urea across the luminal and basolateral membranes into the interstitial fluid.

III Renal Handling of Organic Anions (Para-aminohippuric acid, Urate, Bile salts, Fatty acids, Hydroxybenzoates, Acetazolamide, Chlorothiazide, Penicillin, Salicylates, Sulfonamides).

Because most organic anions are bound to large plasma proteins (that are not filtered), organic anions are NOT freely-filtered from the glomerular capillaries → Bowman's space but instead are **prolifically secreted** by the **proximal convoluted tubule.** In organic anion secretion, the key factor is that the secretion of all organic anions occurs by a transport mechanism very similar to that of para-aminohippuric acid.

A. **Proximal Convoluted Tubule (PCT).** The PCT secretes **100%** of the non-filtered organic anions. The carrier proteins for most organic anions involved include:
   1. **Na^+-K^+ATPase**
   2. **Na^+-Dicarboxylate/Tricarboxylate Cotransporter**
   3. **Organic Anion-Dicarboxylate/Tricarboxylate Exchanger**
   4. **Organic Anion-X^- Exchanger**
   5. The situation for the organic anion, **urate,** is a little different. Elevated plasma levels of urate cause **gout.** Urate is freely-filtered from the glomerular capillaries → Bowman's space. As urate flows through the proximal convoluted tubule, reabsorption of urate occurs (tubular fluid → plasma) by **active transport ("uphill").** In addition, secretion of urate by **active transport ("uphill")** may also occur in the proximal convoluted tubule. In other words, there are two processes working in opposite directions. Normally, reabsorption of urate is much greater than secretion of urate. However, if plasma levels of urate increase (due to increased urate production) then the secretion of urate increases, which leads to increased urate excretion in the urine.

B. No other portion of the nephron is involved in organic anion secretion.

IV Renal Handling of Organic Cations (Acetylcholine, Creatinine, Dopamine, Epinephrine, Norepinephrine, Histamine, Serotonin, Atropine, Isoproterenol, Cimetidine, Morphine, etc.).

Because most organic cations are bound to large plasma proteins (that are not filtered), organic cations are NOT freely-filtered from the glomerular capillaries → Bowman's space but instead are prolifically secreted by the proximal convoluted tubule. In organic cation secretion, the key factor is that the secretion of all organic cations occurs by a transport mechanism that is not yet fully elucidated.

A. **Proximal Convoluted Tubule (PCT).** The PCT secretes **100%** of the non-filtered organic cations. The carrier proteins involved include:

1. **Na^+-K^+ ATPase**
2. **Organic Cation-? Exchanger**
3. **Organic Cation-X^+ Exchanger.**

B. No other portion of the nephron is involved in organic cation secretion.

V Summary Table of Renal Handling of Organic Substances (Table 17-1).

TABLE 17-1	SUMMARY TABLE OF RENAL HANDLING OF ORGANIC SUBSTANCES			
	Organic Nutrient Reabsorption	Protein, Polypeptide, Urea Reabsorption	Organic Anion Secretion	Organic Cation Secretion
PCT	**Luminal Membrane**	**Luminal Membrane**	**Luminal Membrane**	**Luminal Membrane**
	Na^+- Nut Cotransporters	Specific Protein Receptor Peptidases	An^--X^- Exchanger	Cat^+-X^+ Exchanger
	Basolateral Membrane	**Basolateral Membrane**	**Basolateral Membrane**	**Basolateral Membrane**
	Na^+-K^+ ATPase Nut Transporters	None	Na^+-K^+ ATPase Na^+-Di/Tri Cotransporter An^--Di/Tri Exchanger	Na^+-K^+ ATPase Cat^+-? Exchanger
		50% of filtered urea is reabsorbed by diffusion		
PST	X	X	X	X
DTL	X	X	X	X
ATL	X	X	X	X
DST	X	X	X	X
DCT	X	X	X	X

TABLE 17-1	SUMMARY TABLE OF RENAL HANDLING OF ORGANIC SUBSTANCES (*continued*)		
	Organic Nutrient Reabsorption	Protein, Polypeptide, Urea Reabsorption	Organic Anion Secretion	Organic Cation Secretion
Med CD		**Luminal Membrane** Urea Transporter		
	X	**Basolateral Membrane** Urea Transporter 10% of filtered urea is reabsorbed by facilitated diffusion	X	X

PCT = proximal convoluted tubule; PST = proximal straight tubule; DTL = descending limb of the loop of Henle; ATL = ascending thin limb of the loop of Henle; DST = distal straight tubule; DCT = distal convoluted tubule; medCD = medullary collecting duct; Shaded region = loop of Henle; Nut = organic nutrient; An⁻ = an organic anion; Di/Tri = dicarboxylates/tricarboxylates; X⁻ = any of a large number of organic anions; X⁺ = any of a large number of organic cations; ? = specific substance unknown; **X** = no reabsorption or secretion.

18

Renal Handling of Na$^+$, Cl$^-$, and H$_2$O

I **Renal Handling of Na$^+$.** Na$^+$ is freely-filtered from the glomerular capillaries → Bowman's space and then is reabsorbed by particular segments of the nephron. In Na$^+$ reabsorption, the key factor is **Na$^+$-K$^+$ATPase** that transports Na$^+$ across the basolateral membrane into the interstitial fluid (i.e., "pumps" Na$^+$ out of the cell) keeping cytoplasmic [Na$^+$] low.

A. **Early Proximal Convoluted Tubule (PCT).** The PCT (early and late) reabsorbs **65%** of the filtered Na$^+$ isosmotically (i.e., Na$^+$ and H$_2$O are reabsorbed exactly proportionately). The transport of Na$^+$ occurs via carrier (or transporter) proteins. The carrier proteins involved include:
   1. **Na$^+$-K$^+$ATPase.**
   2. **Na$^+$-organic nutrient Cotransporters**
   3. **Na$^+$-H$^+$ Exchanger**
   4. **Na$^+$-HCO$_3$$^-$ Cotransporter. Acetazolamide (Diamox)** inhibits carbonic anhydrase by acting primarily on the early PCT resulting in decreased reabsorption of HCO$_3$$^-$. It is used clinically to treat glaucoma and altitude sickness.

B. **Late Proximal Convoluted Tubule (PCT).** The transport of Na$^+$ in the late PCT is related to Cl$^-$ reabsorption which will be discussed later.

C. **Ascending Thin Limb of the Loop of Henle (ATL).** The ATL reabsorbs **10%** of the filtered Na$^+$ by **passive transport ("downhill")**, the mechanism of which is poorly understood. Note that the ATL is **impermeable to H$_2$O**.

D. **Distal Straight Tubule of the Loop of Henle (DST).** The DST reabsorbs **15%** of the filtered Na$^+$. The transport of Na$^+$ occurs via carrier (or transporter) proteins and by diffusion via the paracellular route across a zonula occludens. Note that the DST is **impermeable to H$_2$O**. Note that the ATL and DST reabsorb Na$^+$ but not H$_2$O because these segments are impermeable to H$_2$O. Therefore, the tubular fluid entering the DCT is **hyposmotic (hypotonic)** or **more dilute** compared to plasma. Therefore, the ATL and DST are frequently called the **diluting segment**. The carrier proteins involved include:
   1. **Na$^+$-K$^+$ATPase**
   2. **Na$^+$-K$^+$-2Cl$^-$ Cotransporter. Furosemide (Lasix; last six hours), Bumetanide (Bumex), and Torsemide (Demadix)** inhibit the Na$^+$-K$^+$-2Cl$^-$ cotransporter by acting primarily on the **DST of the loop of Henle ("loop diuretics")**. Loop diuretics are the most efficacious diuretics available and are sometimes called

"**high ceiling diuretics**". They are used clinically to treat edema associated with congestive heart failure, pulmonary edema, and hypertension.

   3. Na$^+$-H$^+$ Exchanger

   4. Na$^+$-HCO$_3^-$ Cotransporter.

E. Distal Convoluted Tubule (DCT). The DCT reabsorbs **5%** of the filtered Na$^+$. The transport of Na$^+$ occurs via carrier (or transporter) proteins and ion channel proteins. The carrier proteins and ion channel proteins involved include:

   1. Na$^+$-K$^+$ATPase

   2. Na$^+$-Cl$^-$ Cotransporter. Hydrochlorothiazide (HydroDIURIL), Chlorthalidone (Hygroton), Indapamide (Lozol) and Metolazone (Mykrox) inhibit the Na$^+$-Cl$^-$ cotransporter by acting primarily on the **DCT** resulting in decreased Na$^+$ reabsorption (**"thiazide diuretics"**). They are used clinically to treat edema associated with congestive heart failure and hypertension.

   3. Na$^+$ ion channel protein

F. Collecting Duct (CD). The CD (mainly the **principal cells** of the CD) reabsorbs **5%** of the filtered Na$^+$. The transport of Na$^+$ occurs via carrier (or transporter) proteins and ion channels proteins. The carrier proteins and ion channel proteins involved include:

   1. Na$^+$-K$^+$ATPase

   2. Na$^+$ ion channel

Renal Handling of Cl$^-$.

Cl$^-$ is freely-filtered from the glomerular capillaries → Bowman's space and then is reabsorbed at particular segments of the nephron mainly dependent on Na$^+$ reabsorption. Consequently, the key factor in Cl$^-$ reabsorption is again **Na$^+$-K$^+$ATPase** that transports Na$^+$ across the basolateral membrane into the interstitial fluid (i.e., "pumps" Na$^+$ out of the cell) keeping cytoplasmic [Na$^+$] low in most nephron segments and **H$^+$ ATPase** that transports H$^+$ across the basolateral membrane into the interstitial fluid in the collecting duct.

A. Early Proximal Convoluted Tubule (PCT). The PCT (early and late) reabsorbs **65%** of the filtered Cl. The transport of Cl$^-$ occurs by diffusion via the paracellular route across a zonula occludens.

B. Late Proximal Convoluted Tubule (PCT). The transport of Cl$^-$ occurs via carrier (or transporter) proteins. The carrier proteins involved include:

   1. Na$^+$-K$^+$ATPase

   2. Na$^+$-H$^+$ Exchanger

   3. Cl$^-$-Base Exchanger

   4. K$^+$-Cl$^-$ Cotransporter

C. Ascending Thin Limb of the Loop of Henle (ATL). The ATL reabsorbs **10%** of the filtered Cl$^-$ by **passive transport ("downhill")**, the mechanism of which is poorly understood. Note that the ATL is **impermeable to H$_2$O.**

D. Distal Straight Tubule of the Loop of Henle (DST). The DST reabsorbs **15%** of the filtered Cl$^-$. The transport of Cl$^-$ occurs via carrier (or transporter) proteins and ion channel proteins. Note that the DST is **impermeable to H$_2$O.** The carrier proteins and ion channel proteins involved are as follows:

   1. Na$^+$-K$^+$ATPase

   2. Na$^+$-K$^+$-2Cl$^-$ Cotransporter

3. **K$^+$-Cl$^-$ Cotransporter**
4. **Cl$^-$ ion channel protein.**

E. **Distal Convoluted Tubule (DCT).** The DCT reabsorbs **5%** of the filtered Cl$^-$. The transport of Cl$^-$ occurs via carrier (or transporter) proteins and ion channel proteins. The carrier proteins and ion channel proteins involved include:
   1. **Na$^+$-K$^+$ATPase**
   2. **Na$^+$-Cl$^-$ Cotransporter**
   3. **Cl$^-$ ion channel protein**

F. **Collecting Duct (CD).** The CD (**Type B intercalated cells**) reabsorbs **5%** of the filtered Cl$^-$. The transport of Cl$^-$ occurs via carrier (or transporter) proteins, ion channel proteins, and by diffusion via the paracellular route across a zonula occludens. The carrier proteins and ion channel proteins include:
   1. **H$^+$-ATPase** transports H$^+$ across the basolateral membrane into the interstitial fluid.
   2. **Cl$^-$-HCO$_3^-$ Exchanger**
   3. **Cl$^-$ ion channel protein**

III. Renal Handling of H$_2$O.

H$_2$O is freely-filtered from the glomerular capillaries → Bowman's space and then is reabsorbed by particular segments of the nephron.

A. **Proximal Convoluted Tubule (PCT).** The PCT reabsorbs **65%** of the filtered H$_2$O. The transport of H$_2$O across the luminal and basolateral membranes into the interstitial fluid occurs by **diffusion** using **aquaporin H$_2$O channels.** The transport of H$_2$O across the luminal membrane into the interstitial fluid also occurs by **diffusion via the paracellular route** across a zonula occludens. The diffusion of H$_2$O occurs because of the osmolarity difference between the tubular fluid and interstitial fluid.

B. **Proximal Straight Tubule of the Loop of Henle (PST).** The PST reabsorbs **5%** of the filtered H$_2$O. The transport of H$_2$O across the luminal and basolateral membranes into the interstitial fluid occurs by **diffusion** using **aquaporin H$_2$O channels.** The transport of H$_2$O across the luminal membrane into the interstitial fluid also occurs by **diffusion via the paracellular route** across a zonula occludens. The diffusion of H$_2$O occurs because of the osmolarity difference between the tubular fluid and interstitial fluid as indicated for the PCT.

C. **Descending Thin Limb of the Loop of Henle (DTL).** The DTL reabsorbs **5%** of the filtered H$_2$O. The transport of H$_2$O across the luminal and basolateral membranes into the interstitial fluid occurs by **diffusion** using **aquaporin H$_2$O channels.** The transport of H$_2$O across the luminal membrane into the interstitial fluid also occurs by **diffusion via the paracellular route** across a zonula occludens. The diffusion of H$_2$O occurs because of the osmolarity difference between the tubular fluid and interstitial fluid. The osmolarity difference is created by the reabsorption of Na$^+$ and Cl$^-$ out of the ascending thin limb of the loop of Henle (ATL) into the interstitial fluid, which raises the osmolarity of the interstitial fluid (i.e., hyperosmotic).

D. **Ascending Thin Limb of the Loop of Henle (ATL).** The ATL is impermeable to H$_2$O.

E. **Distal Straight Tubule of the Loop of Henle (DST).** The DST is impermeable to H_2O.

F. **Distal Convoluted Tubule (DCT).** The DCT is impermeable to H_2O.

G. **Collecting Duct (CD).** The CD reabsorbs **5%–25%** of the filtered H_2O depending on the H_2O balance of the person (well-hydrated person vs. poorly-hydrated person, respectively). The transport of H_2O across the luminal and basolateral membranes into the interstitial fluid occurs by **diffusion** using **aquaporin H_2O channels.** The transport of H_2O across the luminal membrane into the interstitial fluid also occurs by **diffusion via the paracellular route** across a zonula occludens. The H_2O reabsorption by the CD is controlled by **anti-diuretic hormone (ADH),** which acts on the **principal cells** of the cortical and medullary collecting ducts and causes increased H_2O reabsorption.

1. **In a Well-hydrated Person.** ADH levels are low and therefore H_2O reabsorption by the CD is low. Consequently, the hyposmotic tubular fluid entering the cortical and medullary CD from the DCT remains hyposmotic as it flows through the CD. The result is the excretion of a large volume of hyposmotic (dilute) urine known as **water diuresis**.

2. **In a Poorly-hydrated Person.** ADH levels are high and therefore H_2O reabsorption by the CD is high.

Ⅳ Summary Table of Renal Handling of Na⁺, Cl⁻, and H₂O (Table 18-1).

TABLE 18-1	**SUMMARY TABLE OF Na⁺, Cl⁻, AND H₂O HANDLING**		
	Na⁺ Reabsorption	Cl⁻ Reabsorption	H₂O Reabsorption
Early PCT	**Luminal Membrane** Na⁺-Nut Cotransporter Na⁺-H⁺ Exchanger	**Luminal Membrane** Diffusion via paracellular route	Diffusion across the cell (aquaporin H₂O channels)
	Basolateral Membrane Na⁺-K⁺ATPase Na⁺-HCO₃⁻ Cotransporter		Diffusion via paracellular route
Late PCT	**Luminal Membrane** Na⁺-H⁺ Exchanger Cl⁻-Base Exchanger	**Luminal Membrane** Na⁺-H⁺ Exchanger Cl⁻ - Base Exchanger	Diffusion across the cell (aquaporin H₂O channels)
	Basolateral Membrane Na⁺-K⁺ATPase K⁺-Cl⁻ Cotransporter 65%	**Basolateral Membrane** Na⁺-K⁺ATPase K⁺-Cl⁻ Cotransporter 65%	Diffusion via paracellular route 65%
PST*	X	X	Diffusion across the cell (aquaporin H₂O channels)
			Diffusion via paracellular route 5%

TABLE 18-1	SUMMARY TABLE OF Na⁺, Cl⁻, AND H₂O HANDLING *(continued)*		
	Na⁺ Reabsorption	**Cl⁻ Reabsorption**	**H₂O Reabsorption**
DTL*	X	X	Diffusion across the cell (aquaporin H_2O channels) Diffusion via paracellular route 5%
ATL*†	Mechanism ? 10%	Mechanism? 10%	X
DST*†	**Luminal Membrane** Na^+-K^+-$2Cl^-$ Cotransporter Na^+-H^+ Exchanger Diffusion via paracellular route	**Luminal Membrane** Na^+-Cl^--$2K^+$ Cotransporter	X
	Basolateral Membrane Na^+-K^+ATPase Na^+-HCO_3^- Cotransporter 15%	**Basolateral Membrane** Na^+-K^+ATPase K^+-Cl^- Cotransporter Cl^- ion channel protein 15%	
DCT	**Luminal Membrane** Na^+-Cl^- Cotransporter Na^+ ion channel protein	**Luminal Membrane** Na^+-Cl^- Cotransporter	X
	Basolateral Membrane Na^+-K^+ATPase 5%	**Basolateral Membrane** Na^+-K^+ATPase Cl^- ion channel protein 5%	
CD	**Luminal Membrane** Na^+ ion channel protein	**Luminal Membrane** Cl^- -HCO_3^- Exchanger Diffusion via paracellular route	Diffusion across the cell (aquaporin H_2O channels)
	Basolateral Membrane Na^+-K^+ATPase 5%	**Basolateral Membrane** H^+ATPase Cl^- ion channel protein 5%	Diffusion via paracellular route ADH sensitive 5–25%

Nut = organic nutrient;   * = loop of Henle;   † = diluting segment;   **X** = no reabsorption;   ? = mechanism not fully elucidated

19

Concentration of Urine

I   **Concentration of Urine.** As mentioned previously, the isosmotic tubular fluid entering the medullary CD from the cortical CD undergoes more H_2O reabsorption by diffusion because of the osmolarity difference between the isosmotic tubular fluid (300 mOsm/L) and the hyperosmotic medullary interstitial fluid (as high as 1400 mOsm/L). What causes the medullary interstitial fluid to be so hyperosmotic is the countercurrent multiplier system.

II   **The Countercurrent Multiplier System (Figure 19-1A).** The countercurrent multiplier system **creates the hyperosmolarity gradient** within the interstitial fluid in the kidney medulla, which is crucial for urine concentration. The countercurrent multiplier system involves the **loops of Henle** from juxtamedullary nephrons, which extend very long loops of Henle deep into the medulla. In the loops of Henle, tubular fluid flows down the descending limb (PST and DTL) and then back up the ascending limb (ATL and DST); hence the term **countercurrent**. The differences in permeability of the descending limb and ascending limb establish a small osmolarity difference at the higher levels of the loop of Henle so that the tubular fluid entering the next lower level of the loop of Henle is more concentrated. This process is repeated over and over as tubular fluid flows to lower levels of the loop of Henle. Consequently, the countercurrent flow multiplies a small osmolarity difference such that a hyperosmotic gradient of **300–1400 mOsm** is created within the medullary interstitial fluid; hence the term **multiplier**. The permeability differences of the descending limb and ascending limb of the loop of Henle are reviewed below.

    A. **Descending Limb of the loop of Henle (PST and DTL)** is impermeable to Na^+ and Cl^- but permeable to H_2O.

    B. **Ascending Limb of the loop of Henle (ATL and DST)** is permeable to Na^+ and Cl^- but impermeable to H_2O.

III   **The Balancing of Urea (Figure 19-1B).** The discussion of the countercurrent multiplier system may give the false impression that the hyperosmolarity of the medullary interstitial fluid is due solely to Na^+ and Cl^-. However, about 50% of the hyperosmolarity of the medullary interstitial fluid is due to urea such that the 1400 mOsm/L at the tip of the medulla is due to Na^+ and Cl^- (700 mOsm/L) and urea (700 mOsm/L). The concentration of urea within the tubular fluid of the cortical and outer medullary collecting ducts rises progressively as reabsorption of H_2O occurs but urea is retained because these duct segments are impermeable to urea. As a result, the concentration of urea within the tubular fluid delivered to the inner medullary collecting ducts is very high. Consequently, the inner medullary collecting ducts reabsorb urea by facilitated diffusion using the Urea Transporter and simultaneously reabsorb H_2O, which maintains a high concentration of urea within the inner medullary collecting ducts even though urea is being reabsorbed from these ducts. The net result is that the concentration of urea within the tubular fluid of the inner medullary collecting ducts equals the concentration of urea within the inner medullary interstitial fluid, that is, the urea concentration is balanced.

IV — THE COUNTERCURRENT EXCHANGER SYSTEM (Figure 19-10) maintains the hyperosmolarity gradient of the interstitial fluid in the kidney medulla, which is crucial for urine concentration. The countercurrent exchanger system involves the **vasa recta** (capillaries) that arise from the efferent arteriole of juxtamedullary nephrons which extend very long capillaries deep into the medulla. The vasa recta form a hairpin loop in which blood flows down the descending side and then back up the ascending side; hence the term **countercurrent**. If the kidney were supplied by an ordinary capillary bed (i.e., no hairpin loop) containing blood of 300 mOsm/L, H_2O would diffuse out of the capillaries and Na^+ and Cl^- ions would diffuse into the capillaries, thereby destroying the hyperosmolarity gradient. This is exactly what happens as blood flows down the descending side, but then the process is reversed or exchanged as blood flows up the ascending side; hence the term **exchanger**. This unique, hairpin loop arrangement of the vasa recta maintains the hyperosmolarity gradient of the medullary interstitial fluid.

V — The Well-Hydrated Person (Production of a Dilute Urine). After drinking a liter of H_2O, an already well-hydrated person will produce a **dilute, hyposmotic urine** (50 mOsm/L_{urine} < 300 mOsm/L_{blood}). This occurs because ADH levels are low (↓ **ADH**) and therefore H_2O reabsorption by the collecting ducts (CD) is low (↓**H_2O reabsorption**). In this situation, the hyperosmolarity gradient within the interstitial fluid in the kidney medulla is reduced compared to normal (300 mOsm/L → 600 mOsm/L versus 300 mOsm/L → 1400 mOsm/L) because about 15% of the filtered H_2O is not reabsorbed, resulting in a high flow rate of the tubular fluid.

VI — The Poorly-Hydrated Person (Production of a Concentrated Urine). In order to conserve the body store of H_2O, a poorly-hydrated person will produce a **concentrated, hyperosmotic urine** (1440 mOsm/L_{urine} > 300 mOsm/Lblood). This occurs because ADH levels are high (↑**ADH**) and therefore H_2O reabsorption by the collecting ducts (CD) is high (↑ **H_2O reabsorption**). In this situation, the hyperosmolarity gradient within the interstitial fluid in the kidney medulla is normal (300 mOsm/L → 1400 mOsm/L), which assists in the H_2O reabsorption.

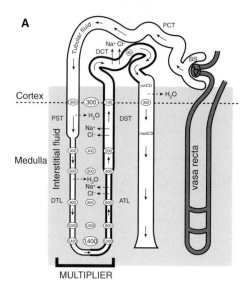

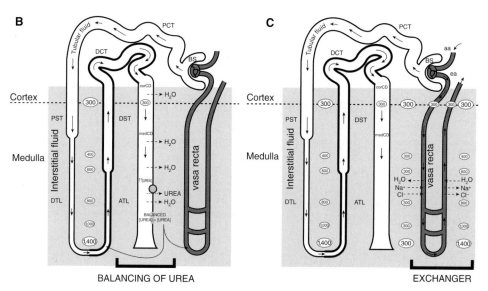

● **Figure 19-1: (A) Diagram of the Countercurrent Multiplier System.** The countercurrent multiplier system involves the loop of Henle. The descending limb of the loop of Henle consists of the proximal straight tubule (PST) and the descending thin limb (DTL). The ascending limb of the loop of Henle consists of the ascending thin limb (ATL) and the distal straight tubule (DST). The PST and DTL are impermeable to Na^+ and Cl^- but permeable to H_2O. The ATL and DST are permeable to Na^+ and Cl^- but impermeable to H_2O. **(B) Diagram of Balancing of Urea.** The balancing of urea involves the reabsorption of H_2O by the cortical and outer medullary collecting ducts, which are impermeable to urea. This results in the delivery of tubular fluid with a very high concentration of urea ($\uparrow\uparrow$ [urea]) to the inner medullary collecting ducts. Note that the inner medullary collecting ducts contain the Urea Transporter (O) which reabsorb urea along with H_2O. The net result in the balancing of urea ([urea]$_{tubular\ fluid}$ = [urea]$_{interstitial\ fluid}$). The urea within the interstitial fluid is either recycled back to the loop of Henle or removed by the vasa recta. **(C) Diagram of the Countercurrent Exchanger System.** The blood (300 mOsm/L) from the efferent arteriole flows down the descending side of the vasa recta within the kidney medulla and is exposed to the hyperosmolarity gradient. This exposure causes the diffusion of H_2O out of the descending side of the vasa recta and diffusion of Na^+ and Cl^- into the descending side of the vasa recta; thereby destroying the hyperosmolarity gradient (Note 300 mOsm/L throughout the medulla). However, when the blood flows up the ascending side of the vasa recta the process is reversed and the hyperosmolarity gradient is reestablished (Note 300–1400 mOsm/L). In reality, the hyperosmolarity gradient is never destroyed because the actions of the descending side and ascending side of the vasa recta occur simultaneously and therefore cancel each other so that the hyperosmolarity gradient is always maintained. BS=Bowman's space; PCT=proximal convoluted tubule; DCT=distal convoluted tubule; corCD=cortical collecting duct; medCD=medullary collecting duct. Dotted lines=diffusion; Dashed lines=facilitated diffusion; aa=afferent arteriole; ea=efferent arteriole. The thick outlining indicates its H_2O impermeability. The numbers in the circles indicate the osmolarity (mOsm/L) of the tubular fluid and the medullary interstitial fluid.

20

Control of Na$^+$ and H$_2$O

Control of Na$^+$ Excretion in the Urine. Even though normal persons have a wide range of Na$^+$ intakes and sporadic occurrences of large losses of Na$^+$ via the skin or GI tract, total body Na$^+$ varies minimally. The amount of Na$^+$ excreted in the urine is given by the formula below:

$$Na^+ \text{ excretion} = Na^+ \text{ filtered} - Na^+ \text{ reabsorbed}$$
$$= (GFR \times [P]_{Na+}) - Na^+ \text{ reabsorbed}$$

where,

GFR = glomerular filtration rate
$[P]_{Na+}$ = plasma concentration of Na$^+$

Consequently, Na$^+$ excretion in the urine can be adjusted by controlling any of three variables: $[P]_{Na+}$, GFR, or Na$^+$ reabsorption as discussed below.

A. [P] $_{Na+}$. In most physiological conditions, $[P]_{Na+}$ changes very little and is not an important control point for Na$^+$ excretion in the urine. The normal plasma concentration of Na$^+$ is 140 mEq/L (**$[P]_{Na+}$ = 140 mEq/L**).

B. GFR. In most physiological conditions, GFR changes very little and is not an important control point of Na$^+$ excretion in the urine.

C. Na$^+$ Reabsorption. Na$^+$ reabsorption is the most important variable in the control of Na$^+$ excretion in the urine. Na$^+$ reabsorption is controlled by a number of factors as indicated below.
   1. **Blood Pressure Monitored by Baroreceptors.** The baroreceptors are stretch receptors that monitor **changes in blood pressure** and are located in the walls of the common carotid arteries (i.e.,**carotid sinus**), great veins, atria, and aortic arch. The baroreceptors are innervated by CN IX and CN X and affect **renin** release.
   2. **Blood Pressure Monitored by Juxtaglomerular (JG) Cells.** The JG complex contains **JG cells** (which act as intrarenal baroreceptors) that monitor **changes in blood pressure** and affect **renin** release.
   3. **Tubular Fluid Concentration of Na$^+$ ([TF]$_{Na+}$).** The JG complex contains **macula densa (MD) cells** that monitor **changes in Na$^+$** within the tubular fluid of the distal straight tubule (DST) and affect **renin** release.

4. **Renin.** Renin is an enzyme that converts **angiotensinogen** (produced by the liver) to **angiotensin I.** Angiotensin I is converted to **angiotensin II** (primarily by endothelium of lung capillaries) by **angiotensin converting enzyme (ACE).**

5. **Angiotensin II.** Angiotensin II has widespread actions (see Chapter 8).

6. **Atrial Natriuretic Peptide (ANP).** ANP is secreted by **myocardial endocrine cells** located within the right and left atria of the **heart.** ANP is secreted in response to increased blood volume or increased venous pressure within the atria (e.g., atrial distention due to left atrial failure). The functions of ANP include the following:

   a. Directly **decreases aldosterone** secretion from the adrenal cortex.

   b. Directly **decreases Na$^+$ reabsorption** by the medullary collecting duct

   c. Directly **increases glomerular filtration rate (GFR)** by vasoconstriction of the efferent arteriole.

   d. Directly **decreases renin** release from juxtaglomerular cells which leads to decreased **angiotensin II**.

II. **Control of Na$^+$ Ingestion in the Diet ("Salt Appetite").** A strong hedonistic appetite is the most important controller of Na$^+$ ingestion in the diet. Most Americans consume about 10–15 g/day even though <0.5 g/day is quite sufficient.

III. **Control of H$_2$O Excretion in the Urine.** Even though normal persons have a wide range of H$_2$O intakes and sporadic occurrences of large losses of H$_2$O via the skin or GI tract, total-body H$_2$O varies minimally. The amount of H$_2$O excreted in the urine is given by the formula below:

$$H_2O \text{ excretion} = H_2O \text{ filtered} - H_2O \text{ reabsorbed}$$
$$= (GFR \times [P]_{H_2O}) - H_2O \text{ reabsorbed}$$

where,
$$GFR = \text{glomerular filtration rate}$$
$$[P]_{H_2O} = \text{plasma concentration of } H_2O$$

Consequently, H$_2$O excretion in the urine can be adjusted by controlling any of three variables: $[P]_{H_2O}$, GFR, Na$^+$ reabsorption as discussed below.

A. [P] $_{H_2O}$. In most physiological conditions, $[P]_{H_2O}$ changes very little and is not an important control point for H$_2$O excretion in the urine.

B. GFR. In most physiological conditions, GFR changes very little and is not an important control point of H$_2$O excretion in the urine.

C. H$_2$O Reabsorption. H$_2$O reabsorption is the most important variable in the control of H$_2$O excretion in the urine. H$_2$O reabsorption is controlled by a number of factors as indicated below.

1. **Blood Pressure Monitored by Baroreceptors.** The baroreceptors are stretch receptors that monitor **changes in blood pressure** and are located in the walls of the common carotid arteries (i.e.,**carotid sinus**), great veins, atria, and aortic arch. The baroreceptors are innervated by CN IX and CN X that relay information to the supraoptic nucleus and paraventricular nucleus of the **hypothalamus**.

2. **Plasma Osmolarity Monitored by Osmoreceptors.** The osmoreceptors are neurons that monitor **changes in plasma osmolarity** and are located in various nuclei within the hypothalamus. These neurons relay information to the supraoptic nucleus and paraventricular nucleus of the **hypothalamus**.

3. **ADH.** ADH is the most important controller of H_2O reabsorption and hence H_2O excretion in urine. ADH is secreted by axon terminals within the **neurohypophysis** whose cell bodies are located in the supraoptic nucleus and paraventricular nucleus of the **hypothalamus**. ADH **increases H_2O reabsorption** from tubular fluid → plasma by the cortical and medullary collecting ducts and thereby decreases H_2O excretion in the urine.

Ⅳ Control of H₂O Ingestion in the Diet ("Thirst").

The **hypothalamic thirst center** is the most important controller of H_2O ingestion in the diet. A decreased blood pressure or increased plasma osmolarity will increase the firing of the hypothalamic thirst center and lead to the subjective feeling of thirst that causes an individual to increase H_2O ingestion in the diet. **Angiotensin II** will also increase the firing of the CNS areas and lead to the subjective feeling of thirst that causes an individual to increase H_2O ingestion in the diet.

Ⅴ Epilogue.

The control of Na^+ and H_2O excretion in the urine is the way the body regulates **plasma volume**. By the same token, control of Na^+ and H_2O excretion in the urine is the way the body regulates **extracellular fluid (ECF) volume** since Na^+ accounts for >90% of all osmotically active extracellular solutes. Note that plasma volume affects blood volume, venous blood pressure, atrial blood pressure, ventricular blood pressure, stroke volume, cardiac output, and finally arterial blood pressure. In order to see the forest through the trees, one must appreciate the relationship between the **control of Na^+ and H_2O excretion in the urine, plasma volume and ECF volume**, and **arterial blood pressure**. Increased arterial blood pressure (i.e., hypertension) will cause a decreased Na^+ reabsorption through the renin-angiotensin II mechanism leading to a marked, rapid increase in Na^+ (and H_2O) excretion in the urine. This is sometimes called **"pressure natriuresis" ("pressure diuresis")** and is the most important long-term blood pressure control.

Ⅵ Physiological Reactions to a Decreased Plasma Volume Due to Low Body Na+ Levels (e.g., low NaCl diet) and Loss of H₂O (e.g., hemorrhage, diarrhea, or severe sweating).

A. **Control of Na^+ Excretion in the Urine.** The low body Na^+ levels and loss of H_2O will result in a **decreased plasma volume**. The low Na^+ levels in the tubular fluid will be monitored by the macula densa cells (MD) of the distal straight tubule (DST), while the decrease in blood pressure will be monitored by baroreceptors and JG cells. This leads to **increased renin release**, which leads to **increased angiotensin II**. Increased angiotensin II stimulates the adrenal cortex, which leads to **increased aldosterone**. Increased ALD stimulates the kidney, which leads to **increased Na^+ reabsorption** by the cortical collecting ducts. This is most important controller of Na^+ reabsorption.

B. **Control of H_2O Excretion in the Urine.** The loss of H_2O will result in a **decreased plasma volume**. The increase in plasma osmolarity will be monitored by hypothalamic osmoreceptors, while the decrease in blood pressure will be monitored by barorecep-tors. The osmoreceptors and baroreceptors stimulate neurons within the supraoptic and paraventricular nuclei, which leads to **increased anti-diuretic hormone (ADH)** release from the neurohypophysis. Increased ADH stimulates the kidney, which leads to **increased H_2O reabsorption** by the cortical and medullary collecting ducts. This is the most important controller of H_2O reabsorption.

VII Physiological Reactions to an Increased Plasma Volume Due to High Body Na^+ Levels (e.g., high NaCl diet) and Gain of H_2O (e.g., excess H_2O ingested).

A. **Control of Na^+ Excretion in the Urine.** The high body Na^+ levels and gain of H_2O will result in an **increased plasma volume**. The high Na^+ levels in the tubular fluid will be monitored by the macula densa cells (MD) of the distal straight tubule (DST), while the increase in blood pressure will be monitored by baroreceptors and JG cells. This leads to **increased atrial natriuretic peptide (ANP)**. ANP **directly decreases aldosterone** secretion from the adrenal cortex, **directly decreases Na^+ reabsorption** by the medullary collecting duct, **directly increases glomerular filtration rate (GFR)** by vasoconstriction of the efferent arteriole, and **directly decreases renin** release from juxtaglomerular cells, which leads to **decreased angiotensin II**. Decreased angiotensin II leads to **decreased aldosterone.**

B. **Control of H_2O Excretion in the Urine.** The gain of H_2O will result in an **increased plasma volume**. The decrease in plasma osmolarity will be monitored by hypothalamic osmoreceptors, while the increase in blood pressure will be moni-tored by baroreceptors. The osmoreceptors and baroreceptors inhibit neurons within the supraoptic and paraventricular nuclei, which leads to **decreased anti-diuretic hormone (ADH)** release from the neurohypophysis. Decreased ADH leads to **decreased H_2O reabsorption** by the cortical and medullary collecting ducts. This is the most important controller of H_2O reabsorption.

21

Renal Handling of K⁺

❶ **Renal Handling of K⁺.** K1 is freely-filtered from the glomerular capillaries $\rightarrow$ Bowman's space and then is reabsorbed or secreted by particular segments of the nephron.

A. **Proximal Convoluted Tubule (PCT).** The PCT reabsorbs **55%** of the filtered K^+ by **diffusion via the paracellular route** across the zonula occludens whether the person is on a low K^+ diet (K^+ depleted) or high/normal K^+ diet.

B. **Distal Straight Tubule of the Loop of Henle (DST).** The DST reabsorbs **30%** of the filtered K^+. The transport of K^+ occurs via carrier (or transporter) proteins and by **diffusion via the paracellular route** across the zonula occludens whether the person is on a low K^+ diet (K^+ depleted) or high/normal K^+ diet. The carrier proteins involved include:
   1. **Na^+-K^+ATPase** transports Na^+ across the basolateral membrane into the interstitial fluid (i.e., "pumps" Na^+ out of the cell) keeping cytoplasmic $[Na^+]$ low by countertransport with K^+ into the cytoplasm (i.e.,"pumps" K^+ into the cell) keeping cytoplasmic $[K^+]$ high.
   2. **Na^+-K^+-$2Cl^-$ Cotransporter**

C. **Distal Convoluted Tubule (DCT).** The DCT reabsorbs filtered K^+ by **diffusion via the paracellular route** across the zonula occludens when a person is on a low K^+ diet (K^+ depleted). The DCT secretes plasma K^+ (plasma $\rightarrow$ tubular fluid) when a person is on a high/normal K^+ diet but its contribution is minimal.

D. **Cortical Collecting Duct (corCD).**
   1. **The corCD (Type A intercalated cells)** reabsorbs filtered K^+ when a person is on a low K^+ diet (K^+ depleted). The reabsorption of K^+ occurs via carrier (transporter) proteins and ion channel proteins. The carrier proteins and ion channel proteins involved include:
      a. **H^+-K^+ATPase** transports K^+ across the luminal membrane into the cytoplasm by countertransport with H^+ into the tubular fluid.
      b. **K^+ ion channel protein**
   2. **The corCD (principal cells)** secretes plasma K^+ (plasma$\rightarrow$ tubular fluid) when a person is on a high/normal K^+ diet. The secretion of K^+ occurs via carrier (transporter) proteins and ion channel proteins. The carrier proteins and ion channel proteins involved include:
      a. **Na^+-K^+ATPase**
      b. **K^+ ion channel protein**.

E. Medullary Collecting Duct (medCD). The medCD reabsorbs filtered K^+ by **diffusion via the paracellular route** across the zonula occludens whether the person is on a low K^+ diet (K$^+$ depleted) or high/normal K^+ diet.

Ⅱ Summary Table of Renal Handling of K⁺. (Table 21-1).

TABLE 21-1	SUMMARY TABLE OF K+ HANDLING	
	K⁺ Reabsorption	**K⁺ Secretion**
PCT	**Luminal Membrane** Diffusion via paracellular route **55%**	X
PST*	X	X
DTL*	X	X
ATL*	X	X
DST*	**Luminal Membrane** Na⁺-K⁺-2Cl⁻ Cotransporter Diffusion via paracellular route **Basolateral Membrane** Na⁺-K⁺ATPase 30%	X
DCT	**Luminal Membrane** Diffusion via paracellular route	Minimal secretion
corCD	**Luminal Membrane** H⁺-K⁺ ATPase **Basolateral Membrane** K⁺ ion channel protein Low K⁺ Diet Type A Intercalated	**Luminal Membrane** K⁺ ion channel protein **Basolateral Membrane** Na⁺-K⁺ATPase High/Normal K⁺ Diet Principal cell
medCD	**Luminal Membrane** Diffusion via paracellular route	

*= loop of Henle;   X=no reabsorption or secretion;   PCT= proximal convoluted tubule;
PST=proximal straight tubule;   DTL=descending limb of the loop of Henle;   ATL=ascending limb of the loop of Henle;
DCT=distal convoluted tubule;   corCD=cortical collecting duct;   medCD=medullary collecting duct.

22

Control of K⁺

❶ **Control of K⁺ Excretion in the Urine.** Even though normal persons have a wide range of K⁺ intakes and sporadic occurrences of large losses of K⁺ via the GI tract (e.g., vomiting or diarrhea), total body K⁺ varies minimally with about 98% of total body K⁺ residing within the intracellular fluid (ICF) because of the action of Na^+-K^+ATPase pumps. The amount of K⁺ excreted in the urine is given by the formula below:

$$K^+ \text{ excretion} = K^+ \text{ filtered} - K^+ \text{ reabsorbed} + K^+ \text{ secreted}$$
$$= (GFR \times [P]_{K+}) - K^+ \text{ reabsorbed} + K^+ \text{ secreted}$$

where,

GFR = glomerular filtration rate

$[P]_{K+}$ = plasma concentration of K⁺

Consequently, K⁺ excretion in the urine can be adjusted by controlling any of four variables: $[P]_{K+}$, GFR, K⁺ reabsorption, or K⁺ secretion as discussed below.

A. **$[P]_{K+}$.** In most physiological conditions, $[P]_{K+}$ changes very little. The normal plasma concentration of K⁺ is 4mEq/L (**$[P]_{K+}$ = 4mEq/L**).

B. **GFR.** In most physiological conditions, GFR changes very little and is not an important control point of K⁺ excretion in the urine.

C. **K⁺ Reabsorption.** In most physiological conditions, K⁺ reabsorption changes very little and is not an important control point of K⁺ excretion in the urine. However, in patients treated with diuretics that decrease Na^+ reabsorption from the PCT or DST, decreased K⁺ reabsorption also occurs at the PCT or DST, thereby causing increased K⁺ excretion in the urine.

D. **K⁺ Secretion.** K⁺ secretion by the **principal cells of the cortical collecting duct** is the most important variable in the control of K⁺ excretion in the urine. K⁺ secretion is controlled by a number of factors as indicated below:

    1. **$[P]_{K+}$ Monitored by Zona Glomerulosa (ZG) Cells of the Adrenal Cortex.** The ZG cells of the adrenal cortex monitor **changes in $[P]_{K+}$** and secrete **aldosterone (ALD)** in response to increased $[P]_{K+}$. ALD **increases K⁺ secretion by the principal cells of the corCD** and thereby increases K⁺ excretion in the urine.

ALD elicits this action (like any other steroid hormone) by binding to an intracellular receptor within the principal cells, entering the nucleus, and causing the translation of proteins that increase the activity and/or number of K^+ ion channel proteins and Na^+-K^+ ATPase.

2. **$[P]_{K+}$ Monitored by Principal Cells of the Cortical Collecting Ducts (corCD).** The principal cells of the corCD monitor **changes in $[P]_{K+}$.** Increased $[P]_{K+}$ enhances the activity of the **Na^+-K^+ATPase** on the basolateral membrane of the principal cells of the corCD, which allows more K^+ to enter the cytoplasm. The **K^+ ion channel protein** transports the increased cytoplasmic K^+ across the luminal membrane into the tubular fluid by forming hydrophilic pores that allow diffusion of K^+. This **increases K^+ secretion by the principal cells of the corCD** and thereby increases K^+ excretion in the urine.

3. **Plasma pH Affects Activity of Na^+-K^+ATPase.** Increased plasma pH (alkalosis) enhances the activity of the **Na^+-K^+ATPase** on the basolateral membrane of the principal cells of the cortical collecting duct (corCD) which allows more K^+ to enter the cytoplasm. The **K^+ ion channel protein** transports the increased cytoplasmic K^+ across the luminal membrane into the tubular fluid by forming hydrophilic pores that allow diffusion of K^+. This **increases K^+ secretion by the principal cells of the corCD** and thereby increases K^+ excretion in the urine.

A Dilemma for K^+ Balance.
It should be remembered that aldosterone (ALD) is the most important controller of Na^+ reabsorption. ALD affects Na^+ reabsorption by the principal cells of the cortical collecting ducts (corCD). But, ALD also affects K^+ secretion by the principal cells of the corCD. So, this question arises: When the body tries to regulate Na^+ balance by ALD secretion, does it cause an inappropriate change in K^+ balance? The answer is no in most physiological conditions as indicated below.

A. **Person on a High NaCl Diet.** A high NaCl diet leads to **decreased ALD,** causing decreased Na^+ reabsorption by the corCD and **decreased anti-diuretic hormone (ADH),** causing decreasing H_2O reabsorption by the corCD and medullary collecting ducts (medCD). This results in an **increased flow of tubular fluid (mL/min)** flowing into the corCD, which causes **increased K^+ secretion.** Why? Because the increased flow of tubular fluid keeps the $[K^+]$ within the tubular fluid very low and thus promotes the final step in K^+ secretion, which is diffusion through K^+ ion channel proteins. However, at the same time, decreased ALD causes **decreased K^+ secretion.** Consequently, the increased K^+ secretion caused by the increased flow of tubular fluid is counterbalanced by the decreased K^+ secretion caused by decreased ALD so that **no change in K^+ excretion in the urine** occurs.

B. **Patient Treated with Loop Diuretics or Thiazide Diuretics.** Treatment with loop diuretics [e.g., Furosemide (Lasix)] or thiazide diuretics [e.g., Hydrochlorothiazide (HydroDIURIL)] leads to decreased Na^+ reabsorption and decreased H_2O reabsorption. This results in an **increased flow of tubular fluid (mL/min)** flowing into the corCD which causes **increased K^+ secretion.** Why? Because the increased flow of tubular fluid (TF) keeps the tubular fluid concentration of K^+ very low ($\downarrow[TF]_{K+}$) and thus promotes the final step in K^+ secretion, which is diffusion through K^+ ion channel proteins. However, loop diuretics or thiazide diuretics do not affect ALD secretion. Consequently, the increased K^+ secretion caused by the increased flow of tubular fluid is not counterbalanced so that **increased K^+ excretion in the urine** occurs, which leads to severe K^+ depletion.

III **Epilogue.** The physiological regulation of the K$^+$ concentration within the extracellular fluid (**[ECF]$_{K+}$**) is very important, due to its role in the excitability of nerve and muscle tissue. The control of K$^+$ excretion in the urine is one way the body regulates [ECF]$_{K+}$. The control of K$^+$ distribution between the extracellular fluid and intracellular fluid (i.e., [ECF]$_{K+}$ versus [ICF]$_{K+}$) is another way the body regulates [ECF]$_{K+}$. [ECF]$_{K+}$ accounts for about 2% of the total body K$^+$, while [ICF]$_{K+}$ accounts for about 98% of the total body K$^+$. Since the amount of K$^+$ within the ECF is so small even minor shifts of K$^+$ into or out of cells can result in large changes in [ECF]$_{K+}$. The three major factors that control K$^+$ distribution are as follows:

A. Epinephrine. During exercise or trauma, epinephrine moves K$^+$ into cells by stimulating Na$^+$-K$^+$ATPase pumps (ECF → ICF).

B. Insulin. After a meal, insulin moves K$^+$ into cells by stimulating Na$^+$-K$^+$ ATPase pumps (ECF → ICF).

C. H$^+$ Concentration Within the Extracellular Fluid ([ECF]$_{H+}$). A decrease in [ECF]$_{H+}$ (i.e., alkalosis) moves K$^+$ into cells by unknown mechanisms (ECF → ICF). An increase in [ECF]$_{H+}$ (i.e., acidosis) moves K$^+$ out of cells by unknown mechanisms (ICF→ ECF).

IV **Physiological Reactions to Low K$^+$ Diet.** A low K$^+$ diet will result in a decreased plasma concentration of K$^+$ ($\downarrow$ [P]$_{K+}$). The $\downarrow$ [P]$_{K+}$ will be monitored by the zona glomerulosa (ZG) cells of the adrenal cortex. This leads to **decreased aldosterone (ALD)**. Decreased ALD leads to **decreased K$^+$ secretion** by the cortical collecting ducts. The $\downarrow$ [P]$_{K+}$ will also be monitored by the principal cells of the cortical collecting ducts (corCD). This leads to **decreased activity of Na$^+$-K$^+$ATPase** on the basolateral membrane of the principal cells of the corCD. Decreased activity of Na$^+$-K$^+$ATPase leads to **decreased K$^+$ secretion.** Note that there are other pathological and pharmacological situations that may lead to decreased K$^+$ secretion [e.g., hypoaldosteronism (due to Addison Disease or Congenital Adrenal Hyperplasia), acidosis, or K$^+$-sparing diuretics]. The net physiological reaction leads to decreased K$^+$ excretion in the urine.

V **Physiological Reactions to High K$^+$ Diet.** A high K$^+$ diet will result in an increased plasma concentration of K$^+$ ($\uparrow$ [P]$_{K+}$). The high K$^+$ levels in the plasma will be monitored by the zona glomerulosa (ZG) cells of the adrenal cortex. This leads to **increased aldosterone (ALD).** Increased ALD leads to **increased K$^+$ secretion** by the cortical collecting ducts. The high K$^+$ levels in the plasma will also be monitored by the principal cells of the cortical collecting ducts (corCD). This leads to **increased activity of Na$^+$-K$^+$ATPase** on the basolateral membrane of the principal cells of the corCD. Increased activity of Na$^+$-K$^+$ATPase leads to **increased K$^+$ secretion.** Note that there are other pathological and pharmacological situations that may lead to increased K$^+$ secretion [e.g., hyperaldosteronism (due to Conn Syndrome), alkalosis, loop diuretics, thiazide diuretics, or luminal anions]. The net physiological reaction leads to increased K$^+$ excretion in the urine.

23

Renal Handling of Ca^{2+} and PO_4^{2-}

① **Renal Handling of Ca^{2+}.** Ca^{2+} (not bound to proteins) is freely-filtered from the glomerular capillaries → Bowman's space and then is reabsorbed by particular segments of the nephron.

A. **Proximal Convoluted Tubule (PCT).** The PCT reabsorbs **80%** of the filtered Ca^{2+} by **diffusion via the paracellular route** across the zonula occludens. The forces driving Ca^{2+} reabsorption are dependent on Na^+ reabsorption. In this regard, a low NaCl diet will increase Ca^{2+} reabsorption by the PCT; whereas, a high NaCl diet will decrease Ca^{2+} reabsorption by the PCT.

B. **Distal Straight Tubule (DST).** The DST reabsorbs **10%** of the filtered Ca^{2+} by **diffusion via the paracellular route** across the zonula occludens. In this regard, a low NaCl diet will increase Ca^{2+} reabsorption by the DST, whereas a high NaCl diet will decrease Ca^{2+} reabsorption by the DST.

C. **Distal Convoluted Tubule (DCT).** The DCT reabsorbs **5%** of the filtered Ca^{2+}. The transport of Ca^{2+} occurs via carrier (transporter) proteins and ion channel proteins. The carrier proteins and ion channel proteins involved include:
   1. **Ca^{2+} ATPase** transports Ca^{2+} across the basolateral membrane into the interstitial fluid.
   2. **Na^+-Ca^{2+} Exchanger**
   3. **Na^+-K^+ ATPase**
   4. **Ca^{2+} ion channel protein**

D. **Collecting Duct (CD).** The CD reabsorbs **5%** of the filtered Ca^{2+}. The transport of Ca^{2+} occurs via carrier (transporter) proteins and ion channel proteins. The carrier proteins and ion channel proteins involved are the same as for the DCT above.

② **Renal Handling of PO_4^{2-}.** PO_4^{2-} (not bound to proteins) is freely-filtered from the glomerular capillaries → Bowman's space and then is reabsorbed solely by the proximal convoluted tubule (PCT).

A. **Proximal Convoluted Tubule (PCT).** The PCT reabsorbs **85%** of the filtered PO_4^{2-}. Since the later nephron segments do not reabsorb PO_4^{2-}, the remaining 15% of PO_4^{2-}

is excreted in the urine. The transport of PO_4^{2-} occurs via carrier (transporter) proteins. The carrier (transporter) proteins include:

1. **Na^+-PO_4^{2-} Cotransporter**
2. **PO_4^{2-} - Anion Exchanger**
3. **Na^+-K^+ ATPase**

B. No other portion of the nephron is involved in PO_4^{2-} reabsorption.

III Summary Table of Renal Handling of Ca^{2+} and PO_4^{2-} (Table 23-1).

TABLE 23-1	SUMMARY TABLE OF Ca^{2+} AND PO_4^{2-} HANDLING	
	Ca^{2+} Reabsorption	PO_4^{2-} Reabsorption
PCT	**Luminal Membrane** Diffusion via paracellular route 80%	**Luminal Membrane** Na^+-PO_4^{2-} Cotransporter **Basolateral Membrane** PO_4^{2-} - Anion Exchanger Na^+-K^+ ATPase 85%
PST*	X	X
DTL*	X	X
ATL*	X	X
DST*	**Luminal Membrane** Diffusion via paracellular route 10%	X
DCT	**Luminal Membrane** Ca^{2+} ion channel protein **Basolateral Membrane** Ca^{2+} ATPase Na^+-Ca^{2+} Exchanger Na^+-K^+ATPase 5%	X
CD	**Luminal Membrane** Ca^{2+} ion channel protein **Basolateral Membrane** Ca^{2+} ATPase Na^+-Ca^{2+} Exchanger Na^+-K^+ATPase 5%	X

* = loop of Henle

24

Control of Ca^{2+} and PO_4^{2-}

I **Control of Ca^{2+} Excretion in the Urine.** The amount of Ca^{2+} excretion in the urine equals the amount of new Ca^{2+} added to the body via absorption by the gastrointestinal (GI) tract. Consequently, the kidneys maintain a stable balance of total body Ca^{2+}. However, the kidneys do not respond to a low/high Ca^{2+} diet as much as they do to a low/high NaCl diet or a low/high K^+ diet because most of the dietary increment never gains entry into the blood because the GI tract fails to absorb the dietary increment. The amount of Ca^{2+} excreted in the urine is given by the formula below:

$$Ca^{2+} \text{ excretion} = Ca^{2+} \text{ filtered} - Ca^{2+} \text{ reabsorbed}$$
$$= (GFR \times [P]_{Ca2+}) - Ca^{2+} \text{ reabsorbed}$$

where,

$$GFR = \text{glomerular filtration rate}$$
$$[P]_{Ca2+} = \text{plasma concentration of } Ca^{2+}$$

Consequently, Ca^{2+} excretion in the urine can be adjusted by controlling any of three variables: $[P]_{Ca2+}$, GFR, or Ca^{2+} reabsorption as discussed below.

A. $[P]_{Ca2+}$. Plasma calcium exists in three forms: ionized calcium (Ca^{2+}; 45%), calcium complexed with anions (e.g., $CaPO_4$; 15%), and calcium reversibly bound to plasma proteins, which is profoundly affected by plasma pH (40%). In most physiological conditions, $[P]_{Ca2+}$ changes very little. The normal plasma concentration of Ca^{2+} is 5mEq/L ($[P]_{Ca2+} = 5mEq/L$).

B. GFR. In most physiological conditions, GFR changes very little and is not an important control point for Ca^{2+} excretion in the urine.

C. Ca^{2+} Reabsorption. Ca^{2+} reabsorption is the most important variable in the control of Ca^{2+} excretion in the urine. Ca^{2+} reabsorption is controlled by a number of factors as indicated below.
   1. **$[P]_{Ca2+}$ Monitored by Chief Cells of the Parathyroid Gland.** The chief cells of the parathyroid gland monitor **changes in $[P]_{Ca2+}$** and secrete **parathyroid hormone (PTH)** in response to decreased $[P]_{Ca2+}$. PTH **increases Ca^{2+} reabsorption** by the distal convoluted tubule (DCT) and collecting duct (CD) and thereby decreases Ca^{2+} excretion in the urine.
   2. **Na^+ Reabsorption.** The forces driving Ca^{2+} reabsorption are dependent on Na^+ reabsorption. In this regard, a low NaCl diet increases Ca^{2+} reabsorption by the PCT and thereby decreases Ca^{2+} excretion in the urine; whereas, a high NaCl diet

decreases Ca^{2+} reabsorption by the PCT and thereby increases Ca^{2+} excretion in the urine. This can be used clinically to either increase or decrease the amount of Ca^{2+} in the body.

3. **Plasma pH.** Decreased plasma pH (acidosis) decreases Ca^{2+} reabsorption and thereby increases Ca^{2+} excretion in the urine. Increased plasma pH (alkalosis) increases Ca^{2+} reabsorption and thereby decreases Ca^{2+} excretion in the urine.

Ⅱ Control of Ca^{2+}: The Rest of the Story.
The control of Na$^+$, H$_2$O, K$^+$, HCO$_3{}^-$, and H$^+$ is accomplished almost entirely by the kidney. However, control of Ca^{2+} is accomplished not only by the kidney but also by the gastrointestinal tract (GI) tract and bone.

A. **GI Tract.** Most of the ingested dietary Ca^{2+} is <u>not</u> absorbed by the GI epithelium from the intestinal lumen into the plasma (intestinal lumen → plasma) but is instead eliminated in the feces. However, the amount of ingested dietary Ca^{2+} absorbed by the GI epithelium from the intestinal lumen → plasma is controlled by **1,25-(OH)$_2$ vitamin D.** Vitamin D sources include dietary intake and production by skin keratinocytes stimulated by ultraviolet light. Vitamin D is hydroxylated by liver hepatocytes to **25-(OH) vitamin D.** 25-(OH) vitamin D is hydroxylated by the PCT to **1,25-(OH)$_2$ vitamin D,** the active metabolite that functions similar to a steroid hormone.

B. **Bone.** About 99% of total body Ca^{2+} resides in bone. Since bone is constantly resorbed and reformed, bone provides a huge source of Ca^{2+} to increase plasma concentration of Ca^{2+} or a huge sink for Ca^{2+} to decrease plasma concentration of Ca^{2+}. A number of hormones are involved in this process as indicated below.

1. **PTH.** PTH acts directly on osteoblasts to secrete **macrophage colony-stimulating factor (M-CSF)** and to express a cell surface protein called **RANKL.** M-CSF stimulates monocytes to differentiate into macrophages and express a cell surface receptor called **RANK.** RANKL (on the osteoblast) and RANK (on the macrophage) interact and cause the differentiation of macrophages into osteoclasts. Osteoclasts increase bone resorption and thereby increase plasma concentration of Ca^{2+} (↑[P]$_{Ca2+}$).

2. **1,25-(OH)$_2$ vitamin D.** 1,25-(OH)$_2$ vitamin D acts directly on osteoblasts to secrete IL-1, which stimulates osteoclasts to increase bone resorption and thereby increase plasma concentration of Ca^{2+} (↑[P]$_{Ca2+}$).

3. **Calcitonin.** The parafollicular cells of the thyroid gland monitor **changes in [P]$_{Ca2+}$** and secrete **calcitonin** in response to increased [P]$_{Ca2+}$. Calcitonin acts directly on osteoclasts to decrease bone resorption and thereby decrease plasma concentration of Ca^{2+} (↓[P]$_{Ca2+}$).

Ⅲ Control of PO$_4{}^{2-}$ Excretion in the Urine.
The control of PO$_4{}^{2-}$ excretion in the urine is interrelated with the control of Ca^{2+}.

25

Renal Handling of HCO_3^- and H^+

Renal Handling of HCO_3^-. HCO_3^- is freely-filtered from the glomerular capillaries→Bowman's space and then is reabsorbed by particular segments of the nephron. It is very important that virtually all of the filtered HCO_3^- be reabsorbed so that the body fluids do not become extremely acidic. In HCO_3^- reabsorption, the key factor is **H^+ ATPase** that transports H^+ across the luminal membrane into the tubular fluid (i.e., "pumps H^+ out of the cell"). HCO_3^- reabsorption is not accomplished in the conventional manner (i.e., by direct reabsorption of HCO_3^- per se by carrier proteins) but instead involves the **secretion of H^+**. In other words, **the renal handling of HCO_3^- is governed by movements of H^+**.

A. **Proximal Convoluted Tubule (PCT).** The PCT reabsorbs **80%** of the filtered HCO_3^-. The transport of HCO_3^- occurs via carrier (or transporter) proteins. The carrier proteins involved include:
   1. H^+ ATPase
   2. Na^+-H^+ Exchanger
   3. Na^+-HCO_3^- Cotransporter

B. **Proximal Straight Tubule of the Loop of Henle (PST).** The PST is not involved in HCO_3^- reabsorption or secretion.

C. **Descending Thin Limb of the Loop of Henle (DTL).** The DTL is not involved in HCO_3^- reabsorption or secretion.

D. **Ascending Thin Limb of the Loop of Henle (ATL).** The ATL is not involved in HCO_3^- reabsorption or secretion.

E. **Distal Straight Tubule of the Loop of Henle (DST).** The DST reabsorbs **10%** of the filtered HCO_3^-. The transport of HCO_3^- occurs via carrier (or transporter) proteins. The carrier proteins involved are the same as for the PCT above.

F. **Distal Convoluted Tubule (DCT).** The DCT is not involved in HCO_3^- reabsorption or secretion.

G. **Collecting Duct (CD). The CD (Type A intercalated cells)** reabsorbs **10%** of the filtered HCO. The transport of HCO_3^- occurs via carrier (or transporter) proteins and ion channel proteins. The carrier proteins and ion channel proteins involved include:
   1. H^+ ATPase
   2. H^+-K^+ATPase
   3. Cl^--HCO_3^-
   4. Cl^- ion channel protein
   5. K^+ ion channel protein

II # General Mechanism of HCO_3^- Reabsorption (Figure 25-1A). It is not intuitively obvious how the reabsorption of HCO_3^- is accomplished by the secretion of H^+. This involves a number of steps as indicated below:

A. The filtered HCO_3^- within the tubular fluid combines with secreted H^+ to form H_2CO_3, which disassociates into CO_2 and H_2O.

B. The CO_2 and H_2O diffuse into the cytoplasm of the tubular cell and form H_2CO_3 catalyzed by **carbonic anhydrase.**

C. The H_2CO_3 disassociates into H^+ and HCO_3^-.

D. The H^+ is secreted and the HCO_3^- is reabsorbed. This process results in a reabsorption of HCO_3^- but does not result in a net secretion of H^+ since H^+ is merely recycled in this process. The key points to remember are that when filtered HCO_3^- combines with secreted H^+ within the tubular fluid: reabsorption of HCO_3^- occurs so that all the filtered HCO_3^- is conserved (a conservation process), which prevents acidosis of the plasma that would occur if the filtered HCO_3^- was not recovered; no new HCO_3^- is added to the plasma during this process so that alkalinization of the plasma does not occur; and the secreted H^+ is recycled so that no H^+ excretion in the urine occurs.

III # Renal Handling of H^+. H^+ is not freely-filtered from the glomerular capillaries→ Bowman's space because the concentration of H^+ at pH 7.4 (the normal pH of plasma and tubular fluid) is $<10^{-7}$ M (an insignificant amount). This means then that any H^+ within the tubular fluid arrived by tubular **secretion of H^+.**

A. Proximal Convoluted Tubule (PCT). The PCT secretes H^+. The transport of H^+ occurs via carrier (or transporter) proteins. The carrier proteins involved include:
1. H^+ ATPase
2. Na^+-H^+ Exchanger
3. Na^+-NH_4^+ Exchanger

B. Distal Straight Tubule of the Loop of Henle (DST). The DST secretes H^+. The transport of H^+ occurs via carrier (or transporter) proteins. The carrier proteins involved include:
1. H^+ ATPase
2. Na^+-H^+ Exchanger

C. Collecting Duct (CD). The CD **(Type A intercalated cells)** secretes H^+. The transport of H^+ occurs via carrier (or transporter) proteins and ion channel proteins. The carrier proteins and ion channel proteins involved include:
1. H^+ ATPase
2. H^+-K^+ ATPase
3. K^+ ion channel protein

General Mechanism of H^+ Secretion That Leads to H^+ Excretion in the Urine (Figure 25-1B,C). It is not intuitively obvious how the secretion of H^+ that leads to H^+ excretion in the urine is accomplished. This is accomplished by two pathways as indicated below:

A. Combination of Secreted H^+ with HPO_4^{2-} Buffer (occurs mainly in the collecting ducts).

  1. The CO_2 and H_2O diffuse into the cytoplasm of the tubular cell and form H_2CO_3 catalyzed by **carbonic anhydrase.**
  2. The H_2CO_3 disassociates into H^+ and HCO_3^-.
  3. The H^+ is secreted into the tubular fluid and combines with filtered HPO_4^{2-} (a buffer) to form $H_2PO_4^-$, which is excreted in the urine. In other words, the secreted H^+ is trapped by the HPO_4^{2-} buffer, remains in the tubular fluid, and therefore is excreted in the urine as $H_2PO_4^-$. This occurs mainly in the collecting ducts after a large majority of the filtered HCO_3^- has already been reabsorbed.
  4. The HCO_3^- generated in this process is reabsorbed and added to the plasma as "new" HCO_3^-, so that alkalinization of the plasma does occur.
  5. Note that when a secreted H^+ combines with a buffer in the tubular fluid other than HCO_3^- (like HPO_4^{2-}), two things happen: the H^+ is excreted in the urine while "new" HCO_3^- is added to the plasma and alkalinizes the plasma.

B. Catabolism of Glutamine and NH_4^+ Secretion (occurs mainly in the proximal convoluted tubule).

  1. The cells of the proximal convoluted tubule (PCT) extract glutamine from both the tubular fluid and interstitial fluid. Glutamine is hydrolyzed to glutamate ion and NH_4^+. The glutamate ion is metabolized to α-ketoglutarate, which liberates another NH_4^+. The α-ketoglutarate is further metabolized and yields $2HCO_3^-$. The overall reaction is: 1 glutamine → $2\ NH_4^+ + 2HCO_3^-$.
  2. The NH_4^+ is secreted into the tubular fluid by the Na^+-NH_4^+ Exchanger located on the luminal membrane of the PCT cells and is excreted in the urine.
  3. The HCO_3^- generated in this process is added to the blood as new HCO_3^-, so that alkalinization of the blood does occur.
  4. Note that when NH_4^+ is secreted, two things happen: the H^+ is excreted in the urine (H^+ combined with NH_3), while new HCO_3^- is added to the blood and alkalinizes the blood.

V **Summary Table of Renal Handling of HCO_3^- and H^+ (Table 25-1).**

TABLE 25-1	SUMMARY OF RENAL HANDLING OF HCO_3^- AND H+	
	HCO_3^- Reabsorption	**H^+ Secretion**
PCT	**Luminal Membrane** H^+ ATPase Na^+-H^+ Exchanger Na^+-NH_4^+ Exchanger **Basolateral Membrane** Na^+-HCO_3^- Cotransporter 80%	**Luminal Membrane** H^+ ATPase Na^+-H^+ Exchanger
PST*	X	X
DTL*	X	X
ATL*	X	X
DST*	**Luminal Membrane** H^+ ATPase Na^+-H^+ Exchanger **Basolateral Membrane** Na^+-HCO_3^- Cotransporter 10%	**Luminal Membrane** H^+ ATPase Na^+-H^+ Exchanger
DCT	X	X
CD (Type A)	**Luminal Membrane** H^+ ATPase H^+-K^+ ATPase **Basolateral Membrane** Cl^--HCO_3^- Exchanger Cl^- ion channel protein K^+ ion channel protein 10%	**Luminal Membrane** H^+ ATPase H^+-K^+ ATPase **Basolateral Membrane** K^+ ion channel protein

A

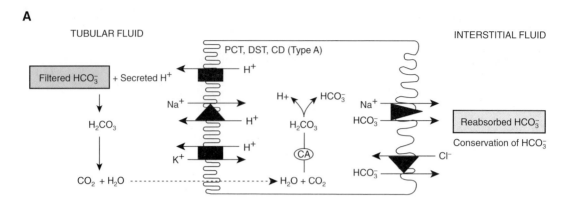

B

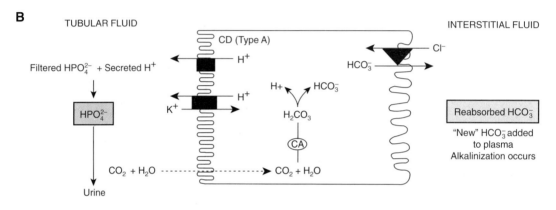

C

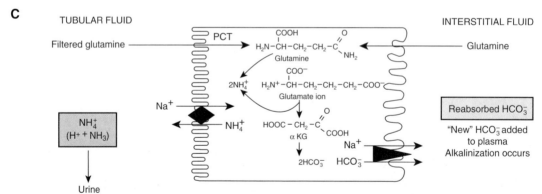

● **Figure 25-1: (A) General Mechanism of HCO$_3^-$ Reabsorption. (B) General Mechanism of H$^+$ Secretion That Leads to H$^+$ Excretion in the Urine.** (1) Combination of Secreted H$^+$ with HPO$_4^{2-}$ Buffer. (2) Catabolism of Glutamine and NH$_4^+$ Excretion.

◆ = Na$^+$-NH$_4^+$ Exchanger   ▶ = Na$^+$-HCO$_3^-$ Cotransporter

■ = H$^+$ ATPase   ▲ = Na$^+$-H$^+$ Exchanger   = Na$^+$-HCO$_3^-$ Cotransporter

▬ = H$^+$-K$^+$ATPase   ▼ = Cl$^-$-HCO$_3^-$ Exchanger

αKG = alpha ketoglutarate   CA = carbonic anhydrase

26

Control of HCO_3^- and H^+

① **Control of HCO_3^- Excretion in the Urine.** The amount of HCO_3^- excreted in the urine is given by the formula below:

$$HCO_3^- \text{ excretion} = HCO_3^- \text{ filtered} - HCO_3^- \text{ reabsorbed} + HCO_3^- \text{ secreted}$$
$$= (GFR \times [P]_{HCO3-}) - HCO_3^- \text{ reabsorbed} + HCO_3^- \text{ secreted}$$

Where,

GFR = glomerular filtration rate
$[P]_{HCO3-}$ = plasma concentration of HCO_3^-

Consequently, HCO_3^- excretion in the urine can be adjusted by controlling any of four variables: $[P]_{HCO3-}$, GFR, HCO_3^- reabsorption, or HCO_3^- secretion as discussed below.

A. $[P]_{HCO3-}$. In most physiological conditions, $[P]_{HCO3-}$ changes very little and is not an important control point for HCO_3^- excretion in the urine. The normal plasma concentration of HCO_3^- is 24 mEq/L. **($[P]_{HCO3-}$ = 24 mEq/L).**

B. GFR. In most physiological conditions, GFR changes very little and is not an important control point for HCO_3^- excretion in the urine.

C. HCO_3^- Reabsorption. HCO_3^- reabsorption is the most important variable in the control of HCO_3^- excretion in the urine. HCO_3^- is freely-filtered from the glomerular capillaries → Bowman's space and then is reabsorbed by particular segments of the nephron. It is very important that virtually all of the filtered HCO_3^- be reabsorbed so that the body fluids do not become extremely acidic. However, HCO_3^- reabsorption is not accomplished in the conventional manner (i.e., by direct reabsorption of HCO_3^- per se by carrier proteins) but instead involves the **secretion of H^+**. So, there are no specific mechanisms that control HCO_3^- reabsorption; but instead, the control mechanisms are placed on the secretion of H^+.

D. HCO_3^- Secretion. The Type B intercalated cells of the cortical collecting ducts secrete HCO_3^- using H^+ATPase located on the basolateral membrane and Cl^--HCO_3^- Exchanger located on the luminal membrane. HCO_3^- secretion plays a minor role in the control of HCO_3^- excretion in the urine. However, a point worth remembering is that: alkalosis stimulates HCO_3^- secretion by which large amounts of HCO_3^- can be excreted in the urine but little is known about the control mechanisms of HCO_3^- secretion.

11 ## Control of H⁺ Excretion in the Urine.

H^+ is <u>not</u> freely-filtered from the glomerular capillaries $\rightarrow$ Bowman's space because the normal plasma concentration of H^+ at pH 7.4 is 40 mEq/L ($[P]_{H+} = \textbf{40 mEq/L}$) which is an insignificant amount. This means then that any H^+ within the tubular fluid arrived by tubular **secretion of H⁺**. The amount of H^+ excreted in the urine is given by the formula below:

$$H^+ \text{ excretion} = (H_2PO_4^- \text{ excretion}) + (NH_4^+ \text{ excretion})$$

Where,

$H_2PO_4^-$ excretion = secreted H^+ combined with HPO_4^{2-}
NH_4^+ excretion = secreted H^+ combined with NH_3 (i.e., NH_4^+)

Consequently, H^+ excretion in the urine can be adjusted by controlling any of two variables: secreted H^+ combined with HPO_4^{2-} or secreted H^+ combined with NH_3 (i.e., NH_4^+) as discussed below. HPO_4^{2-} is the most important non-HCO_3^- buffer.

A. H⁺ Secretion. Whether or not secreted H^+ combines with filtered HCO_3^- in the tubular fluid (which leads to H^+ recycling and HCO_3^- conservation) or combines with filtered HPO_4^{2-} in the tubular fluid (which leads to H^+ excretion in the urine and "new" HCO_3^- addition to the plasma), the control of H^+ secretion is the same. H^+ secretion is controlled by a number of factors as indicated below.

    1. **Partial Pressure of Arterial CO₂ (P_{aCO2}).** There is intrarenal monitoring of P_{aCO2} to maintain acid-base balance. Arterial CO_2 easily diffuses into the cytoplasm of proximal convoluted tubule (PCT) cells, distal straight tubule (DST) cells, and collecting duct (CD; Type A) cells. Intracellular CO_2 affects H^+ concentration and H^+ secretion by a little known mechanism. A **low plasma concentration of H⁺ (i.e., alkalosis; ↓[P]_{H+})** results in a **decreased P_{aCO2}** monitored by the kidney, which decreases H^+ secretion and thereby decreases H^+ excretion in the urine as $H_2PO_4^-$ and no "new" HCO_3^- is added to the plasma. A **high plasma concentration of H⁺ (i.e., acidosis; ↑[P]_{H+})** results in an **increased P_{aCO2}** monitored by the kidney, which increases H^+ secretion and thereby increases H^+ excretion in the urine as $H_2PO_4^-$ and "new" HCO_3^- is added to the plasma.

    2. **Interstitial Fluid pH (pH_{ISF}).** There is intrarenal monitoring of pH_{ISF} to maintain acid-base balance. A change in pH_{ISF} causes a change in the intracellular fluid pH (pH_{ICF}) of PCT cells, DST cells, and collecting duct (CD; Type A) cells. The pH_{ICF} affects H^+ secretion by a little known mechanism. A **low plasma concentration of H⁺ (i.e., alkalosis; ↓[P]_{H+})** results in an **increased pH_{ISF}** monitored by the kidney, which decreases H^+ secretion and thereby decreases H^+ excretion in the urine as $H_2PO_4^-$ and no "new" HCO_3^- is added to the plasma. **High plasma H⁺ levels (i.e., acidosis)** result in a **decreased pH_{ISF}** monitored by the kidney which increases H^+ secretion and thereby increases H^+ excretion in the urine as $H_2PO_4^-$ and "new" HCO_3^- is added to the plasma.

B. NH₄⁺ Secretion. NH_4^+ secretion is controlled by a number of factors as indicated below.

    1. **Interstitial Fluid pH (pH_{ISF}).** There is intrarenal monitoring of pH_{ISF} to maintain acid-base balance. A change in pH_{ISF} causes a change in the intracellular fluid pH (pH_{ICF}) of PCT cells that effects the transport activity of the Na^+-NH_4^+ Exchanger and glutamine metabolism. A **low plasma concentration of H⁺ (i.e., alkalosis; ↓[P]_{H+})** results in **increased pH_{ISF}** monitored by the kidney, which decreases

transport activity of the Na$^+$-NH$_4^+$ Exchanger and decreases glutamine metabolism by the PCT, and thereby decreases H$^+$ excretion in the urine as NH$_4^+$ and no "new" HCO$_3^-$ is added to the plasma. A **high plasma concentration of H$^+$ (i.e., acidosis; ↑[P]$_{H+}$)** results in **decreased pH$_{ISF}$** monitored by the kidney, which increases transport activity of the Na$^+$-NH$_4^+$ Exchanger and increases glutamine metabolism by the PCT, and thereby increases H$^+$ excretion in the urine as NH$_4^+$, and "new" HCO$_3^-$ is added to the plasma.

2. **Other factors.** Other factors have not been clearly elucidated as yet.

27

Acid-Base Balance

I **General Features.** The maintenance of acid-base balance in the body can be broadly divided into a **respiratory component** involving the lung, which expires CO_2, and a **metabolic component** involving the kidney, which conserves HCO_3^- and generates "new" HCO_3^-.

II **Respiratory Component.**

   A. Intracellular Production of Volatile Acid. All cells of the body produce CO_2 (a volatile acid; H_2CO_3) by the aerobic metabolism of carbohydrates, fats, and proteins. A massive amount of CO_2 (15,000 mmol/day) is produced and this volatile acid must be eliminated by the lungs or the acid-base balance will be skewed.

   B. Intravascular Transport of CO_2. The CO_2 produced by the cells freely diffuses into red blood cells (RBCs). In RBCs, CO_2 combines with H_2O to form H^+ and HCO_3^- ($CO_2 + H_2O \rightarrow H_2CO_3 \rightarrow H^+ + HCO_3^-$) in a reaction catalyzed by **carbonic anhydrase (CA).** HCO_3^- leaves the RBC in exchange for Cl^- (called the **chloride shift**) using **band III protein.** CO_2 is transported to the lung as HCO_3^- in the plasma. The H^+ is buffered by combining with deoxyHb to form deoxyHb-H^+.

   C. CO_2 Exhaled by the Lungs. In the lung, HCO_3^- reenters the RBC and combines with H^+ from deoxyHb-H^+ to form CO_2 and H_2O ($CO_2 + H_2O \leftarrow H_2CO_3 \leftarrow H^+ + HCO_3^-$) in a reaction catalyzed by CA. CO_2 diffuses to lung alveoli and is exhaled. In the normal steady-state, the brain regulates alveolar ventilation (V_A) so that $P_{aCO2} = 40$ mmHg. Hypoventilation occurs when $P_{aCO2} > 45$ mmHg (hypercapnia). Hyperventilation occurs when $P_{aCO2} < 35$ mmHg (hypocapnia).

III **Metabolic Component.**

   A. Intracellular Production of Non-Volatile Acids. All cells of the body produce H_2SO_4, H_2PO_4, **ketoacids, lactic acid, and salicylic acid (non-volatile acids)** by the anaerobic metabolism of carbohydrates and aerobic metabolism of fats and proteins. A comparatively small amount of non-volatile acid (50–70 mEq/day) is produced and these non-volatile acids must be eliminated by the kidneys or the acid-base balance will be skewed.

B. **Intravascular Transport of Non-volatile Acids.** The non-volatile acids produced by the cells freely diffuse into the plasma, where they disassociate into H^+ and respective anion (A^-). The A^- are excreted in the urine. In the plasma, the H^+ combine with HCO_3^- to form CO_2 and H_2O ($CO_2 + H_2O \leftarrow H_2CO_3 \leftarrow H^+ + HCO_3^-$) in a reaction catalyzed by **carbonic anhydrase (CA).** The CO_2 produced is eliminated by the lungs. Note that in this process a HCO_3^- is consumed and must be replenished.

C. **Plasma HCO_3^- Conserved and "New" HCO_3^- Added to Plasma by the Kidney.** The kidney conserves HCO_3^- when secreted H^+ combines with filtered HCO_3^- within the tubular fluid of the proximal convoluted tubule, distal straight tubule, or collecting duct. The kidney adds "new" HCO_3^- to the plasma when secreted H^+ combines with filtered HPO_4^- within the tubular fluid of the collecting duct (mainly) or when NH_4^+ secretion occurs by the proximal convoluted tubule (mainly). See Chapter 26 for details.

IV Primary Acid-Base Disorders (Figure 27-1A).

A. **Respiratory Acidosis.** A respiratory acidosis is a disorder whose primary disturbance is an **increase in partial pressure of arterial CO_2 ($\uparrow P_{aCO2}$; hypercapnia).** The $\uparrow P_{aCO2}$ drives the equation $CO_2 + H_2O \rightarrow H_2CO_3 \rightarrow H^+ + HCO_3^-$ to the right, thus causing high plasma H^+ levels (i.e., acidosis). Although HCO_3^- also increases in this process, the amount of HCO_3^- produced is relatively insignificant when compared to the large amount of HCO_3^- present in the extracellular fluid (ECF). **A respiratory acidosis may be caused by:** respiratory depression by drugs (e.g., opiates, sedatives, anesthetics); cerebral disease; cardiopulmonary arrest response; neuromuscular disease (e.g., Guillain-Barre syndrome, polio, amyotrophic lateral sclerosis (ALS), multiple sclerosis, myasthenia gravis); and poor ventilation secondary to disease (e.g., asthma, pneumonia, bronchitis, emphysema). **Clinical signs include:** hypercapnia, confusion, blunted sensation and pain, asterixis (intermittent lapse of assumed posture), and papilledema (edema of optic disk).
   1. **Respiratory Compensation.** None
   2. **Renal Compensation.** The $\uparrow P_{aCO2}$ and $\downarrow pH_{ISF}$ are both monitored by the kidney and cause increased H^+ secretion by the proximal convoluted tubule (PCT), distal straight tubule (DST), and Type A cells of the collecting duct (CD). The H^+ combines with HPO_4^-, which leads to **increased H^+ excretion in the urine as $H_2PO_4^-$ and "new" HCO_3^- added to the plasma.** The $\downarrow pH_{ISF}$ is monitored by the kidney and causes increased activity of the Na^+-NH_4^+ Exchanger and increased glutamine metabolism. This leads to increased NH_4^+ secretion by the PCT and **increased NH_4^+ excretion in the urine** and **"new" HCO_3^- added to the plasma.**

B. **Metabolic Acidosis.** A metabolic acidosis is a disorder whose primary disturbance is a **decrease in plasma concentration of HCO_3^- ($\downarrow [P]_{HCO3}-$).** In a metabolic acidosis, a nonvolatile acid (e.g., lactic acid or ketoacids) is added directly to the acid-base balance or indirectly (e.g., inappropriate wasting of HCO_3^- by the kidney or GI tract; essentially the addition of HCl). The addition of the acid drives the equation $CO_2 + H_2O \leftarrow H_2CO_3 \leftarrow H^+ + HCO_3^-$ to the left, thus causing a $\downarrow [P]_{HCO3-}$ (i.e., the HCO_3^- is consumed to buffer the added acid). **A metabolic acidosis may be caused by:** chronic renal failure; lactic acidosis; uremia; ketoacidosis; intoxication (salicylate, methanol/formaldehyde, ethylene glycol); diarrhea*; renal tubular acidosis (RTA)*; and acetazolamide* (* indicates a normal anion gap acidosis; all other acidosis items have an elevated anion gap). **Clinical signs include:** fatigue, shortness of breath, abdominal pain, vomiting, Kussmaul breathing, hypotension, and tachycardia.

1. **Respiratory Compensation.** Hyperventilation (Kussmaul breathing).
2. **Renal Compensation.** The $\downarrow pH_{ISF}$ is monitored by the kidney and causes increased H^+ secretion by the PCT, DST, and Type A cells of the CD. The H^+ combines with HPO_4^- which leads to **increased H^+ excretion in the urine as $H_2PO_4^-$ and "new" HCO_3^- added to the plasma.** The $\downarrow pH_{ISF}$ is monitored by the kidney and causes increased activity of the Na^+-NH_4^+ Exchanger and increased glutamine metabolism. This leads to increased NH_4^+ secretion by the PCT and **increased NH_4^+ excretion in the urine** and "new" HCO_3^- added to the plasma.
3. **Types of Metabolic Acidosis (Figure 27-1B,C)**
   a. **Elevated-gap Metabolic Acidosis.** The serum anion gap represents the unmeasured serum anions (e.g., SO_4^{2-}, PO_4^{2-}, citrate, formate, and protein). The normal serum anion gap equals **12 mEq/L.** For electroneutrality to be maintained during a metabolic acidosis, the concentration of an unmeasured serum anion may increase **(20 mEq/L)** to replace the HCO_3^- that is consumed to buffer the added acid.
   b. **Normal-gap Metabolic Acidosis (Hyperchloremic Acidosis).** For electroneutrality to be maintained during a metabolic acidosis, the concentration of Cl^- may increase to replace the HCO_3^- that is consumed to buffer the added acid. Hence, the serum anion gap remains normal **(12 mEq/L).**

C. **Respiratory Alkalosis.** A respiratory alkalosis is a disorder whose primary disturbance is a **decrease in partial pressure of arterial CO_2 ($\downarrow P_{aCO2}$; hypocapnia).** The $\downarrow P_{aCO2}$ drives the equation $CO_2 + H_2O \leftarrow H_2CO_3 \leftarrow H^+ + HCO_3^-$ to the left, thus causing low plasma H^+ levels (i.e., alkalosis). Although HCO_3^- also decreases in this process, the amount of HCO_3^- consumed is relatively insignificant when compared to the large amount of HCO_3^- present in the extracellular fluid (ECF). **A respiratory alkalosis may be caused by:** asthma, pneumonia, pulmonary edema, heart disease with cyanosis, pulmonary fibrosis, salicylate intoxication, gram-negative sepsis, fever, anxiety, pregnancy, drugs, and high altitude. **Clinical signs include:** hyperventilation, numbness, tingling, paresthesia, and tetany (if severe).

1. **Respiratory Compensation.** None
2. **Renal Compensation.** The $\downarrow P_{aCO2}$ and $\uparrow pH_{ISF}$ are both monitored by the kidney and cause decreased H^+ secretion by the PCT, DST, and Type A cells of the CD. The decreased H^+ does not combine with HPO_4^-, which leads to **decreased H^+ excretion in the urine as $H_2PO_4^-$ and no "new" HCO_3^- added to the plasma.** In addition, the decreased H^+ causes a decrease in the amount of HCO_3^- conserved, and therefore leads to increased HCO_3^- excretion in the urine. Furthermore, HCO_3^- secretion by the Type B intercalated cells of the CD is increased, which leads to **increased HCO_3^- excretion in the urine.** The $\uparrow pH_{ISF}$ is monitored by the kidney and causes decreased activity of the Na^+-NH_4^+ Exchanger and decreased glutamine metabolism. This leads to decreased NH_4^+ secretion by the PCT and **decreased NH_4^+ excretion in the urine** and no "new" HCO_3^- added to the plasma.

D. **Metabolic Alkalosis.** A metabolic alkalosis is a disorder whose primary disturbance is an **increase in plasma concentration of HCO_3^- ($\uparrow [P]_{HCO3-}$).** In a metabolic alkalosis, a nonvolatile acid (e.g., HCl) is lost from the acid-base balance or an inappropriate amount of HCO_3^- is added to the acid-base balance (e.g., vomiting where HCl is lost and HCO_3^- remains behind). The loss of the acid drives the equation $CO_2 + H_2O \rightarrow H_2CO_3 \rightarrow H^+ + HCO_3^-$ to the right, thus causing a $\uparrow [P]_{HCO3-}$. **A metabolic alkalosis may be**

caused by: loop or thiazide diuretics, vomiting, milk alkali syndrome, large intake of alkaline substance, Cushing syndrome, and primary hyperaldosteronism. **Clinical signs include:** no specific signs or symptoms; can cause apathy, stupor, and confusion; tetany if coupled with low calcium.

1. **Respiratory Compensation.** Hypoventilation.
2. **Renal Compensation.** The $\uparrow pH_{ISF}$ is monitored by the kidney and causes decreased H^+ secretion by the PCT, DST, and Type A cells of the CD. The decreased H^+ does not combine with HPO_4^-, which leads to **decreased H^+ excretion in the urine as $H_2PO_4^-$** and **no "new" HCO_3^- added to the plasma.** In addition, the decreased H^+ causes a decrease in the amount of HCO_3^- conserved and therefore leads to increased HCO_3^- excretion in the urine. Furthermore, HCO_3^- secretion by the Type B intercalated cells of the CD is increased, which leads to **increased HCO_3^- excretion in the urine.** The $\uparrow pH_{ISF}$ is monitored by the kidney and causes decreased activity of the Na^+-NH_4^+ Exchanger and decreased glutamine metabolism. This leads to decreased NH_4^+ secretion by the PCT and **decreased NH_4^+ excretion in the urine** and no "new" HCO_3^- added to the plasma.
3. **Metabolic Alkalosis in Euvolemia and Normal Renal Function.** Even in the face of a greatly elevated loss of a non-volatile acid or a greatly elevated addition of HCO_3^-, it is difficult to maintain a significant metabolic alkalosis if the patient has normal kidney function and is not ECF volume depleted. This is because the kidney has a remarkable ability to eliminate all extra HCO_3^-.
4. **Metabolic Alkalosis in ECF Volume Depletion (Saline-Responsive Alkalosis).** In the face of ECF volume depletion (e.g., hemorrhage and a decrease in blood pressure), **increased angiotensin II** causes increased Na^+ reabsorption by the PCT. Normally, Cl^- is the anion reabsorbed along with Na^+, but in ECF volume depletion Cl^- is very low, so HCO_3^- is reabsorbed in its place and results in a metabolic alkalosis. In addition, in the face of ECF volume depletion, **increased aldosterone (ALD)** causes increased H^+ secretion by the PCT, DST, and Type A cells of the CD. The H^+ combines with HPO_4^-, which leads to increased H^+ excretion in the urine as $H_2PO_4^-$ and "new" HCO_3^- added to the plasma, and results in a metabolic alkalosis. Administration of a saline solution to an ECF–volume-depleted patient with a metabolic alkalosis rapidly reverses the metabolic alkalosis; hence the name saline-responsive alkalosis.
5. **Metabolic Alkalosis in Hyperaldosteronism (Saline-Nonresponsive Alkalosis).** In the face of hyperaldosteronism (e.g., Cushing syndrome, primary hyperaldosteronism, ACTH-secreting tumor), **increased ALD** causes increased Na^+ reabsorption by the cortical CD, and therefore increased H_2O reabsorption resulting in **ECF volume excess.** In addition, increased ALD causes increased H^+ secretion by the PCT, DST, and Type A cells of the CD. The H^+ combines with HPO_4^-, which leads to increased H^+ excretion in the urine as $H_2PO_4^-$ and "new" HCO_3^- added to the plasma, and results in a metabolic alkalosis. Administration of a saline solution to a hyperaldosteronism patient with a metabolic alkalosis does not reverse the metabolic alkalosis because there is already an ECF volume excess present, hence the name saline-nonresponsive alkalosis.

A

$$pH \cong \frac{[HCO_3^-]}{P_{aCO_2}}$$

Controlled by kidney

Controlled by lung

Acid-Base Disorder		Compensation	
Respiratory acidosis	$\dfrac{[HCO_3^-]}{P_{aCO_2}\uparrow} = pH\downarrow$	Renal	$\dfrac{[HCO_3^-]\Uparrow}{P_{aCO_2}\uparrow} = pH\downarrow\Uparrow$
Metabolic acidosis	$\dfrac{[HCO_3^-]\downarrow}{P_{aCO_2}} = pH\downarrow$	Respiratory	$\dfrac{[HCO_3^-]\downarrow}{P_{aCO_2}\Downarrow} = pH\downarrow\Uparrow$
Respiratory alkalosis	$\dfrac{[HCO_3^-]}{P_{aCO_2}\downarrow} = pH\uparrow$	Renal	$\dfrac{[HCO_3^-]\Downarrow}{P_{aCO_2}\downarrow} = pH\uparrow\Downarrow$
Metabolic alkalosis	$\dfrac{[HCO_3^-]\uparrow}{P_{aCO_2}} = pH\uparrow$	Respiratory	$\dfrac{[HCO_3^-]\uparrow}{P_{aCO_2}\Uparrow} = pH\uparrow\Downarrow$

$\uparrow\downarrow$ = Primary disturbance $\Uparrow\Downarrow$ = Compensation

B

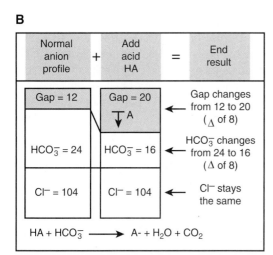

C

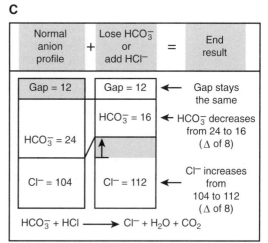

● **Figure 27-1: (A) Acid-Base Disorders.** This table shows the primary disturbance in each acid-base disorder and the compensatory changes. **(B) Elevated-gap Metabolic Acidosis.** When a strong nonvolatile acid is added to the plasma (e.g., ketoacids), HCO_3^- is consumed. For electroneutrality to be maintained, an unmeasured anion is added to the plasma, so that the serum anion gap increases. **(C) Normal-gap Metabolic Acidosis (Hyperchloremic Acidosis).** When a strong nonvolatile acid is added to the plasma (e.g., ketoacids), HCO_3^- is consumed. For electroneutrality to be maintained, Cl^- is added to the plasma, so that the serum anion gap remains normal.

28

General Principles of the Gastrointestinal System

Ⅰ   **Gastrointestinal Motility in General (Figure 28-1).** The smooth muscle of the GI tract is **single-unit smooth muscle** containing **gap junctions** (see Chapter 3). The smooth muscle contraction of the inner circular layer of the muscularis externa leads to a **decrease in diameter** of the GI tract. The smooth muscle contraction of the outer longitudinal layer of the muscularis externa leads to a **decrease in length** of the GI tract. The inner circular layer of the muscularis externa comprises the bulk of the smooth muscle in the stomach and small intestines and is the main generator of propulsive contractions.

A. **Slow Waves.** Single-unit smooth muscle demonstrates spontaneous rhythmic cycles of depolarization and repolarization called **slow waves**. Slow waves are **not** action potentials. The slow waves originate in the **interstitial cells of Cajal,** which serve as the pacemaker of GI smooth muscle.

B. **Production of Slow Waves.** The depolarization phase of slow waves is caused by the cyclic entry of Ca^{2+} into the smooth muscle cell through Ca^{2+} **channels.** The repolarization phase of slow waves is caused by the entry of K^+ into the smooth muscle cell through K^+ **channels.** The depolarization phase of the slow wave brings the smooth muscle cell closer to threshold. This increases the probability that action potentials will occur at the crest of the depolarization phase of the slow wave. When an action potential occurs, the smooth muscle cell undergoes phasic contraction. As the number of action potentials increase at the crest of the depolarization phase, the strength of the phasic contraction increases.

C. **Frequency of Slow Waves.** The frequency of slow waves **sets the maximum frequency of smooth muscle contractions** for each part of the GI tract. The frequency of slow waves is characteristic for each part of the GI tract and ranges from 3–12 slow waves/minute. The stomach has the lowest frequency, with 3 slow waves/minute, whereas the duodenum has the highest frequency, with 12 slow waves/minute. The frequency of slow waves is **not** modified by neural or hormonal input. In contrast, the frequency of action potentials and strength of contractions are modified by neural and hormonal input.

D. **Tonic and Phasic Contractions.** Even sub-threshold slow waves produce a weak smooth muscle contraction such that GI smooth muscle is never completely relaxed. This is called **tonic contraction or tonus.** When action potentials occur at the crest of the depolarization phase of the slow wave, a stronger smooth muscle contraction occurs. This is called **phasic contraction.**

II **Innervation of the Gastrointestinal (GI) Tract.** The GI tract is innervated by the autonomic nervous system (ANS), which consists of two components: the **intrinsic component (or enteric nervous system)** and the **extrinsic component.**

A. Intrinsic Component (or Enteric Nervous System). The phyla-genetically primitive enteric nervous system is an entirely separate nervous system in the body, since most functions of the GI tract are controlled by the enteric nervous system even in the absence of the extrinsic component, that is, the enteric nervous system can function autonomously. Many different neurotransmitters have been localized in the enteric nervous system: **acetylcholine (ACh; the "traditional" postganglionic parasympathetic neuron), nitric oxide (NO), vasoactive intestinal polypeptide (VIP), ATP, serotonin, and somatostatin.** The enteric nervous system is composed of **two distinct** interconnected neuronal circuits as indicated below:

1. **Submucosal Plexus of Meissner.** The neuronal cell bodies of the submucosal plexus are found in the submucosa. This plexus extends from the small intestine to the upper anal canal.
   a. **Motor Component.** The motor component of this plexus controls primarily **mucosal and submucosal gland secretion and blood flow.**
   b. **Sensory Component.** The sensory component of this plexus consists of **mucosal mechano-sensitive neurons.**

2. **Myenteric Plexus of Auerbach.** The neuronal cell bodies of the myenteric plexus are found between the inner circular and outer longitudinal layer of the muscularis externa. This plexus extends from the esophagus to the upper anal canal.
   a. **Motor Component.** The motor component of this plexus controls primarily **GI motility (contraction/relaxation of GI smooth muscle).**
   b. **Sensory Component.** The sensory component of this plexus consists of **tension-sensitive neurons** and **chemo-sensitive neurons.**

B. Extrinsic Component (Parasympathetic and Sympathetic Nervous Systems). The extrinsic component **modulates** the activity of the enteric nervous system, although specific functions are hard to detail. The extrinsic component is composed of two distinct pathways:

1. **Parasympathetic Nervous System.**
   a. The motor component involves **CN X (vagus nerve)** and the **pelvic splanchnic nerves (S2–S4).** These nerves synapse in the complex circuitry of the enteric nervous system. Hence, it is difficult to detail specific parasympathetic motor functions, although they are usually considered **excitatory** in nature.
   b. The sensory component involves the **nodose (inferior) ganglion of CN X** and the **dorsal root ganglia at S2–S4 spinal cord levels.** These neurons transmit the sensations of **visceral pressure, visceral movement, visceral stretch, visceral osmolarity, and visceral temperature.** Reflexes in which the sensory and motor components travel in CN X are called **vagovagal reflexes.**

2. **Sympathetic Nervous System.**
   a. The motor component involves the **greater splanchnic nerve, lesser splanchnic nerve, least splanchnic nerve,** and **lumbar splanchnic nerves,** which synapse in the **celiac ganglion, superior mesenteric ganglion, inferior mesenteric ganglion,** and the **superior hypogastric plexus.** Postganglionic axons synapse in the complex circuitry of the enteric nervous system. Hence, it is difficult to detail specific sympathetic motor functions, although they are usually considered **inhibitory** in nature. However, one motor function that is fairly well established is the **regulation of GI blood flow.**

b. The sensory component involves the **dorsal root ganglia at T5–L2/L3 spinal cord levels.** These neurons transmit the sensation of **visceral pain.**

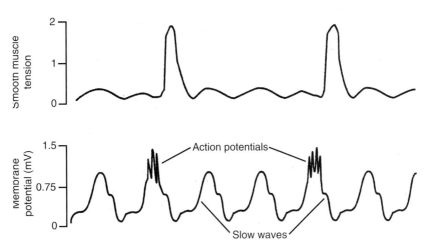

● **Figure 28-1: Slow Waves in GI Motility.** The slow waves are shown with action potentials at the crest of two slow waves (bottom trace). The action potentials trigger phasic contraction of the GI smooth muscle (top trace). A latent period separates the action potentials and the onset of contraction.

29
Oral Cavity and Esophagus

① Salivation.

A. Functions of Saliva. These functions of saliva include: cleanses the oral cavity, moistens the oral cavity for speech, participates in digestion due to the presence of digestive enzymes (e.g., amylase, lipase), lubricates ingested food by adding mucus, protects the oral cavity and esophagus by diluting and buffering ingested food, provides bacterial protection to the teeth due to the presence of lysozyme, promotes healing of the GI mucosa due to the presence of EGF, and provides immunological protection for the body due to the presence of IgA, IgG, and IgM.

B. Composition of Saliva. The average rate of saliva production is **1–1.5 L/day.** The composition of saliva includes: Na^+, Cl^-, HCO_3^-, K^+, amylase, lipase, mucins, ribonuclease, lysozyme, R protein (protects vitamin B_{12}), secretory IgA, IgG, IgM (from plasma cell within the connective tissue of the salivary glands), kallikrein (an enzyme that cleaves kininogens to form bradykinin, which is a vasodilator), epidermal growth factor (EGF), vasoactive intestinal polypeptide (VIP). In addition, testosterone, estrogen, progesterone, poisons, and viruses can be excreted in the saliva.

C. Concentration of Saliva Versus Salivary Flow Rate (Figure 29-1A,B). The concentration of the major electrolytes (Na^+, Cl^-, HCO_3^-, K^+) varies with the salivary flow rate. The initial saliva from the acini is **isotonic** (i.e., with similar $[Na^+]$, $[Cl^-]$, $[HCO_3^-]$, and $[K^+]$ as plasma). However, the intercalated and striated ducts modify the **initial isotonic saliva** by **reabsorption of Na^+ and Cl^-** (saliva → plasma), while being **H_2O impermeable**, and **secretion of HCO_3^- and K^+** (plasma →saliva). The result of these duct modifications is a **final hypotonic saliva** that is released into the oral cavity because Na^+ and Cl^- is reabsorbed while H_2O remains in the ductal lumen. The effect of flow rate on the saliva concentration of Na^+, Cl^-, and K^+ is due to the contact time between the initial isotonic saliva and the ducts for reabsorption and secretion to occur. The contact time explanation does not pertain to HCO_3^- because HCO_3^- secretion is selectively stimulated when saliva flow rate is increased.

1. **At the lowest flow rates,** the initial isotonic saliva undergoes the most modifications by the ducts and hence becomes hypotonic with $\downarrow Na^+$, $\downarrow Cl^-$, $\downarrow HCO_3^-$, $\uparrow K^+$.

2. **At the highest flow rates (4 mL/min),** the initial isotonic saliva undergoes the least modifications by the ducts and hence remains isotonic with $\uparrow Na^+$, $\uparrow Cl^-$, $\uparrow HCO_3^-$, $\downarrow K^+$.

D. Regulation of Saliva Production. Saliva production is unique in that it is increased by both the parasympathetic nervous system and the sympathetic nervous system. However, the parasympathetic nervous system plays a much more dominant role. The GI hormones do not play a role.

II Esophagus.

A. **General Features.** The **upper 5%** of the esophagus consists of skeletal muscle only. The **middle 45%** of the esophagus consists of both skeletal muscle and smooth muscle interwoven together. The **distal 50%** of the esophagus consists of smooth muscle only. The esophagus has two sphincters as indicated below.

1. The **upper esophageal sphincter (UES)** separates the pharynx from the esophagus. The UES is composed of **opening muscles,** specifically the **thyrohyoid muscle** and **geniohyoid muscle,** both of which are innervated by C1 via CN XII. In addition, the UES is composed of **closing muscles,** specifically the **inferior pharyngeal constrictor muscle** and the **cricopharyngeus muscle** (main player), both of which are innervated by CN X via the pharyngeal plexus. The UES is **skeletal muscle.** The UES relaxes (opens) during swallowing (deglutition), belching, and vomiting. The UES maintains closure of the upper end of the esophagus, prevents air from entering the esophagus and, with severe gastric acid reflux, prevents refluxed material from entering the pharynx.

2. The **lower esophageal sphincter (LES)** separates the esophagus from the stomach and **prevents gastroesophageal reflux,** which is the reflux of acidic gastric contents into the esophagus [i.e., gastroesophageal reflux disease (GERD)]. The LES is composed of **smooth muscle,** with the inner circular layer of smooth muscle the major determinant of LES tone. At rest, the LES is tonically contracted at a pressure 12–30 mm Hg > gastric pressure, which is maintained even in the absence of neural input (e.g., a bilateral vagotomy does not eliminate LES tonic contraction). Isolated LES muscle strips have a higher contractility than isolated muscle strips from other areas of the esophagus, which is probably due to the enhanced use of intracellular Ca^{2+} mediated by a **PKC_β–dependent pathway.** On the baseline of LES tonic contraction, the LES can be further contracted and then relaxed.

   a. **LES contraction** involves CN X and postganglionic enteric neurons that release **ACh,** which binds to M_3 muscarinic acetylcholine receptors (mAChRs) located on the smooth muscle cells. The LES contraction is mediated by a **calmodulin-dependent pathway.**

   b. **LES relaxation** involves CN X and postganglionic enteric neurons that release either **nitric oxide (NO)** or **vasoactive intestinal polypeptide (VIP).**

B. **Gastroesophageal (GE) Junction (Figure 29-1C-F).** The histological GE junction does NOT correspond to the gross anatomical GE junction. The mucosal lining of the cardiac portion of the stomach **extends about 2cm into the esophagus,** such that the distal 2cm of the esophagus is lined by a simple columnar epithelium. The junction where stratified squamous epithelium changes to simple columnar epithelium (or the mucosal GE junction) can be seen macroscopically as a **zig-zag line** (called the **Z-line**). This distinction is clinically very important, especially when dealing with Barrett's esophagus.

C. **Swallowing.** Swallowing is coordinated by the swallowing center located in the medulla, which receives sensory information via CN V, IX, and X. Humans swallow about 600 times/day. Swallowing occurs in two phases, as indicated below.

1. **Oropharyngeal Phase.** A number of events occur during this phase.
   a. The bolus of food is pushed upward and backward against the hard palate, which forces the bolus of food into the pharynx.
   b. The soft palate elongates to close off the nasopharynx.
   c. The epiglottis tips over to close off the larynx.
   d. The hyoid bone and larynx move upward.
   e. Respiration is stopped.
   f. The UES relaxes and opens for about 0.5–1 second to allow the bolus of food to pass into the esophagus. Subsequently, the UES contracts tightly.

2. **Esophageal Phase.** A number of events occur during this phase, which lasts about **6–10 seconds.**
   a. A **primary peristaltic wave** sweeps down the entire esophagus and pushes the food bolus toward the stomach, aided by gravity.
   b. A **secondary peristaltic wave** clears the esophagus of any residual food.
   c. The LES relaxes within 2 seconds after swallowing, at a time when the primary peristaltic wave is observed in the middle portion of the esophagus.
   d. When the food bolus reaches the LES, the LES is relaxed but closed. The food bolus, with the aid of peristalsis, forces the LES open.

D. **Vomiting (Emesis) Figure 29-2.** Vomiting is coordinated by the **vomiting center** located in the medulla (dorsolateral reticular formation), which receives sensory information from the **vestibular system** (e.g., motion sickness), **limbic system** (sights, smells, and emotions can induce vomiting), **chemoreceptor trigger zone** in the area postrema (activated by certain chemicals, drugs like emetics, radiation, certain metabolic states, and the vestibular system), **touch receptors in the pharynx,** and **CN X sensory neurons and sympathetic sensory neurons** from the GI tract that sense distention and mucosal irritation. Vomiting occurs in a number of steps, as indicated below.

1. Nausea, accompanied by sweating, pallor, and hypersalivation, is experienced.
2. **Reverse peristalsis** is observed in the small intestine and moves intestinal contents toward the stomach.
3. A **forced inspiration** occurs so that the epiglottis tips over to close off the larynx. At the same time, a **giant retrograde contraction** begins in the small intestine and moves the intestinal contents into the stomach.
4. The **abdominal muscles contract** while the breath is held, thereby increasing the intra-abdominal pressure.
5. The **UES and LES relax,** which allows the expulsion of gastric contents through the oral cavity as vomitus. If the UES remains closed, **retching** occurs.

Ⅲ Clinical Considerations.

A. **Gastroesophageal Reflux Disease (GERD).** GERD is described as the symptoms or mucosal damage produced by the abnormal reflux of gastric contents through the LES into the esophagus. The most common symptoms of GERD are **heartburn (or pyrosis),** which may worsen when bending or lying down, **regurgitation,** and **dysphagia.** Heartburn is typically described as a retrosternal burning discomfort that radiates towards the neck, most commonly experienced in the postprandial period. Regurgitation is the effortless return of gastric contents into the pharynx without nausea, retching, or abdominal contractions. Dysphagia is common in the setting of long-standing heartburn. The most dreaded cause of dysphagia is esophageal cancer (e.g., either adenocarcinoma arising from Barrett's metaplasia, or squamous cell carcinoma).

B. Barrett's Esophagus (see earlier Figure 29-1E,F). Barrett's esophagus can be defined as the replacement of esophageal stratified squamous epithelium with metaplastic "intestinalized" simple columnar epithelium with Goblet cells extending **at least 3 cm** into the esophagus. This metaplastic invasion is most commonly caused by GERD. The clinical importance of this metaplastic invasion is that virtually all lower esophageal adenocarcinomas occur as a sequelae.

C. Achalasia occurs due to the loss of ganglion cells in the myenteric plexus of Auerbach and is characterized by the failure to relax the lower esophageal sphincter (LES), which will cause progressive dysphagia and difficulty in swallowing. The most effective treatment is **pneumatic dilation,** in which high air pressure stretches the constricted LES to induce relaxation. A barium swallow radiograph shows a dilated esophagus above the LES and distal stenosis at the LES ("bird beak appearance"). Chagas disease caused by Trypanosoma cruzi may lead to achalasia.

D. Forceful vomiting is commonly seen in alcoholism, bulimia, and pregnancy, which may tear the posterior wall of the esophagus. Clinical findings include: severe retrosternal pain after vomiting and extravasated contrast medium. **Mallory-Weiss tears** involve only the mucosal and submucosal layers. **Boerhaave Syndrome** involve tears through all layers of the esophagus.

E. Esophageal Varices refer to the dilated subepithelial and submucosal venous plexuses of the esophagus that drain into the **left gastric (coronary) vein.** The left gastric vein empties into the portal vein from the distal esophagus and proximal stomach. Esophageal varices are caused by **portal hypertension** due to cirrhosis of the liver.

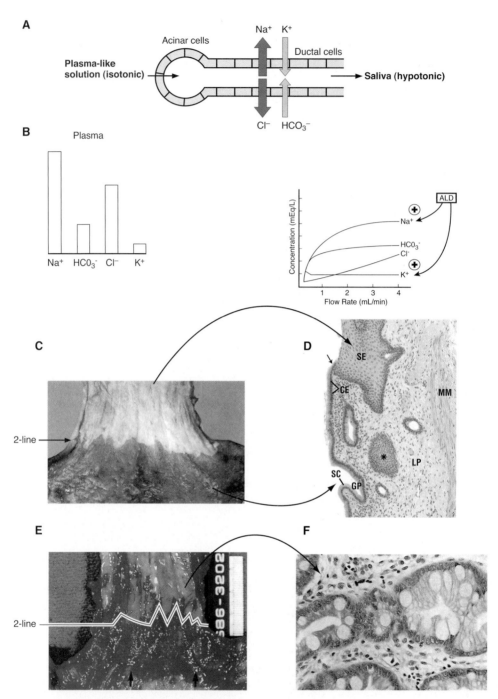

● **Figure 29-1: Saliva Characteristics. (A)** Modification of Initial Isotonic Saliva by Ductal Cells. **(B)** Concentration of Saliva versus Salivary Flow Rate. Note the comparison on the ionic concentration of saliva to plasma. Aldosterone (ALD) secreted from the zona glomerulosa of the adrenal gland will increase Na^+ reabsorption from the ducts and increase the K^+ secretion by the ducts. **(C,D) Gastroesophageal Junction.** (C) Photograph shows the Z line where the stratified squamous epithelium changes to simple columnar epithelium (or the mucosal GE junction). (D) LM shows the mucosal GE junction where the stratified squamous epithelium of the esophagus abruptly changes to simple columnar epithelium similar to the stomach. **(E,F) Barrett's Esophagus.** (E) Photograph shows the pathological disruption of the Z line. (F) LM shows the metaplastic "intestinalized" simple columnar epithelium with Goblet cells extending above the Z line.

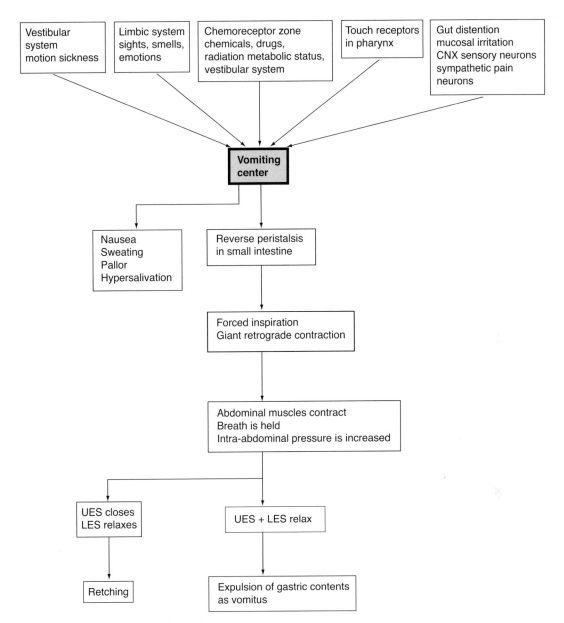

● **Figure 29-2: A flow chart of vomiting.**

30
Stomach

I **General Features.** The function of the stomach is to macerate, homogenize, and partially digest the swallowed food to produce a semi-solid paste called **chyme.** The stomach is also a reservoir, capable of holding **2–3 liters of food.** The stomach receives food from the esophagus and releases its contents into the duodenum. The stomach is divided gross anatomically into four regions: **cardia, fundus, body,** and **pyloric antrum.** The pyloric orifice is surrounded by the **pyloric sphincter (or pylorus).** The stomach is divided physiologically into two regions: **orad region** (i.e., cardiac, fundus, and proximal body) and **caudad region** (distal body and pylorus). The innervation of the stomach is by the **enteric nervous system,** which in the stomach consists of the myenteric plexus of Auerbach only. The enteric nervous system is modulated by the parasympathetic and sympathetic nervous systems.

II **Stomach Motility (Figure 30-1).**

A. Receptive Relaxation. With each swallow of food, the thin muscularis externa of the orad stomach relaxes to receive the food bolus (called **receptive relaxation**) so that the stomach can accommodate ≈1.5 L of food. Receptive relaxation is a **vagovagal reflex,** whereby visceral stretch sensory information from mechanoreceptors in the stomach travels with CN X to the CNS, and motor impulses (i.e., preganglionic parasympathetic axons) travel with CN X to the muscularis externa. The neurotransmitter **vasoactive intestinal polypeptide (VIP)** released from postganglionic axons seems to play an important role in receptive relaxation.

B. Gastric Mixing.
   1. Fed State. In the fed state after a large meal, the stomach enters a **lag phase** where contractions are absent but gastric secretion is high. After the lag phase, the thick muscularis externa of the caudad stomach contracts to grind the food bolus into smaller particles and to mix the food bolus with the gastric secretions to form **chyme.** The frequency of slow waves (3 slow waves/minute in the stomach) sets the maximum frequency of smooth muscle contractions. Strong peristaltic contractions begin in the caudad stomach and sweep distally toward the pyloric antrum where the contractions are the strongest, thereby moving the chyme toward the pyloric sphincter. The contractions occur at a rate of **3–5 contractions/min** and last between **2–20 seconds.** Chyme with small particles of food is emptied into the duodenum through the pyloric sphincter. Chyme with large particles of food is propelled back into the stomach (called **retropulsion**).

The peristaltic contractions involved in gastric mixing are increased by the parasympathetic nervous system (CN X). The peristaltic contractions involved in gastric mixing are decreased by the sympathetic nervous system.

2. **Fasting or Interdigestive State.** In the fasting or interdigestive state, periodic peristaltic contractions are observed called **migrating motor complexes (MMCs),** which occur at **90–120 minute intervals** and are mediated by **motilin** (secreted by enterochromaffin-like cells in the small intestine). The MMCs move chyme through the small intestines to the ileocecal valve during an overnight fast. The MMCs also move gastric HCl through the small intestines to control bacterial growth. The pyloric sphincter is open during the MMC.

C. **Gastric Emptying.** After a meal, the stomach contains $\approx$**1.5 L** and it takes $\approx$**3 hours** to empty this amount into the duodenum. The processes of gastric mixing and gastric emptying are a continuum. As retropulsion occurs, chyme with small particles of food is emptied into the duodenum through the pyloric sphincter. The amount of chyme emptied into the duodenum through the pyloric sphincter is determined by the strength of the peristaltic contractions and the pressure gradient between the pyloric antrum and duodenum.

1. When the stomach contents is **isotonic**, the rate of emptying is **fast.**
2. When the stomach contents is **hypertonic or hypotonic,** the rate of emptying is **slow.**
3. When the stomach contents contains ↑**fat,** the rate of empting is **slow.** This is mediated by **cholecystokinin (CCK)** that is secreted by **I cells** when fatty acids arrive in the duodenum. This provides adequate time for fat's digestion and absorption by the small intestine. CCK also stimulates enzyme secretion from the pancreas and stimulates bile release from the gall bladder.
4. When the duodenal contents contains ↑**H^+ ions (low pH),** the rate of emptying is **slow.** Chemo-sensitive receptors in the duodenum sense H^+ ions and relay this information back to the muscularis externa of the stomach via the myenteric plexus of Auerbach. This provides adequate time for H^+ ion's neutralization by pancreatic HCO_3^-.

III **Gastric Secretion.** The cells of the gastric mucosa secrete a fluid called **gastric juice,** which consists mainly of **mucus, HCO_3^-, intrinsic factor, pepsinogen,** and **HCl.** The average adult produces $\approx$**2–3 L /day** of gastric juice. The resting gastric juice is an **acidic (pH 2–2.5) isotonic solution.** HCl secretion from the parietal cell is maintained at $\approx$10% of its maximum rate to ensure that the resting juice is acidic. After a meal, the buffering capacity of the food raises the pH of the gastric juice to $\approx$**pH 4–5.**

A. **Contents of the Gastric Juice.**
1. **Gastric Mucus.** Gastric mucus is secreted by surface mucous cells and mucous neck cells in the stomach. Mucus consists of a mucus glycoprotein (a heavily glycosylated polymeric protein), phospholipids, sphingolipids, glyceroglucolipids, and HCO_3^-, all of which combine to form an alkaline, viscous gel that coats the luminal surface of the stomach. Mucus in the lumen of the stomach is in solution (rather than gel form) and adheres to food particles.
    a. **Function of Gastric Mucus.** Gastric mucus acts as a **lubricant** for the mucosa and the food to minimize frictional forces and prevent tissue injury. Mucus acts as a **protectant** against the acidic and proteolytic properties of the gastric juice by: **trapping HCO_3^-** and thereby creating a pH gradient between the gastric

juice in the lumen and mucosal epithelium; **preventing direct contact between the gastric juice in the lumen and the mucosal epithelium.**

b. **Regulation of Gastric Mucus Secretion.** Gastric mucus secretion is increased by both the **parasympathetic nervous system (CN X),** which increases **soluble mucus** secretion from mucous neck cells and **chemical/mechanical irritation,** which increases **gel-forming mucus** from surface mucus cells. The production of gel-forming mucus as a result of chemical/mechanical irritation is mediated via the generation of **prostaglandins (PGE_1, PGE_2, $PGF_{2\alpha}$).** Prostaglandin biosynthesis involves phospholipase A_2 and cyclooxygenase (COX). The ability of **non-steroidal anti-inflammatory drugs (NSAIDs;** e.g., aspirin, ibuprofen, naproxen, indomethacin) to inhibit COX may explain the ulcerogenic side effect of NSAIDs.

2. **HCO_3^-.** HCO_3^- is secreted by surface mucus cells in the stomach. The surface mucus cells can uptake HCO_3^- at the basolateral membrane and secrete HCO_3^- at the apical membrane. In addition, **carbonic anhydrase,** which generates HCO_3^- ($CO_2 + H_2O \rightarrow H^+ + HCO_3^-$) has been localized at the apical portion of surface mucus cells. HCO_3^- is mediated by a Cl^- and HCO_3^- exchange. In addition to active secretion, passive efflux of HCO_3^- occurs via the paracellular route.

   a. **Function of HCO_3^-.** Gastric HCO_3^- becomes trapped in the gel mucus and forms part of the mucus-HCO_3^- barrier, thereby maintaining a **pH gradient** of pH 2 of gastric acid in the lumen→pH7 at mucosal epithelium.

   b. **Regulation of HCO_3^- Secretion.** HCO_3^- secretion is increased by the **parasympathetic nervous system (CN X), chemical irritation** (i.e., presence of HCl in the lumen), and **prostaglandins.**

3. **Intrinsic Factor (IF).** IF is secreted by parietal cells in the stomach.

   a. **Functions of IF.** IF binds to and promotes the absorption of **vitamin B_{12}** in the terminal ileum by receptor-mediated endocytosis. **Pernicious anemia** may result from vitamin B_{12} deficiency caused by atrophic gastritis with decreased IF production.

   b. **Regulation of IF Secretion.** IF secretion is increased by **parasympathetic nervous system (CN X), gastrin,** and **histamine** (i.e., the same factors that increase gastric HCl secretion).

4. **Pepsinogen.** Pepsinogen (inactive) represents a family of related isozymes that have been divided into two groups. **Group I pepsinogen isozymes** are secreted by chief cells, mucus neck cells, and surface mucus cells of gastric glands. **Group II pepsinogen isozymes** are secreted by mucus-secreting cells of the pyloric glands (antrum of the stomach) and the submucosal glands of Brunner in the proximal duodenum.

   a. **Function of Pepsinogen.** Pepsinogen isozymes are converted to **pepsin isozymes (active)** on contact with the acid pH of the gastric juice. The pH optimum for pepsin isozymes falls between pH 1.5 → 5.0. Pepsin isozymes are endopeptidases that cleave peptide bonds between hydrophobic amino acids and are particularly active in the proteolysis of collagen, a major constituent of meat. The small peptides generated by this proteolytic process serve as signals for the secretion of GI hormones (e.g., gastrin, CCK).

   b. **Regulation of Pepsinogen Secretion.** Pepsinogen secretion is increased by **parasympathetic nervous system (CN X)** mediated by ACh and GRP (gastrin-releasing peptide, **chemical irritation** (i.e., presence of HCl in the lumen), **secretin,** and **CCK.**

5. **HCl (Figure 30-2).** Gastric HCl is secreted by the parietal cells in the stomach. The resting parietal cell contains a collapsed **canalicular membrane system** that is continuous with the surface cell membrane and many small vesicles called

tubulovesicles located close to the canicular membrane system, but separate. **Cl⁻ ion channels** are present on the canalicular membrane system and **H⁺-K⁺ ATPases** are present on the tubulovesicles. The activated parietal cell contains an interdigitating canalicular membrane system with microvilli to which the tubulovesicles have fused. The fusion of the canalicular membrane system and the tubulovesicles brings the Cl⁻ ion channels and H⁺-K⁺ ATPases together bordering the luminal space. The parietal cells contain **carbonic anhydrase,** which generates H^+ (CO_2 + $H_2O \rightarrow H^+ + HCO_3^-$). The key event in HCl secretion is the **cAMP-dependent opening of Cl⁻ ion channels,** which allows both Cl⁻ and K⁺ to move into the luminal space. K⁺ plays an important role because a **K⁺ gradient** in the opposite direction of H⁺ movement is necessary in order for the H⁺-K⁺ ATPase to pump H⁺.

a.   **Function of HCl.** Gastric HCl aids in the digestion of food, converts pepsinogen (inactive) → pepsin (active), and provides a defense mechanism by killing ingested microorganisms.

b.   **Stimulation of HCl Secretion.** Gastric HCl secretion is increased by the **parasympathetic nervous system (CN X; acetylcholine), gastrin,** and **histamine.** Acetylcholine (ACh) released from postganglionic parasympathetic neurons binds to the M_3 muscarinic acetylcholine receptor (mAChR) and activates the parietal cell through the IP_3 + DAG pathway. Gastrin (endocrine mechanism) released from the G cells binds to the CCK2 receptor and activates the parietal cell and the ECL cell through the IP_3 + DAG pathway. Histamine (paracrine mechanism) released from ECL cells binds to the H_2 receptor and activates the parietal cell through the ↑cAMP pathway. The major stimulus for HCl secretion seems to be histamine.

c.   **Inhibition of HCl Secretion.** Gastric HCl secretion is decreased by **CCK, secretin, GIP, somatostatin, prostaglandins (PGE₁), hypertonic solutions, emptying of the stomach, and distention of the duodenum.** CCK released by I cells in the duodenum in response to fatty acids in the duodenum deactivates the parietal cell. Secretin released from S cells in the duodenum in response to acid in the duodenum <pH 2.0 inhibits the release of gastrin by G cells. GIP released from K cells in the duodenum in response to fatty acids in the duodenum inhibits the release of gastrin by G cells. Somatostatin (paracrine mechanism) released from D cells in the stomach inhibits the release of histamine from ECL cells through the ↓cAMP + open K⁺ channel pathway. PGE_1 released from inflammatory cells deactivates the parietal cell through the ↓cAMP pathway. Hypertonic solutions within the stomach lumen inhibit HCl secretion via enteric nervous system reflexes. Emptying of the stomach inhibits HCl secretion via enteric nervous system reflexes. Distention of the duodenum inhibits HCl secretion via enteric nervous system reflexes.

d.   **Phases of HCl Secretion.**

   i)   **Cephalic Phase.** The cephalic phase is initiated by **sight, smell, taste,** and **conditioned reflexes.** The cephalic phase accounts for **30%** of the total HCl secreted in response to a meal and lasts ≈**30 minutes** into the meal. The cephalic phase is controlled by the **parasympathetic nervous system (CN X). ACh** released from postganglionic parasympathetic neurons binds to the M_3 muscarinic acetylcholine receptor (mAChR) and activates the parietal cell through the IP_3 + DAG pathway. **GRP (gastrin-releasing peptide)** released from postganglionic enteric neurons binds to receptors on the G cells and stimulates gastrin secretion, which then activates the parietal cell.

   ii)   **Gastric Phase.** The gastric phase is initiated by **stomach distention** and the presence of **amino acids/small peptides** in the stomach lumen. The gastric phase accounts for **60%** of the total HCL secreted in response to a meal and lasts ≈**2.5 hours** after the start of the meal. The gastric phase is controlled by the **parasympathetic nervous system (CN X)** and a **direct effect on G cells. ACh** released from postganglionic parasympathetic neurons binds to the M_3 muscarinic acetylcholine receptor (mAChR) and activates the parietal cell through the IP_3 + DAG pathway. **GRP (gastrin-releasing peptide)** released from postganglionic enteric neurons binds to receptors on the G cells and stimulates gastrin secretion which then activates the parietal cell. Amino acids/small peptides directly affect G cells and stimulate gastrin secretion, which then activates the parietal cell.

iii) **Intestinal Phase.** The intestinal phase is initiated by the **presence of chyme in the duodenum.** The intestinal phase accounts for **10%** of the total HCL secreted in response to a meal. Amino acids/small peptides within the duodenum directly affect G cells and stimulate gastrin secretion, which then activates the parietal cell. However, the intestinal phase can also inhibit HCl secretion via somatostatin, secretin, GIP, and CCK.

B. Other Gastric Secretions.
1. **HCO_3^-.** HCO_3^- is secreted into the bloodstream by the parietal cells in the stomach. This causes a rise in blood pH called the **alkaline tide.** For every H^+ that is pumped into the stomach lumen during the formation of gastric HCl, an OH^- remains in the parietal cell cytoplasm. In order to prevent intracellular alkalization and cell death, the enzyme carbonic anhydrase ($CO_2 + H_2O \rightarrow H^+ + HCO_3^-$) generates the formation of HCO_3^- from CO_2 and the OH^-. The HCO_3^- is transported across the basolateral cell membrane in exchange for Cl^-. Thus, an HCO_3^- enters the bloodstream for every H^+ produced. In addition, some of this HCO_3^- may find its way into the mucus–HCO_3^- barrier via the paracellular route.

2. **Gastrin.** Gastrin is secreted into the bloodstream (endocrine mechanism) by G cells in the pyloric antrum of the stomach/proximal duodenum. Two major forms of gastrin are secreted called **G17** (containing 17 amino acids; little gastrin) and **G34** (containing 34 amino acids; big gastrin). The common feature of all gastrins is a **C-terminal tetrapeptide (Try-Met-Asp-Phe)** which has full biological activity. Gastrin binds to the CCK2 receptor, which is a G protein-linked receptor using the IP_3 + DAG pathway.

a. **Functions of Gastrin.** Gastrin stimulates HCl secretion from parietal cells, stimulates histamine release from ECL cells, and promotes growth of the gastric mucosa.

b. **Regulation of Gastrin Secretion.** Gastrin secretion is increased by the **parasympathetic nervous system (CN X; GRP), stomach distention,** and the presence of **amino acids/small peptides** in the stomach lumen. GRP released from postganglionic enteric neurons binds to receptors on the G cells and stimulates gastrin secretion. Stomach distention stimulates gastrin secretion via a vagovagal reflex whereby the sensory component (from stretch receptors) travels with the CN X and the motor component preganglionic neurons travel with CN X and synapse on postganglionic enteric neurons that use ACh as a neurotransmitter. Amino acids/small peptides (phenylalanine and tryptophan are the most potent) directly affect G cells and stimulate gastrin secretion, which then activates the parietal cell. Gastrin secretion is decreased by the presence of HCl in the stomach lumen, which serves as a negative feedback loop to control HCl secretion.

3. **Histamine.** Histamine is secreted into the extracellular space (paracrine mechanism) by ECL cells in the stomach. Histamine is derived from the amino acid histidine and contains an imidazole containing a characteristic five membered ring with two nitrogen atoms. Histamine binds to the H_2 receptor, which is a G protein-linked receptor using the $\uparrow$cAMP pathway.

    a. **Functions of Histamine.** Histamine stimulates HCl secretion from parietal cells.

    b. **Regulation of Histamine Secretion.** Histamine secretion is increased by **gastrin** released from G cells in the stomach/proximal duodenum. Histamine secretion is decreased by **somatostatin** released from D cells in the stomach.

4. **Somatostatin.** Somatostatin is secreted into the extracellular space (paracrine mechanism) by D cells in the stomach. Two major forms of somatostatin are secreted called **SS-14** and **SS-28**. SS-14 is a 14-amino acid peptide with a cyclic structure. SS-28 (or prosomatostatin) is identical to SS-14 but with 14 additional amino acids. Both SS-14 and SS-28 are found in human circulation, but SS-14 seems to be the main player. SS-14 binds to the somatostatin receptor, which is a G protein-linked receptor, using the $\downarrow$cAMP + open K^+ channel pathway.

    a. **Functions of SS-14.** SS-14 inhibits histamine secretion from ECL cells and thereby inhibits HCl secretion. In general, SS-14 is a major inhibitory peptide and inhibits the secretion of all GI hormones.

    b. **Regulation of SS-14.** SS-14 secretion is increased by the presence of HCl in the stomach lumen and by gastrin. This suggests that the major function of SS-14 is to modulate HCl secretion in response to gastrin.

Ⅳ Clinical Considerations.

A. **Gastric Ulcers (Figure 30-3A)** most often occur within the **body of the stomach** along the **lesser curvature** above the **incisura angularis** at a histological transition zone where the gastric glands change from predominately parietal cells (HCl-producing) to G cells (gastrin-producing). They are caused by **damage to the mucosal barrier** (resulting in decreased mucus and bicarbonate production) due to smoking, salicylate or non-steroidal anti-inflammatory drugs (NSAID) ingestion, type B chronic atrophic gastritis, mucosal ischemia due to reduced PGE production, or bile reflux. About 80% of patients with gastric ulcers have associated *Helicobacter pylori* infection. Clinical findings include: burning epigastric pain **soon after eating;** pain increases with food intake; pain is relieved by antacids; patient is afraid to eat and loses weight.

B. **Duodenal ulcers (Figure 30-3B)** most often occur on the anterior wall of the first part of the duodenum (i.e., at the **duodenal cap**) followed by the posterior wall (danger of perforation into the pancreas). They are caused by **damage to the mucosal barrier** (resulting in decreased mucus and bicarbonate production) and **gastric acid hypersecretion** due to increased parietal cell mass, increased secretion to stimuli, increased nocturnal secretion, or rapid gastric emptying. About 95% of patients have associated *Helicobacter pylori* infection. Clinical findings include: burning epigastric pain **1–3 hours after eating;** pain decreases with food intake; pain is relieved by antacids; patient does not lose weight; patient wakes at night due to pain.

C. **Dumping Syndrome** refers to the abnormally rapid emptying of **hyperosmotic** stomach contents (especially high carbohydrate foods) into the jejunum within 30 minutes after a meal ("early dumping") or 1–3 hours ("late dumping"). The dumping syndrome usually occurs after a partial gastrectomy or vagotomy for treatment of obesity or an ulcer. Clinical findings include: epigastric discomfort, borborygmi (rumbling sounds due to gas movement), palpitations, dizziness, diarrhea, and hypoglycemia.

D. Gastroparesis. Gastroparesis is delayed gastric emptying in the absence of mechanical obstruction and is the most common gastric motor dysfunction. The failure to generate enough force to empty the stomach may be caused by: abnormal slow wave progression, vagotomy, or peripheral neuropathy due to diabetes. The most common cause of delayed gastric emptying in adults is pyloric antrum obstruction caused by scarring from a peptic ulcer.

E. Zollinger-Ellison Syndrome is due to a gastrin-secreting tumor of the pancreas that causes increased HCl secretion from parietal cells. The HCl secretion from parietal cells continues unabated since the tumor cells are not subject to feedback inhibition.

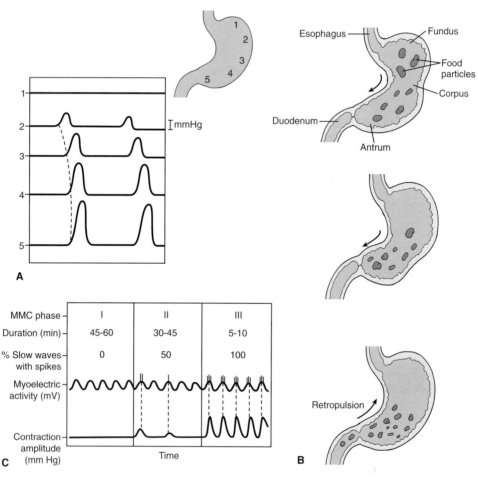

● **Figure 30-1: Stomach Motility. (A)** Intraluminal pressures measured from five regions of the stomach (1–5). The increase in intraluminal pressure is caused by peristaltic contractions of the muscularis externa. In region 1, no increase in intraluminal pressure is observed. In region 2, periodic spikes in intraluminal pressure are first observed. The periodic spikes increase in intensity as they sweep distally toward the pyloric antrum (region 5). **(B)** Diagram of Retropulsion. Chyme with large particles of food is propelled back into the stomach. **(C)** Stomach Motility in the Fasting or Interdigestive State. The migrating motor complexes (MMCs) have three phases. In Phase I (quiescent phase), no action potentials at the crest of the slow waves are observed and therefore, no smooth muscle contraction occurs. In Phase II, action potentials at the crest of ≈50% of the slow waves are observed and therefore some smooth muscle contraction occurs. In Phase III, action potentials at the crest of 100% of the slow waves are observed and therefore, strong smooth muscle contraction occurs that lasts ≈5–10 minutes. In Phase III, gastric contents is moved a long distance.

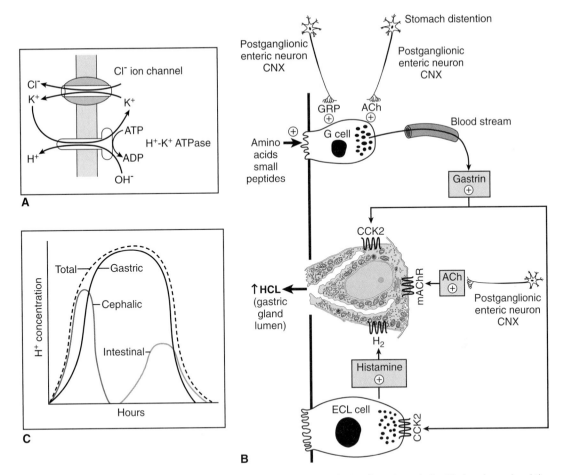

● **Figure 30-2: Parietal Cell and HCl Secretion. (A)** Diagram shows the ion flow through the Cl⁻ ion channel and the H⁺-K⁺ ATPase. **(B)** Diagram shows the factors that increase HCl secretion from the parietal cell. ACh = acetylcholine; GRP = gastrin-releasing peptide; ECL = enterochromaffin-like cell; CCK2 = cholecystokinin 2 receptor; H₂ = histamine 2 receptor; mAChR = muscarinic acetylcholine receptor. **(C)** Graph shows the three phases of HCl secretion.

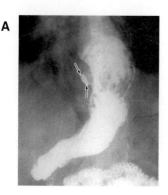
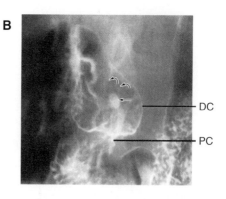

Comparison of Gastric and Duodenal Ulcers

	Gastric Ulcer	Duodenal Ulcer
% of ulcer cases	25%	75%

Epidemiology	Male : Female ratio = 1:1
	Increased risk with blood Type A
	No association with MEN I or II
	COPD
	Renal failure
		Male :Female ratio= 2:1
		Increased risk with blood Type O
		Associated with Zollinger-Ellison syndrome
		  (MEN I)
		Liver cirrhosis/alcohol
		COPD
		Renal failure
		Hyperparathyroidism
		Family history with an autosomal dominant
		  pattern

Pathogenesis	*H. pylori* infection in 80% of cases Damage to mucosal barrier due to smoking, salicylate or NSAID ingestion, type B chronic atrophic gastritis, mucosal ischemia due to reduced PGE production, or bile reflux	*H. pylori* infection in 95% of cases Damage to mucosal barrier Gastric acid hypersecretion due to increased parietal cell mass, increased secretion to stimuli, increased nocturnal secretion, or rapid gastric emptying

Location	Single ulcer within the body of the
	stomach along the lesser curvature
	above the incisura angularis
		Single ulcer on the anterior wall of the first
		  part of the duodenum (i.e., at the
		  duodenal cap) most common
		Single ulcer on the posterior wall (danger
		  of perforation into the pancreas)

Malignant Potential	No malignant potential Cancer may be associated with a benign ulcer in 1-3% of cases (biopsy necessary)	No malignant potential

Complications	Bleeding from left gastric artery
	Perforation
	Both are less common than seen
	  in duodenal ulcers
		Bleeding from gastroduodenal artery
		Perforation (air under diaphragm, pain
		  radiates to left shoulder)
		Gastric outlet obstruction
		Pancreatitis

Clinical Findings	Burning epigastric pain **soon after
	  eating**
	Pain increases with food intake
	Pain is relieved by antacids
	Patient is afraid to eat and loses weight
		Burning epigastric pain **1-3 hours after
		  eating**
		Pain decreases with food intake
		Pain is relieved by antacids
		Patient does not lose weight
		Patient wakes at night due to pain

COPD=chronic obstructive pulmonary disease; MEN=mulitiple endocrine neoplasia; PGE= prostaglandin E.

● **Figure 30-3: Ulcers. (A)** Radiograph shows a gastric ulcer (arrows) along the lesser curvature of the stomach. **(B)** Radiograph shows a duodenal ulcer (straight arrow) located in the duodenal cap (DC). The duodenal mucosal folds (curved arrows) radiate toward the ulcer crater. PC = pyloric canal **(C)** Comparison table of gastric and duodenal ulcers. Treatment for gastric or duodenal ulcers includes: Sucralfate (Carafate or Sulcrate) is a drug that forms a polymer in an acidic environment that protects ulcers from further irritation and damage. The antibiotic regimens of bismuth subsalicylate (Pepto-Bismol), Tetracycline, and Metronidazole or Amoxicillin and Clarithromycin are effective in eradication of *Helicobacter pylori*. Omeprazole (Prilosec), Esomeprazole (Nexium), Lansoprazole (Prevacid) are irreversible H^+-K^+ ATPase inhibitors that inhibit HCl secretion from parietal cells. Atropine is a muscarinic acetylcholine receptor (mAChR) antagonist that blocks the stimulatory effects of ACh released from postganglionic parasympathetic neurons (CN X) on HCl secretion. Cimetidine (Tagamet), Ranitidine (Zantac), Nizatidine (Axid), and Famotidine (Pepcid) are H_2-receptor antagonists that block the stimulatory effects of histamine released from inflammatory cells or mast cells on HCl secretion. The H_2 –receptor is a G-protein linked receptor that increases cAMP levels. Misoprostol (Cytotec) is a PGE_1 analog that inhibits HCl secretion and stimulates secretion of mucus and HCO_3^- from surface mucous cells of the stomach. Proximal Gastric Vagotomy (PGV). A PGV transects the vagus nerve (CN X) fibers only to the distal esophagus and fundus of the stomach and results in decreased gastric acid secretion.

31

Small Intestine

I. General Features. The function of the small intestine is **to continue digestion of chyme** received from the stomach using enzymes of the glycocalyx, pancreatic enzymes, and liver bile; and **to absorb nutrients derived from the digestive process, H_2O, electrolytes, and minerals.** The small intestine extends from the stomach (pyloric sphincter) to the colon (ileocecal valve) and is $\approx$**6–7 m long.** The small intestine is divided into the **duodenum, jejunum,** and **ileum.** The innervation of the small intestine is by the **enteric nervous system,** which in the small intestine consists of the submucosal plexus of Meissner and the myenteric plexus of Auerbach. The enteric nervous system is modulated by the parasympathetic and sympathetic nervous systems.

II. Small Intestine Motility (Figure 31-1). Small intestine motility mixes the chyme, brings the chyme into contact with the absorptive mucosal surface, and propels the chyme forward. Chyme takes about 2–3 hours to pass through the small intestine. As in the stomach, the frequency of slow waves (12 slow waves/minute in the duodenum $\rightarrow$ 8 slow waves/minute in the ileum) sets the maximum frequency of smooth muscle contractions.

A. Fed State. In the fed state after a large meal, two types of contractions are observed in the small intestine: **segmentation (mixing) contractions** and **peristaltic (propulsion) contractions.** In a segmentation contraction, a small section of small intestine contracts (i.e., the inner circular layer of smooth muscle) which sends chyme in both the orad and caudad directions. Subsequently, the same section then relaxes and the chyme returns with no net caudad movement of chyme. In a peristaltic contraction, a small section of small intestine contracts (i.e., the outer longitudinal layer of smooth muscle) behind a bolus of chyme while simultaneously a small section of small intestine relaxes ahead of the bolus of chyme. This results in a rapid caudad movement of chyme at a rate of 2–25 cm/second. In the fed state, smooth muscle contraction is modulated by the **parasympathetic nervous system (CN X)** whereby postganglionic parasympathetic neurons release **ACh** and other postganglionic enteric neurons release **substance P.** In the fed state, smooth muscle relaxation is modulated by the **parasympathetic nervous system (CN X)** whereby postganglionic enteric neurons release **NO** and **VIP.**

B. Fasting or Interdigestive State. In the fasting or interdigestive state, periodic peristaltic contractions are observed called **migrating motor complexes (MMCs),** which are a continuation of the MMCs initiated in the stomach. MMCs occur at **90–120 minute intervals** and are mediated by **motilin** (secreted by enterochromaffin-like cells in the small intestine). The MMCs sweep the small intestine clean of undigestible food residua, bacteria, and desquamated epithelial cells. As soon as feeding occurs, the MMCs stop and the fed-pattern of motility returns.

C. **Ileocecal Sphincter.** The ileocecal sphincter separates the terminal ileum from the cecum. This sphincter is normally closed. When it opens, small amounts of chyme enter the colon at a rate that is compatible with the ability of the colon to absorb H_2O and electrolytes. This sphincter is incompetent so that the build up of gas or feces in the colon is prevented. The ileocecal sphincter opens in response to the following: distension of the terminal ileum, peristaltic contractions in the terminal ileum, and the **gastroileal reflex,** which causes the emptying of the ileum after a meal.

Ⅲ Small Intestine Secretion (Table 31-1).

A. **Aqueous Solution.** The enterocytes of the small intestine secrete an aqueous solution during the course of digestion. Under normal circumstances, the enterocytes absorb more than they secrete. Under pathological circumstances (e.g., cholera infection), aqueous secretion greatly exceeds absorption and diarrhea results.

B. **Mucus.** Mucus is secreted by Goblet cells in the small intestine. Mucus consists of a mucus glycoprotein (a heavily glycosylated polymeric protein), phospholipids, sphingolipids, glyceroglucolipids, which combine to form a gel that coats the luminal surface of the small intestine. Small intestinal mucus acts as a lubricant for the mucosa to minimize frictional forces and prevent tissue injury.

C. **Cholecystokinin (CCK).** CCK is secreted into the bloodstream (endocrine mechanism) by the enteroendocrine I-cells in the intestinal glands (crypts of Lieberkuhn). CCK is a 33-amino acid peptide and is a member of the gastrin-CCK family. The C-terminal five amino acids of CCK (CCK-5) are identical to those of gastrin and include the tetrapeptide that is minimally necessary for gastrin activity, which means that CCK has some gastrin activity. The minimum fragment of CCK necessary for biological activity is the C-terminal heptapeptide (CCK-7). CCK binds selectively to the CCK1 receptor, whereas CCK and gastrin bind to the CCK2 receptor.
    1. **Functions of CCK.** CCK increases bile release by the contraction of the gall bladder and relaxation of the sphincter of Oddi, increases pancreatic enzyme and HCO_3^- secretion, decreases HCl secretion by parietal cells, inhibits gastric emptying, and exerts a growth effect on the pancreas and gall bladder.
    2. **Regulation of CCK Secretion.** CCK secretion is increased by the presence of amino acids (tryptophan and phenylalanine)/small peptides and fatty acids/monoglycerides in the small intestinal lumen.

D. **Secretin (SEC; called "nature's antacid).** SEC is secreted into the bloodstream (endocrine mechanism) by the enteroendocrine S cells in the intestinal glands (crypts of Lieberkuhn). SEC is a 27-amino acid peptide and is a member of the secretin-glucagon family. All 27 amino acids are necessary for biological activity.
    1. **Functions of Secretin.** SEC increases HCO_3^- release from the pancreas and liver biliary tract and inhibits the effect of gastrin on the parietal cell. The neutralization of acidic chyme by HCO_3^- is essential for fat digestion because pancreatic lipases have a pH 6–8 optimum.
    2. **Regulation of Secretin Secretion.** SEC secretion is increased by the presence of H^+ (<pH 4.5) and fatty acids in the intestinal lumen.

E. Gastric Inhibitory Peptide or Glucose Insulinotropic Peptide (GIP). GIP is secreted into the bloodstream (endocrine mechanism) by the enteroendocrine K cells in the intestinal glands (crypts of Lieberkuhn). GIP is a 42-amino acid peptide and is a member of the secretin-glucagon family.

   1. **Functions of GIP.** GIP inhibits the effect of gastrin on the parietal cell and increases insulin secretion under conditions of hyperglycemia by pancreatic β cells. The action of GIP to increase insulin secretion explains why an oral glucose load is utilized by cells more rapidly than an intravenous glucose load. An oral glucose load stimulates insulin secretion from pancreatic β cells via both GIP and blood glucose levels. An intravenous glucose load stimulates insulin secretion from pancreatic β cells via only blood glucose levels.

   2. **Regulation of GIP Secretion.** GIP secretion is increased by the presence of glucose, amino acids/small peptide, and fatty acids in the small intestinal lumen.

F. Glucagon-like Peptide-1 (GLP-1). GLP-1 is secreted into the bloodstream (endocrine mechanism) by the enteroendocrine L cells in the intestinal glands (crypts of Lieberkuhn). GLP-1 is a 30-amino acid peptide with a 50% sequence homology to glucagon. The glucagon gene is composed of six exons that yield preproglucagon. In the pancreatic α cells, preproglucagon is processed to glucagon and glucagon-related polypeptide (GRPP). In the intestinal L cells, preproglucagon is processed to GLP-1, GLP-2, and glycentin (which is a large peptide that contains glucagon).

   1. **Functions of GLP-1.** GLP-1 increases insulin secretion under conditions of hyperglycemia, decreases postprandial glucagon secretion, inhibits gastric emptying, reduces food intake, and stimulates pancreatic β cell growth. GLP-1 has a 1–2 minute half-life due to the rapid degradation of the N-terminus by **dipeptidyl peptidase IV (DPP-IV).** A naturally occurring peptide in the saliva of the Gila monster called **exendin-4** shares sequence homology with GLP-1. However, exendin-4 has a prolonged half-life because it is resistant to DPP-IV degradation. The drug **exenatide** is synthetic exendin-4 and is the first GLP-1 based diabetes therapy approved in the US by the FDA.

   2. **Regulation of GLP-1 Secretion.** GLP-1 secretion is increased the presence of glucose, amino acids/small peptide, and fatty acids in the small intestinal lumen.

IV Digestion and Absorption of Carbohydrates (Figure 31–2A).

A. Digestion. The majority of calories in the US diet are derived from carbohydrates, the majority of which are in the form of starch (a polymer of glucose). The digestion of carbohydrates begins in the oral cavity and then continues in the small intestine. Starch contains both α-1,4 and α-1,6 glycosidic bonds. The α-1,4 glycosidic bonds are hydrolyzed by salivary amylase in the oral cavity (plays a minor role because salivary amylase is inactivated by ↓pH in the stomach) and pancreatic amylase in the small intestine. This yields three disaccharides: **α-dextrins, maltose, and maltotriose.** These three disaccharides are further digested to **glucose** by **α-dextrinase, maltase,** and **sucrase.** There are three main disaccharides in the US diet; **trehalose, lactose,** and **sucrose.** Trehalose is digested to two molecules of glucose by **trehalase.** Lactose is digested to glucose and galactose by **lactase.** Sucrose is digested to glucose and fructose by **sucrase.** The enzymes α-dextrinase, maltase, sucrase, trehalase, and lactase are all located in the glycocalyx of the enterocytes. In short, carbohydrates are digested to the monosaccharides called **glucose, galactose,** and **fructose.**

TABLE 31-1		SUMMARY TABLE OF GASTROINTESTINAL HORMONES	
Hormone	Cell	Functions	Regulation
Gastrin	G cell in stomach	Stimulates HCl secretion from parietal cells Stimulates histamine release from ECL cells Promotes growth of gastric mucosa	Increased by CN X (GRP), stomach distention, presence of amino acids in the stomach lumen
Histamine	ECL cell in stomach (paracrine mechanism)	Stimulate HCl secretion from parietal cells	Increased by gastrin released from G cells Decreased by somatostatin released from D cells
Somatostatin	D cell in stomach (paracrine mechanism)	Inhibits histamine secretion from ECL cells A major inhibitory peptide	Increased by the presence of HCL in the stomach lumen Increased by gastrin
CCK	I cell in small intestine	Increases bile release by contraction of the gall bladder and relaxation of the sphincter of Oddi Increases pancreatic enzyme and HCO_3^- secretion Decreases HCL secretion by parietal cells Inhibits gastric emptying Exerts a growth effect on pancreas and gall bladder	Increased by presence of amino acids/small peptides and fatty acids/monoglycerides in the small intestinal lumen
Secretin	S cell in small intestine	Increases HCO3- release from the pancreas and liver biliary tract Inhibits the effect of gastrin on the parietal cell.	Increased by the presence of H^+ (<pH 4.5) and fatty acids in the intestinal lumen
GIP	K cell in small intestine	Inhibits the effect of gastrin on the parietal cell Increases insulin secretion under conditions of hyperglycemia	Increased by the presence of glucose, amino acids/small peptide, and fatty acids in the small intestinal lumen
GLP-1	L cell in small intestine	Increases insulin secretion under conditions of hyperglycemia Decreases postprandial glucagon secretion Inhibits gastric emptying Reduces food intake Stimulates pancreatic β cell growth	Increased by the presence of glucose, amino acids/small peptide, and fatty acids in the small intestinal lumen

B. Absorption. Only monosaccharides can be absorbed by enterocytes. Glucose and galactose enter enterocytes by secondary active transport using a **Na$^+$ dependent-glucose transporter (SGLT-1).** The energy for this process is derived from a Na$^+$ gradient across the apical membrane, which is created by the **Na$^+$-K$^+$ ATPase** located on the basolateral membrane. Fructose enters enterocytes by facilitated diffusion using **GLUT5.** Glucose, galactose, and fructose exit enterocytes by facilitated diffusion using **GLUT2** to enter portal blood.

Ⅴ Digestion and Absorption of Proteins (Figure 31-2B).

A. Digestion. The protein requirement for a normal healthy adult is ≈40g of protein/day. Humans do not have a storage mechanism for proteins (like, for example, glycogen) and therefore we synthesize about 300 g of protein/day. The digestion of protein begins in the stomach by the action of pepsin, which has an optimum pH of 1.5 → 5.0. However, the action of pepsin is terminated in the small intestine as the pH rises above 5.0. However, the digestion of protein continues in the small intestine by the action of pancreatic proteases and proteases in the glycocalyx of enterocytes. **Trypsinogen (inactive)** is secreted by the exocrine pancreas and is converted to its active form **trypsin (active)** by **enterokinase** located in the glycocalyx of enterocytes. Trypsin then converts all other inactive pancreatic precursors to their active form **(trypsinogen → trypsin, chymotrypsinogen → chymotrypsin, proelastase → elastase, procarboxypeptidase A → carboxypeptidase A, and procarboxypeptidase B → carboxypeptidase B).** These five active pancreatic proteases then hydrolyze dietary protein to **amino acids, dipeptides, tripeptides,** and **oligopeptides.** Oligopeptides are further digested to amino acids, dipeptides, and tripeptides by **aminopeptidases** located in the glycocalyx of enterocytes. Most of the dipeptides and tripeptides are further hydrolyzed to amino acid by **cytoplasmic peptidases** within enterocytes. In short, proteins are digested to **amino acids, dipeptides,** and **tripeptides.**

B. Absorption. Only amino acids, dipeptides, and tripeptides can be absorbed by enterocytes. Dipeptides and tripeptides are absorbed faster than amino acids by enterocytes. L-amino acids enter enterocytes by secondary active transport using **Na$^+$-amino acid cotransporters.** There are four separate Na$^+$-amino acid cotransporters that handle either neutral, acidic, basic, or imino amino acids. The energy for this process is derived from a Na$^+$ gradient across the apical membrane which is created by **Na$^+$-K$^+$ ATPase** located on the basolateral membrane. Dipeptides and tripeptides enter enterocytes by secondary active transport using **H$^+$-dipeptide/tripeptide cotransporters.** The energy for this process is derived from a H$^+$ gradient across the apical membrane, which is created by the **Na$^+$-H$^+$ exchanger** located on the apical membrane. Amino acids exit enterocytes by facilitated diffusion to enter portal blood. Dipeptides and tripeptides exit enterocytes to enter portal blood.

Ⅵ Digestion and Absorption of Lipids (Figure 31-2C).

A. Digestion. Triacylglycerols are the main lipid in the human diet. The digestion of lipids begins in the stomach by the action of **lingual lipase** and **gastric lipase** and then continues in the small intestine by the action of **pancreatic lipase** and **colipase** (which is necessary to stabilize pancreatic lipase at the surface of the lipid droplet), **cholesterol ester hydrolase,** and **phospholipase A$_2$.** 10% of ingested triacylglycerols are hydrolyzed in the stomach to **fatty acids** and **glycerol** by lingual lipase and gastric lipase. The remaining 90% of ingested triacylglycerols are hydrolyzed in the small intestine to **monoacylglycerols** and **fatty acids** by pancreatic lipase/colipase. Ingested **cholesterol esters** are hydrolyzed in the small intestine to **cholesterol** and **fatty acids** by cholesterol ester hydrolase. **Phospholipids** are hydrolyzed in the small intestine to **lysolecithin** and **fatty acids** by phospholipase A_2. Lipid digestion in the small intestine is aided by **bile salts** that are secreted into the small intestine from the gall bladder. Bile salts surround and emulsify lipids (i.e., produce small droplets of lipid dispersed in an aqueous solution), which assists pancreatic enzyme action. In short, lipids are digested to **monoacylglycerols, short, medium, and long chain fatty acids, cholesterol, lysolecithin,** and **glycerol.**

B. **Absorption.** The hydrophobic products of lipid digestion (i.e., monoacylglycerol, >12 carbon long chain fatty acids, cholesterol, and lysolecithin) are packaged into the center of the **micelles** that travel to the microvillus border of the enterocytes. The hydrophobic products enter enterocytes by diffusion assisted by **fatty acid transporters (FATs).** Within the enterocytes, **reesterification** occurs in the **smooth endoplasmic reticulum (sER)** to form triacylglycerols, cholesterol esters, and phospholipids. Within the enterocytes, the reesterified lipids are packaged with **apoproteins** (e.g., ApoB) into **chylomicrons.** The chylomicrons are processed by the **Golgi** into **secretory vesicles,** which bind to the basolateral membrane. The hydrophobic products exit enterocytes by **exocytosis** of chylomicrons into **lacteals** of the lymph system. The hydrophilic product of lipid digestion (i.e., glycerol), along with short and medium chain fatty acids, enters the enterocyte directly by diffusion and exits the enterocyte by diffusion to enter portal blood.

VII Absorption of Vitamins.

A. **Fat–Soluble Vitamins (A, D, E, K).** The fat soluble vitamins A, D, E, and K are processed in the same manner as other lipids in the diet (see Chap 31 VI above).

B. **Water-Soluble Vitamins (B_1, B_2, B_6, B_{12}, biotin, C, folic acid, nicotinic acid, pantothenic acid).**
1. All water-soluble vitamins (except B_{12}) enter enterocytes by secondary active transport using **Na^+-amino acid cotransporters.** All water-soluble vitamins exit enterocytes probably by diffusion to enter portal blood.
2. **Vitamin B_{12} (cobalamin).** In the stomach, vitamin B_{12} binds to **R protein** (secreted by the salivary glands). In the duodenum, pancreatic proteases degrade R protein so that B_{12} then binds to **intrinsic factor (IF)** secreted by parietal cells forming B_{12} + IF that is resistant to pancreatic proteases. Vitamin B_{12} enters enterocytes when a **B_{12} + IF dimer** binds to the **cubilin receptor** located on enterocytes in the **ileum.** Vitamin B_{12} exits enterocytes by diffusion to enter portal blood, where it circulates bound to **transcobalamin II.** The B_{12} + transcobalamin II complex has a half-life of 6–9 minutes and enters vitamin B_{12}-requiring cells (i.e., cells undergoing rapid turnover like hematopoietic cells) by receptor-mediated endocytosis. A vitamin B_{12} deficiency results in **pernicious anemia.**

VIII Absorption of Calcium (Ca^{2+}).
Ca^{2+} enters enterocytes by diffusion and then binds to a cytoplasmic vitamin D-dependent Ca^{2+} binding protein called **calbindin D-28K.** Ca^{2+} exits enterocytes by active transport involving a **Ca^{2+}ATPase** on the basolateral membrane to enter portal blood. Ca^{2+} absorption is dependent on **1,25-$(OH)_2$ vitamin D (a steroid hormone),** which induces the synthesis of calbindin D-28K. Vitamin D sources include

dietary intake and production by skin keratinocytes stimulated by ultraviolet light. Vitamin D is hydroxylated by liver hepatocytes to **25-(OH) vitamin D.** 25-(OH) vitamin D is hydroxylated in the kidney to **1,25-(OH)$_2$ vitamin D,** the active metabolite that functions similar to a steroid hormone.1,25-(OH)$_2$D stimulates absorption of Ca^{2+} and $PO4^{2-}$ from the ileum, thereby elevating blood Ca^{2+} and PO_4^{2-} levels.

IX   # Absorption of Iron (Fe^{2+}).   The total amount of iron in the body is $\approx$3–4 g, which is found in the following sites: hemoglobin (2.5 g), iron-containing proteins (e.g., myoglobin, cytochromes; 400mg), bound to transferrin (3–7 mg), and the remainder is stored as ferritin or hemosiderin. The average US diet contains $\approx$20 mg of iron of which only $\approx$10% can be absorbed. Most dietary iron is in the form of **Fe^{3+}.** Fe^{3+} enters enterocytes by attachment to integrin and some of the Fe^{3+} is reduced to Fe^{2+} by **ascorbic acid** or **ferrireductase.** Fe^{2+} enters enterocytes by binding to **DMT-1 (divalent metal transporter-1).** Heme **Fe^{2+}** (Fe^{2+} bound to hemoglobin or myoglobin) enters enterocytes by binding to **HCP-1 (heme carrier protein-1)** and undergoes receptor-mediated endocytosis. Heme Fe^{2+} is digested to Fe^{2+} by lysosomal enzymes. Fe^{2+} exits enterocytes by transport across the basolateral membrane using **ferroportin-1.** When Fe^{2+} exits enterocytes, Fe^{2+} is oxidized to Fe^{3+} by **ceruloplasmin** (a known ferrooxidase), which then binds to **transferrin** and travels in the plasma as **transferrrin + Fe^{3+}.** The main function of transferrin is to deliver iron to cells, particularly red blood cell precursors, which need iron for hemoglobin synthesis. The transferrin + Fe^{3+} binds to the transferrin receptor located on erythroid precursors cells and is internalized by receptor-mediated endocytosis. The endocytic vesicles bind to an endosome where the pH 5 environment causes the release of iron into the cytoplasm. **Ferritin** is a very large protein that can bind up to 4500 atoms of iron and acts as the **cellular storage protein for iron.** Small amounts of ferritin normally circulate in the plasma, making plasma ferritin a good indicator of the adequacy of body iron stores.

A. **In iron deficiency,** serum ferritin is less than 12 mg/L. Male and females lose $\approx$1 mg of iron/day in the urine and desquamated cells. Females of reproductive age lose $\approx$3 mg of iron/day, the additional amount coming from the menstrual flow. Iron deficiency is the most common cause of anemia.

B. **In iron overload,** serum ferritin approaches 5000 mg/L. Also during iron overload, intracellular ferritin undergoes lysosomal degradation, in which the ferritin protein is degraded and the iron aggregates within the cell as **hemosiderin** (a golden brown hemoglobin-derived pigment) in a condition called **hemosiderosis.** The more extreme accumulation of iron is called **hemochromatosis,** which is associated with liver and pancreas damage. Hemosiderosis can be observed in patients with **increased absorption of dietary iron, impaired utilization of iron, hemolytic anemias, and blood transfusions.**

X   # Absorption and Secretion of Fluid and Electrolytes (Figure 31-3).   The enterocytes of the GI tract (small intestine and colon) absorb fluids ($\approx$9 L of fluid/day) and electrolytes. The source of the 9L of fluid is $\approx$2 L from the diet and $\approx$7 L from salivary, gastric, pancreatic, biliary, and intestinal secretions. $\approx$100–200 mL of fluid is not absorbed and is excreted in the feces. In addition, epithelial cells lining the intestinal glands (crypts of Lieberkühn) secrete fluids and electrolytes. In normal circumstances, absorption is greater than secretion so that any disturbance in absorption can lead to excessive fluid loss via the GI tract, causing diarrhea.

A. **Absorption of Fluid and Electrolytes**. Absorption occurs by enterocytes lining the villi of the small intestine. The absorption of NaCl occurs by an **electroneutral mechanism** (versus the electrogenic mechanism in the small intestine and proximal colon whereby the net reaction is the absorption of Na^+ and Cl^- in exchange for H^+ and HCO_3^- efflux.

1. **Absorption of Na^+ in the Jejunum.** Na^+ is absorbed in the jejunum by various transporters, which include:

   a. **Na^+-K^+ ATPase** transports Na^+ across the basolateral membrane into the interstitial fluid (i.e., "pumps" Na^+ out of the cell) keeping cytoplasmic $[Na^+]$ low by countertransport with K^+ into the cytoplasm (i.e., "pumps" K^+ into the cell) keeping cytoplasmic $[K^+]$ high.

   b. **Glucose Transporter 4 (GLUT4)** transport Na^+ across the luminal membrane into the cytoplasm by cotransport with glucose or galactose into the cytoplasm, ,which occurs because cytoplasmic $[Na^+]$ is kept low by Na^+-K^+ ATPase.

   c. **Na^+-amino acid Cotransporters** transport Na^+ across the luminal membrane into the cytoplasm by cotransport with various amino acids into the cytoplasm, which occurs because cytoplasmic $[Na^+]$ is kept low by Na^+-K^+ ATPase.

   d. **Na^+-H^+ Exchanger** transports Na^+ across the luminal membrane into the cytoplasm by countertransport with H^+ into intestinal fluid. The H^+ are supplied by the reaction $H_2CO_3 \rightarrow H^+ + HCO_3^-$, which is catalyzed by **carbonic anhydrase.**

   e. **HCO_3^- Transporter** transports HCO_3^- across the basolateral membrane into the interstitial fluid.

2. **Absorption of Na^+ in the Ileum.** Na^+ is absorbed in the ileum by various transporters, which include:

   a. **Na^+-K^+ ATPase.**

   b. **Glucose Transporter 4 (GLUT4)**

   c. **Na^+-amino acid Cotransporters**

   d. **Na^+-H^+ Exchanger**

   e. **Cl^--HCO_3^- Exchanger** transports Cl^- across the luminal membrane into the cytoplasm by countertransport with HCO_3^- into the intestinal fluid. The HCO_3^- is supplied by the reaction $H_2CO_3 \rightarrow H^+ + HCO_3^-$, which is catalyzed by **carbonic anhydrase.**

   f. **Cl^- Transporter** transports Cl^- across the basolateral membrane into the interstitial fluid.

3. **Absorption of Cl^-.** Cl^- is absorbed in the small intestine via the paracellular route and by various transporters which include:

   a. **Na^+-K^+ ATPase**

   b. **Na^+-Cl^- Cotransporter** transports Cl^- across the luminal membrane into the cytoplasm by cotransport with Na^+ into the cytoplasm, which occurs because cytoplasmic $[Na^+]$ is kept low by Na^+-K^+ ATPase.

   c. **Cl^--HCO_3^- Exchanger**

   d. **Cl^- Transporter**

4. **Absorption of H_2O.** H_2O is absorbed in the small intestine by **diffusion** using **aquaporin H_2O channels** and by **diffusion via the paracellular route** across a zonula occludens between enterocytes. The absorption of electrolytes and H_2O occur in proportion to each other (i.e., in an **isosmotic fashion**). The diffusion of H_2O occurs because of the osmolarity difference between the intestinal fluid and interstitial fluid. The osmolarity difference is created by the reabsorption of solutes (e.g., Na^+). At the start, the intestinal fluid is isosmotic with the interstitial fluid. Then, solutes are reabsorbed from the intestinal fluid, which lowers the osmolarity of the intestinal fluid (i.e., hyposmotic or raises H_2O concentration) compared with the interstitial fluid, and also raises the osmolarity of the interstitial fluid

(i.e., hyperosmotic or lowers H_2O concentration) compared with the intestinal fluid. The osmolarity difference causes net diffusion of H_2O.

5. **Absorption of HCO_3^- in the Jejunum.** HCO_3^- is absorbed in the jejunum by various transporters, which include:
   a. **Na^+-K^+ ATPase**
   b. **Na^+-H^+ Exchanger**
   c. **HCO_3^- Transporter**
6. **Absorption of K^+.** K^+ is absorbed ($\approx$85% of ingested K^+) in the small intestine by **diffusion via the paracellular route** across the zonula occludens between enterocytes.

B. **Secretion of Fluid and Electrolytes.** Secretion occurs by epithelial cells lining the intestinal glands (crypts of Lieberkuhn).
   1. **Secretion of Cl^-.** Cl^- is the primary ion secreted by the small intestine. Cl^- is secreted into the intestinal fluid of the small intestine by transporter proteins and two ion channel proteins, which include:
      a. **Na^+-K^+ ATPase**
      b. **Na^+-K^+-$2Cl^-$ Cotransporter** transports Na^+ across the basolateral membrane into the cytoplasm by cotransport with K^+ and Cl^- into the cytoplasm, which occurs because cytoplasmic [Na^+] is kept low by Na^+-K^+ ATPase.
      c. **Cl^- ion-channel protein (cystic fibrosis transmembrane conductance regulator; CFTR;** also found in the upper airways of the lung) transports Cl^- across the luminal membrane into the intestinal fluid by forming hydrophilic pores that allow diffusion of Cl^-. CFTR is usually closed but can be opened by ↑cAMP elicited by hormones, neurotransmitters, or **cholera toxin.**
      d. **Cl^- ion-channel protein** transports Cl^- across the luminal membrane into the intestinal fluid by forming hydrophilic pores that allow diffusion of Cl^-. This Cl^- ion channel protein is usually closed but can be opened by ↑cytoplasmic Ca^{2+}.
   2. **Secretion of Na^+.** Na^+ is secreted via the paracellular route by passively following Cl^- into the intestinal fluid.
   3. **Secretion of H_2O.** H_2O is secreted via the paracellular route by passively following Na^+ and Cl^- into the intestinal fluid.
   4. **Secretion of HCO_3^- in the Duodenum and Ileum.** HCO_3^- is secreted into the intestinal fluid of the duodenum and ileum by various transporter proteins and ion channel proteins, which include:
      a. **Na^+-K^+ ATPase**
      b. **Na^+-H^+ Exchanger** transports Na^+ across the luminal membrane into the cytoplasm by countertransport with H^+ into intestinal fluid. The H^+ are supplied by the reaction $H_2CO_3 \rightarrow H^+ + HCO_3^-$, which is catalyzed by **carbonic anhydrase.**
      c. **Cl^--HCO_3^- Exchanger**
      d. **Cl^- ion-channel protein (cystic fibrosis transmembrane conductance regulator; CFTR);** also found in the upper airways of the lung) can also transport HCO_3^- across the luminal membrane into the intestinal fluid by forming hydrophilic pores that allow diffusion of HCO_3^-.

XI **Clinical Considerations.**

A. **Lactose intolerance.** Lactose intolerance is an intolerance to lactose-containing foods, primarily dairy products. Primary causes of lactose intolerance are: racial/ethnic lactose malabsorption (most common) due to a genetic reduction in lactase activity; developmental lactase deficiency due to low lactase levels in the premature infant; and congenital lactase deficiency (autosomal recessive) due to the absence of lactase activity. Secondary causes of lactose intolerance are: bacterial overgrowth in the small intestine; infectious enteritis (e.g., giardiasis), and mucosal injury (e.g., celiac disease, Crohn disease, drug- or radiation-induced enteritis). The unabsorbed lactose passes in the colon where it is converted to short chain fatty acids and hydrogen gas. Clinical findings include: abdominal pain (crampy in nature localized to the periumbilical or lower quadrant), bloating, flatulence, diarrhea, and vomiting (particularly in adolescents), borborygmi may be audible, and bulky, frothy, watery stools.

B. **Abetalipoproteinemia (Bassen-Kornzweig syndrome).** Abetalipoproteinemia is an autosomal recessive disorder due to a mutation in the gene encoding **microsomal triacylglyceride transfer protein (MTP).** MTP transfers triacylglycerides into the lumen of the endoplasmic reticulum for very low density lipoproteins (VLDL) assembly and is required for the synthesis of apo B from the liver. This results in malabsorption of lipids in the small intestine, low levels of serum cholesterol and VLDL, and the **absence of serum apo B.** Clinical findings include: lipid malabsorption, steatorrhea, acanthocytes (spiny red blood cells; Spurr cells), retinitis pigmentosa that results in progressive retinal degeneration, peripheral neuropathy, ataxia, sensory motor neuropathy that typically presents at two to six years of age with hypoesthesia, hypalgesia, proprioceptive loss, and absent tendon reflexes.

C. **Secretory versus Osmotic Diarrhea.** A secretory diarrhea occurs when the secretion of fluid and electrolytes (Cl^-, Na^+, K^+ and H_2O; see X, B) from enterocytes is increased (e.g., cholera). A secretory diarrhea is characterized by: a continued diarrhea despite fasting; stool volumes >1 L/day; and occurs during the daytime and nighttime (these characteristics are uncommon in an osmotic diarrhea). An osmotic diarrhea occurs when an osmotically active substance (e.g., sorbitol present in sugarless candies or lactose for lactose intolerant patients) is present in the intestinal lumen and causes an osmotic imbalance so that H_2O diffuses into the intestinal lumen. Generally, the osmotic agent can be identified and removed from the diet.

D. **Cholera.** *Vibrio cholerae* are comma-shaped, gram-negative bacteria that have caused many pandemics of secretory diarrheal disease. These bacteria never enter the enterocytes but instead remain in the intestinal lumen and secrete an endotoxin called **cholera toxin.** Cholera toxin ADP-ribosylates a G protein (called G_s), which in turn stimulates adenylate cyclase. ADP-ribosylated G_s protein is permanently in an active GTP-bound state, resulting in persistent activation of **adenylate cyclase and ↑cAMP levels. The ↑cAMP levels keep the** Cl^- ion channel protein permanently open, resulting in the diffusion of Cl^- into the small intestinal lumen; Na^+ and H_2O follow. This overwhelms the absorptive function of the colon and liters of "ricewater" diarrhea containing flecks of mucus are produced.

E. **Steatorrhea.** Steatorrhea occurs when there is a malabsorption of lipids. The gold standard for diagnosis of steatorrhea is a quantitative estimate of stool fat. Steatorrhea may be caused by the following:
   1. **Pancreatic disease** (e.g., pancreatitis or cystic fibrosis) which reduces the amount of pancreatic enzymes necessary for lipid digestion.
   2. **Hypersecretion of gastrin,** which increases HCl secretion, ↓pH in intestinal **lumen, and inactivates pancreatic lipase.**
   3. **Ileal** resection, which reduces the bile acid pool and thereby impairs lipid digestion.
   4. **Bacterial overgrowth** which reduces the presence of bile acids throughout the small intestine and thereby impairs lipid digestion.

5. Tropical sprue, which reduces the number in enterocytes and thereby impairs lipid absorption.
6. **Abetalipoproteinemia (Bassen-Kornzweig syndrome)** which reduces the ability to form chylomicrons and thereby impairs lipid absorption.

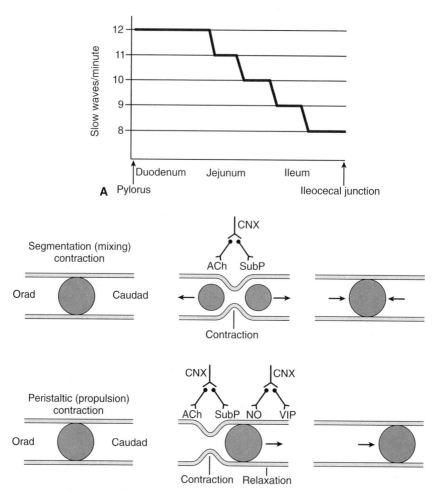

● **Figure 31-1: Small Intestine Motility. (A)** Graph shows the slow wave frequency decreasing in a step-wise pattern from the duodenum to the ileum. **(B)** Diagram shows a segmentation contraction and a peristaltic contraction. Note the neurotransmitters involved in the contraction and relaxation of the smooth muscle. ACh = acetylcholine; Sub P = substance P; NO = nitric oxide; VIP = vasoactive intestinal polypeptide.

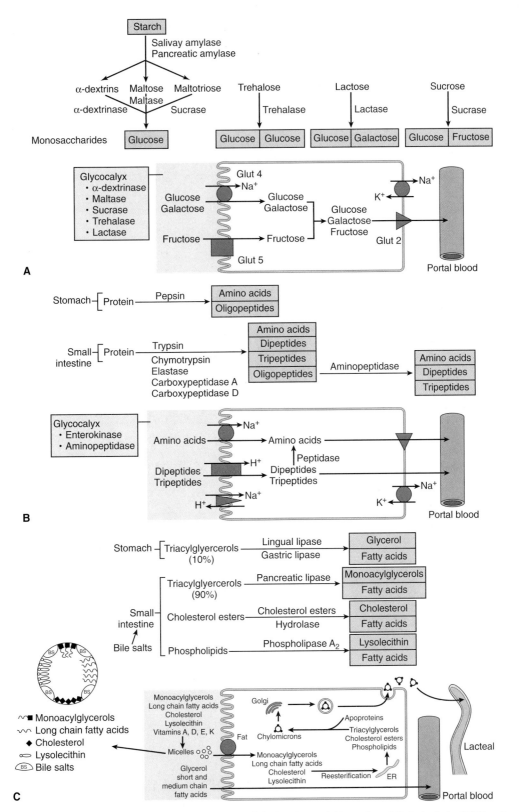

● **Figure 31-2: Digestion and Absorption of Nutrients. (A)** Digestion and Absorption of Carbohydrates **(B)** Digestion and Absorption of Proteins **(C)** Digestion and Absorption of Lipids. GLUT = glucose transporter; FAT = fatty acid transporter; sER = smooth endoplasmic reticulum.

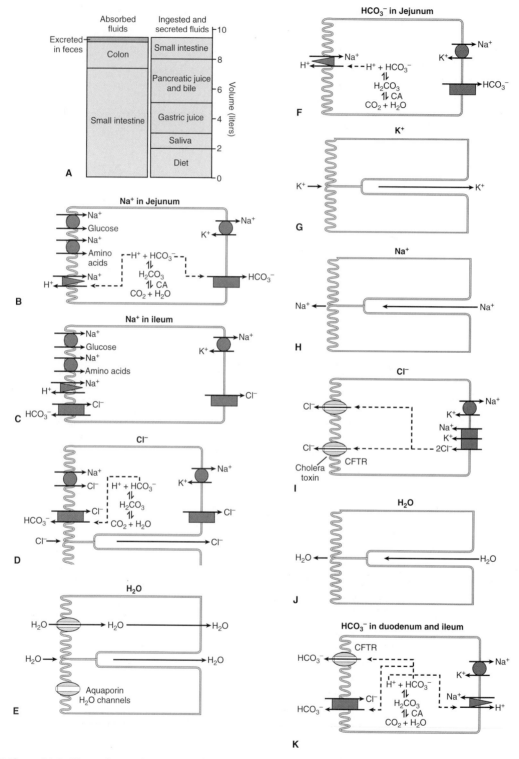

● **Figure 31-3: Absorption and Secretion of Fluid and Electrolytes. (A)** Graph shows a comparison of the volume of fluid ingested and secreted versus that which is absorbed by the intestine. **(B-G) Absorption of Fluid and Electrolytes.** (B) Absorption of Na^+ in the jejunum. (C) Absorption of Na^+ in the ileum. (D) Absorption of Cl^-. (E) Absorption of H_2O (F) Absorption of HCO_3^- (G) Absorption of K^+ **(H-K) Secretion of Fluid and Electrolytes.** (H) Secretion of Na^+ (I) Secretion of Cl^- (J) Secretion of H_2O (K) Secretion of HCO_3^- in duodenum and ileum. CA = carbonic anhydrase; CFTR = cystic fibrosis transmembrane conductance regulator.

32

Large Intestine

I **General Features.** The function of the large intestine is to: absorb Na^+, Cl^- and H_2O from the lumen, soften the fecal mass by addition of mucus, store the fecal mass, support the fecal mass, and eliminate the fecal mass. The large intestine is divided into the **cecum, ascending colon, transverse colon, descending colon, sigmoid colon, rectum**, and **upper anal canal.** The innervation of the large intestine is by the **enteric nervous system,** which in the large intestine consists of the submucosal plexus of Meissner and the myenteric plexus of Auerbach. The enteric nervous system is modulated by the parasympathetic and sympathetic nervous systems.

II **Large Intestine Motility (Figure 32-1).** Material that is not absorbed in the small intestine enters the large intestine, where it is called **feces.** The colon receives $\approx$500–1500 mL of chyme/day from the ileum. A majority of the fluid and electrolytes that enter the colon are absorbed such that the fecal mass contains $\approx$**50–100 mL of H_2O/day.** The fecal mass then moves through the cecum $\rightarrow$ ascending colon $\rightarrow$ transverse colon $\rightarrow$ descending colon $\rightarrow$ sigmoid colon $\rightarrow$ rectum $\rightarrow$ anal canal for defecation. The movement of the fecal mass through the colon is 5–10 cm/hour versus 2–25 cm/second in the small intestine. There are three types of contractions seen in the large intestine, which include:

A. Segmentation (Mixing) and Peristaltic Contractions. In a segmentation contraction, **haustra** are formed by the contraction of the **tenia coli.** The haustra fill with fecal mass and the distention causes the haustra to contract (i.e., inner circular layer of smooth muscle), which sends the fecal mass in both proximal and distal directions. The fecal mass returns with no net movement. This causes a mixing action, which brings the fecal mass in contact with the mucosal surface, thereby facilitating absorption. Segmentation contractions occur predominately in the cecum and proximal colon and last $\approx$12–60 seconds. In a peristaltic contraction, a small section of large intestine contracts (i.e., tenia coli) behind the fecal mass, while simultaneously a small section of large intestine relaxes ahead of the fecal mass. This results in movement of the fecal mass toward the anal canal. Smooth muscle contraction is modulated by the **parasympathetic nervous system (CN X),** whereby postganglionic parasympathetic neurons release **ACh** and other postganglionic enteric neurons release **substance P.** Smooth muscle relaxation is modulated by the **parasympathetic nervous system (CN X),** whereby postganglionic enteric neurons release **NO** and **VIP.**

B. Mass Movement Contractions. Mass movement contractions (a wave of peristaltic contractions) begin mid-transverse colon and move the fecal mass a long distance toward the anal canal. Mass movement contractions occur 1–3 times/day, are responsible for colonic evacuation, and are associated with cramps. During mass movement contractions, segmentation contractions and haustra temporarily disappear. Mass movement contractions occur shortly after a meal (particularly after breakfast) and stimulate the urge to defecate if some fecal mass is present in the rectum. This is a result of the **gastrocolic reflex,** whereby distention of the stomach by food increases the frequency of mass movement contractions in the large intestine. The gastrocolic reflex involves visceral stretch sensory information from **mechanoreceptors** in the stomach, which travel with CN X to the CNS and motor impulses mediated by the hormones **gastrin** and **CCK.**

Ⅲ **Anal Canal.**   The anal canal is surrounded by the **internal anal sphincter** (a continuation of smooth muscle from the rectum with involuntary control via parasympathetic and sympathetic innervation) and the **external anal sphincter** (striated muscle under voluntary control via the pudendal nerve). The anal canal is divided into the upper and lower anal canal by the **pectinate line.**

Ⅳ **Defecation Reflex.**   The rectum is usually empty because it is more active in segmental contractions than the sigmoid colon so that the fecal mass tends to move into the sigmoid colon. The internal anal sphincter (smooth muscle) is usually tonically contracted. When mass movement contractions occur, the fecal mass distends the rectum to >25% of capacity and initiates a reflexive relaxation of the internal anal sphincter and a reflexive contraction of the external anal sphincter (striated muscle). This is called the **retrosphincteric reflex.** Sensory impulses from **pressure-sensitive receptors** travel to sacral spinal cord levels. Motor impulses travel with the **pelvic splanchnic nerves (parasympathetic; S2–S4) and** relax the internal anal sphincter. This causes the urge to defecate.

A. If the person decides to defecate, relaxation of the external anal sphincter (via the **pudendal nerve**) and puborectalis muscle (via the **nerve to the levator ani**) occurs. Evacuation is preceded by a deep breath, which moves the diaphragm down. The glottis closes and contraction of the respiratory muscles with full lungs elevates both intrathoracic and intraabdominal pressures. The abdominal muscles also contract, which further raises the intraabdominal pressure. The increased pressure helps to force the fecal mass through the relaxed external anal sphincter. The muscles of the pelvic diaphragm also relax, allowing the pelvic floor to drop and straighten out the rectum.

B. If the person decides not to defecate, contraction of the external anal sphincter (via the **pudendal nerve**) and puborectalis muscle (via the **nerve to the levator ani**) occurs, pressure-sensitive receptors accommodate relieving the sensation to defecate, the fecal mass moves back into the rectum, and the tone of the internal anal sphincter is regained by the **hypogastric plexus** and **lumbar splanchnic nerves (sympathetic).**

Ⅴ **Absorption and Secretion of Fluid and Electrolytes (Figure 32-2).**   The enterocytes of the GI tract (small intestine and large intestine) absorb ≈9 L of fluid/day. The enterocytes of the small intestine absorb ≈7 L of fluid/day so that normally ≈2 L of fluid/day is delivered to the large intestine. If >2.5 L of fluid/day is delivered to the large intestine, diarrhea will occur.

A. Absorption of Fluid and Electrolytes. In the small intestine and proximal colon, the absorption of NaCl occurs by an **electroneutral mechanism,** whereby the net reaction is the absorption of Na^+ and Cl^- in exchange for H^+ and HCO_3^- efflux. In the distal colon, the absorption of NaCl occurs by an **electrogenic mechanism.**

1. **Absorption of Na$^+$ in the Proximal Colon.** Na$^+$ is absorbed in the proximal colon (by an electroneutral mechanism identical to that of the ileum) by various transporters, which include:
   a. **Na$^+$-K$^+$ ATPase** transports Na$^+$ across the basolateral membrane into the interstitial fluid (i.e., "pumps" Na$^+$ out of the cell) keeping cytoplasmic [Na$^+$] low by countertransport with K$^+$ into the cytoplasm (i.e., "pumps" K$^+$ into the cell) keeping cytoplasmic [K$^+$] high.
   b. **Glucose Transporter 4 (GLUT4)** transport Na$^+$ across the luminal membrane into the cytoplasm by cotransport with glucose or galactose into the cytoplasm, which occurs because cytoplasmic [Na$^+$] is kept low by Na$^+$-K$^+$ ATPase.
   c. **Na$^+$-amino acid Cotransporters** transport Na$^+$ across the luminal membrane into the cytoplasm by cotransport with various amino acids into the cytoplasm, which occurs because cytoplasmic [Na$^+$] is kept low by Na$^+$-K$^+$ ATPase.
   d. **Na$^+$-H$^+$ Exchanger** transports Na$^+$ across the luminal membrane into the cytoplasm by countertransport with H$^+$ into intestinal fluid. The H$^+$ are supplied by the reaction $H_2CO_3 \rightarrow H^+ + HCO_3^-$, which is catalyzed by **carbonic anhydrase.**
   e. **Cl$^-$-HCO$_3$$^-$ Exchanger** transports Cl$^-$ across the luminal membrane into the cytoplasm by countertransport with HCO$_3$$^-$into the intestinal fluid. The HCO$_3$$^-$ is supplied by the reaction $H_2CO_3 \rightarrow H^+ + HCO_3^-$, which is catalyzed by **carbonic anhydrase.**
   f. **Cl$^-$ Transporter** transports Cl$^-$ across the basolateral membrane into the interstitial fluid.
2. **Absorption of Na$^+$ in the Distal Colon.** Na$^+$ is absorbed in the distal colon (by an electrogenic mechanism) by various transporter proteins and ion-channel proteins which include:
   a. **Na$^+$-K$^+$ ATPase**
   b. **Electrogenic Na$^+$ ion-channel protein** transports Na$^+$ across the luminal membrane into the cytoplasm by forming hydrophilic pores that allow diffusion of Na$^+$, which occurs because cytoplasmic [Na$^+$] is kept low by Na$^+$-K$^+$ ATPase. Because the tight junctions in the colon are very tight, electrogenic Na$^+$ transport produces an electrochemical potential of $\approx$**30 mV** across the mucosa. **Aldosterone** increases Na$^+$ reabsorption by enterocytes in the colon by inducing the synthesis of electrogenic Na$^+$ ion channel proteins.
   c. **K$^+$ ion-channel protein** transports K$^+$ across the basolateral membrane into the interstitial fluid in order to compensate for the K$^+$ entry into the cytoplasm and the resulting charge imbalance.
3. **Absorption of Cl$^-$ in the Proximal Colon.** Cl$^-$ is absorbed in the proximal colon (by an electroneutral mechanism identical to that of the small intestine) via the paracellular route and by various transporters which include:
   a. **Na$^+$-K$^+$ ATPase**
   b. **Na$^+$-Cl$^-$ Cotransporter** transports Cl$^-$ across the luminal membrane into the cytoplasm by cotransport with Na$^+$ into the cytoplasm, which occurs because cytoplasmic [Na$^+$] is kept low by Na$^+$-K$^+$ ATPase.
   c. **Cl$^-$-HCO$_3$$^-$ Exchanger**
   d. **Cl$^-$ Transporter**
4. **Absorption of Cl$^-$ in the Distal Colon.** Cl$^-$ is absorbed in the distal colon via the paracellular route driven by the electrogenic Na$^+$ absorption.
5. **Absorption of H$_2$O in the Colon.** H$_2$O is absorbed in the colon by the **standing osmotic gradient mechanism**. This is in contrast to the absorption of H$_2$O in the small intestine, which occurs in an isosmotic fashion whereby the absorption of electrolytes and H$_2$O occur in proportion to each other. The standing osmotic

gradient mechanism involves **Na$^+$-K$^+$ ATPase** located in the basolateral membrane of enterocytes near the apical end of the lateral intercellular space. Na$^+$ is pumped from the cytoplasm into the intercellular space and Cl$^-$ and HCO$_3^-$ follow to preserve electroneutrality. The hyperosmotic solution of NaCl near the apical end of the intercellular space causes the osmotic flow of H$_2$O into the intercellular space from the intestinal fluid and neighboring enterocytes.

6. **Absorption of K$^+$ in the Colon.** K$^+$ is absorbed in the colon by a transporter protein and ion channel protein, which include:
    a. **H$^+$-K$^+$ ATPase** transports K$^+$ across the luminal membrane into the cytoplasm by countertransport with H$^+$ into the intestinal fluid.
    b. **K$^+$ ion-channel protein** transports K$^+$ across the basolateral membrane into the interstitial fluid by forming hydrophilic pores that allow diffusion of K$^+$, which occurs because K$^+$ is kept high by H$^+$-K$^+$ ATPase.

B. **Secretion of Electrolytes.**
    1. **Secretion of Cl$^-$ in the Colon.** Cl$^-$ is secreted in the colon in a manner identical to that in the small intestine. Cl$^-$ is secreted into the intestinal fluid of the colon by transporter proteins and two ion channel proteins, which include:
        a. **Na$^+$-K$^+$ ATPase**
        b. **Na$^+$-K$^+$-2Cl$^-$ Cotransporter** transports Na$^+$ across the basolateral membrane into the cytoplasm by cotransport with K$^+$ and Cl$^-$ into the cytoplasm, which occurs because cytoplasmic [Na$^+$] is kept low by Na$^+$-K$^+$ ATPase.
        c. **Cl$^-$ ion-channel protein (cystic fibrosis transmembrane conductance regulator; CFTR;** also found in the upper airways of the lung) transports Cl$^-$ across the luminal membrane into the intestinal fluid by forming hydrophilic pores that allow diffusion of Cl$^-$. CFTR is usually closed but can be opened by ↑cAMP elicited by hormones, neurotransmitters, or **cholera toxin.**
        d. **Cl$^-$ ion-channel protein** transports Cl$^-$ across the luminal membrane into the intestinal fluid by forming hydrophilic pores that allow diffusion of Cl$^-$. This Cl$^-$ ion channel protein is usually closed but can be opened by ↑cytoplasmic Ca^{2+}.
    2. **Secretion of HCO$_3^-$ in the Colon.** HCO$_3^-$ secretion in the colon is somewhat of an enigma. Some HCO$_3^-$ secretion in the colon is stimulated by the short chain fatty acids and seems to involve HCO$_3^-$ diffusion into the intestinal fluid in response to a pH gradient. In addition, some HCO$_3^-$ is secreted in the colon in a manner identical to that in the small intestine. HCO$_3^-$ is secreted into the intestinal fluid of the colon by various transporter proteins and ion channel proteins, which include:
        a. **Na$^+$-K$^+$ ATPase**
        b. **Na$^+$-H$^+$ Exchanger** transports Na$^+$ across the luminal membrane into the cytoplasm by countertransport with H$^+$ into intestinal fluid. The H$^+$ are supplied by the reaction H$_2$CO$_3$ → H$^+$ + HCO$_3^-$, which is catalyzed by **carbonic anhydrase.**
        c. **Cl$^-$-HCO$_3^-$ Exchanger**
        d. **Cl$^-$ ion-channel protein (cystic fibrosis transmembrane conductance regulator; CFTR;** also found in the upper airways of the lung) can also transport HCO$_3^-$ across the luminal membrane into the intestinal fluid by forming hydrophilic pores that allow diffusion of HCO$_3^-$.
    3. **Secretion of K$^+$ in the Colon.** K$^+$ is secreted in the colon by transporter proteins and ion channel proteins, which include:
        a. **Na$^+$-K$^+$ ATPase**
        b. **Na$^+$-K$^+$-2Cl$^-$ Cotransporter**

c. **K^+ ion channel protein** transports K^+ across the luminal membrane into the intestinal fluid by forming hydrophilic pores that allow diffusion of K^+. In diarrhea, K^+ secretion is increased due to a flow-dependent mechanism so that **hypokalemia** may result.

VI **Intestinal Gas (Flatus).** Flatus is passed 10–14 times/day. The composition and frequency of flatus is a result of dietary intake of fermentable substrates (e.g., carbohydrates, nonabsorbable carbohydrates like stachyose and raffinose in beans and legumes, poorly absorbable carbohydrates like fructose and sorbitol in fruit, and starches) and the activity of the colonic bacterial flora. The principal gases of flatus are O_2, N_2, CO_2, H_2, and CH_4 **(methane).** The O_2 and N_2 in flatus is derived mainly from swallowed air during eating and drinking and also by diffusion from the bloodstream. The CO_2 in flatus is derived from bacterial fermentation of dietary substrates and perhaps from the neutralization of HCl by HCO_3^- in the GI tract. The H_2 in flatus is derived from bacterial fermentation of dietary carbohydrates particularly. The CH_4 (methane) in flatus is derived from bacterial fermentation (by *Methanobrevibacter smithii*) of dietary carbohydrates and proteins. The majority of the gas within flatus is odorless (i.e., O_2, N_2, CO_2, H_2, and CH_4 (methane). The gases within flatus that cause odor and are socially unacceptable include H_2S (hydrogen sulphide), NH_3 (ammonia), and volatile fatty acids and amino acids. Flatulence can be treated by controlling aerophagia (i.e., the amount of swallowed air) by elimination of gum or candy chewing, stopping smoking, improving oral hygiene, and treating anxiety. Flatulence can also be treated by restricting the diet (i.e., reducing consumption of beans, legumes, fruits, and starches). Flatulence can also be treated by taking activated charcoal or simethicone before meals.

VII **Clinical Considerations.**

A. **Familial Adenomatous Polyposis (FAP; Figure 32-3 A,B)** is the archetype of adenomatous polyposis syndromes, whereby patients develop 500–2000 polyps that most commonly carpet the mucosal surface of the **rectosigmoid colon** (60% of all cases) and invariably become malignant. Malignant polyps are irregular in shape, sessile, >2 cm in diameter, exhibit sudden growth, and the base is broader than height. FAP is an autosomal dominant disease and involves a mutation in the **APC anti-oncogene.** The progression from a small polyp to a large polyp is associated with a mutation in the ***ras*** **proto-oncogene.** The progression from a large polyp to metastatic carcinoma is associated with mutations in the **DCC anti-oncogene** (deleted in colon carcinoma) and the **p53 anti-oncogene. Gardner syndrome** is a variation of FAPC whereby patients demonstrate adenomatous polyps and multiple osteomas. **Turcot syndrome** is a variation of FAPC whereby patients demonstrate adenomatous polyps and gliomas.

B. **Adenocarcinoma of the Colon (Figure 32-3 C, D)** will invariably develop in patients with FAP and accounts for 98% of all cancers in the large intestine. Clinical findings include: fatigue, weakness, change in bowel habits, weight loss. Right-sided tumors are associated with iron deficiency anemia. Left-sided tumors are associated with obstruction and bloody stools. It is a clinical maxim that iron-deficiency anemia in an older man means adenocarcinoma of the colon until shown otherwise. Metastasis occurs most commonly to the **liver** since the sigmoid veins and superior rectal veins drain into the hepatic portal system. A posterior metastasis may involve the **sacral nerve plexus,** causing sciatica.

VIII **Summary of overall fluid balance in the small and large intestine (Figure 32-3E).**

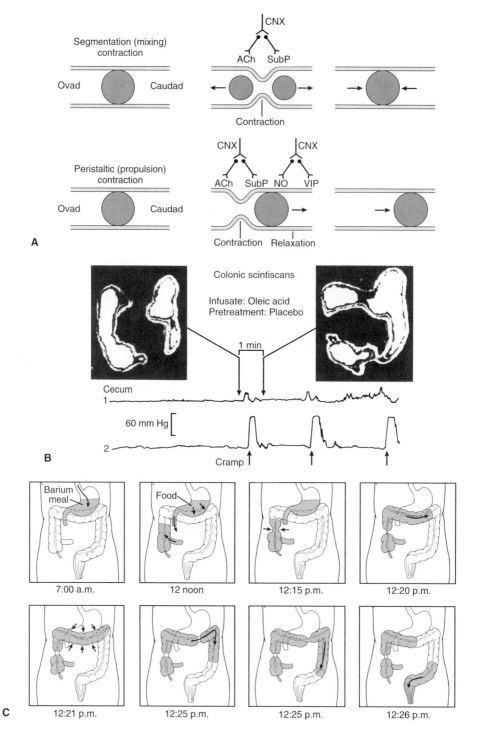

● **Figure 32-1: Large Intestine Motility .** **(A)** Diagram shows a segmentation contraction and a peristaltic contraction. Note the neurotransmitters involved in the contraction and relaxation of the smooth muscle. ACh = acetylcholine; Sub P = substance P; NO = nitric oxide; VIP = vasoactive intestinal polypeptide. **(B)** Diagram shows mass movement contractions. The colonic scintiscans show a movement of the fecal mass from the ascending colon (on the left) to the splenic flexure (on the right). The pressure tracing (below) demonstrates the mass movement contractions associated with this fecal mass movement and abdominal cramps. **(C)** Time course of mass movement contractions in the large intestine. At 7AM, a barium breakfast is ingested (1). At noon, the barium breakfast is in the lower ileum and cecum and the ingestion of lunch accelerates the emptying of the ileum (2). At 12:15, the tip of the barium breakfast is choked off (3). At 12:20, the barium breakfast fills the transverse colon (4). At 12:21, segmentation contractions begin (haustra form) and mix the contents (5). At 12:25 (still during the consumption of lunch), mass movement contractions occur around the leading end of the large intestinal contents and rapidly propel the contents to the sigmoid colon (6–8).

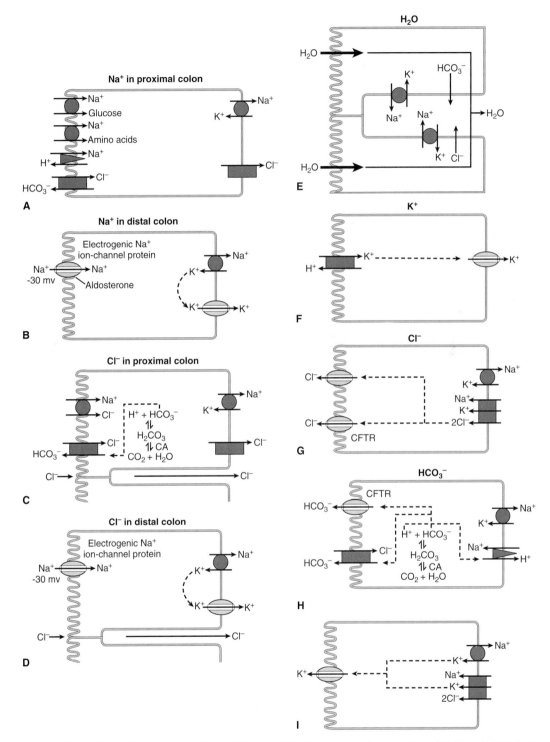

● **Figure 32-2: Absorption and Secretion of Fluid and Electrolytes. (A-F)** Absorption of Fluid and Electrolytes.
(A) Absorption of Na^+ in proximal colon. (B) Absorption of Na^+ in distal colon. (C) Absorption of Cl^- in proximal colon.
(D) Absorption of Cl^- in distal colon. (E) Absorption of H_2O. (F) Absorption of K^+. **(G-I)** Secretion of Fluid and Electrolytes.
(G) Secretion of Cl^- (H) Secretion of HCO_3^- (I) Secretion of K^+
CA = carbonic anhydrase; CFTR = cystic fibrosis transmembrane conductance regulator.

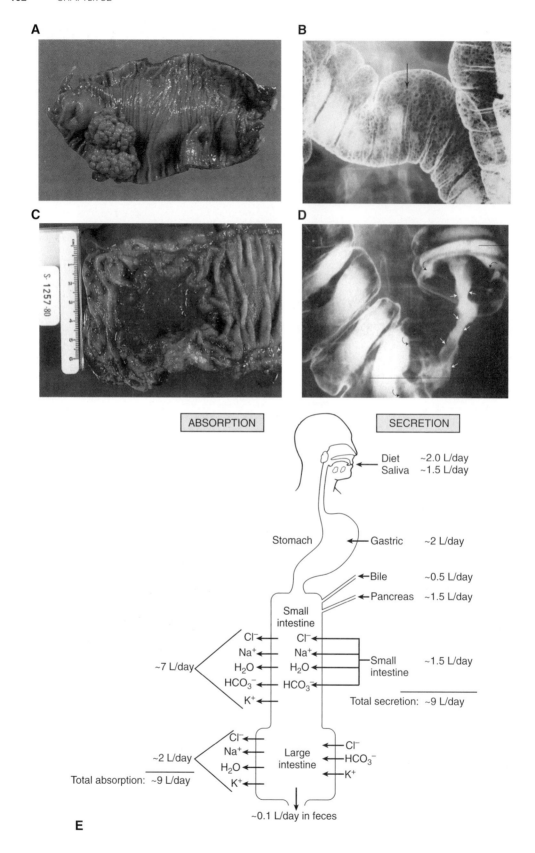

● **Figure 32-3: (A,B)** Adenomatous Polyps. (A) Photograph of a gross specimen of the colon shows a tubulovillous adenoma with a prominent villous architecture. The lesion has a sessile nature, a smooth surface, and a lobulated appearance. (B) Radiograph after barium enema shows the entire colonic mucosa to be carpeted with innumerable small polyps seen as tiny filling defects (arrows) **(C,D)** Adenocarcinoma of the Colon. (C) Photograph of a gross specimen of the colon shows the ulcerated center of the cancerous lesion with heaped up edges. (D) Radiograph of the transverse colon shows the classic "apple core" appearance. The core represents the patent portion of the bowel lumen. Note the irregular mucosa of the narrowed lumen (straight white arrows). The mass creates a shouldering deformity in the neighboring transverse colon both proximally and distally (curved arrows). **(E)** Summary Diagram of the overall fluid balance in the small and large intestine. A total of ≈9 L/day enters the GI tract with 2 L/day from the diet and 7 L/day from various secretions. Of this ≈9 L/day total, the small intestine absorbs ≈7 L/day, which delivers ≈2 L/day to the large intestine. The large intestine absorbs ≈2 L/day, leaving ≈100 mL/day to be excreted with the feces. If >2.5 L/day is delivered to the large intestine, diarrhea will occur.

33

Liver

Functions of the Liver. The functions of the liver are due mainly to the actions of the hepatocytes, which contain the Golgi complex, rough endoplasmic reticulum, smooth endoplasmic reticulum, mitochondria, lysosomes, peroxisomes, lipid droplets, glycogen, and iron.

A. Lymph Production. The liver produces 50% of the lymph in the body. Plasma that remains in the space of Disse travels to the periphery of the classic hepatic lobule and enters the **space of Mall** when the lymph then enters the lymphatic vessels found in the portal triad.

B. Uptake and Release of IgA. IgA binds to the **poly-Ig receptor** on hepatocytes to form a IgA + poly-Ig receptor complex, which is endocytosed and transported toward the bile canaliculus. At the bile canaliculus, the complex is cleaved such that IgA is released into the bile canaliculus and joined with the secretory piece of the receptor and is known as **secretory IgA (sIgA).** sIgA binding to microorganisms/antigens/toxins within the lumen of the GI tract reduces their ability to penetrate the epithelial lining of the GI tract.

C. Storage of Iron. The hepatocytes store iron bound to **ferritin,** which is a very large protein that can bind up to 4500 atoms of iron. In iron overload, ferritin undergoes lysosomal digestion and iron aggregates as **hemosiderin** (a golden brown hemoglobin-derived pigment). The more extreme accumulation of iron is called **hemochromatosis,** which is associated with liver and pancreas damage.

D. Storage of Vitamin A. The hepatic stellate cells (fat-storing cells; Ito cells) store vitamin A (retinol) as **retinyl ester.** When vitamin A levels in the blood are low, retinyl ester is hydrolyzed to form retinol. Retinol binds to **retinol-binding protein** and is released into the blood. Vitamin A is necessary for the light reaction of vision, growth of bone at the epiphyseal growth plate, reproduction, and differentiation and maintenance of epithelial tissues.

E. Carbohydrate Metabolism.
   1. Glycogen Synthesis. After a meal, hepatocytes uptake glucose, which is received from the nutrient-rich portal vein blood using **glucose transporter 2 (GLUT2).** The glucose is phosphorylated to **glucose 6-phosphate** using **glucokinase,** which is converted to **glucose 1-phosphate** by **phosphoglucomutase.** Glucose 1-phosphate reacts with UTP (uridine triphosphate), forming **UDP-glucose,** which adds

glucosyl units to the glycogen chain using **glycogen synthase.** Liver glycogen is synthesized due to an **increase in the insulin: glucagon ratio.** Glycogen is the storage form of glucose and is composed of glucose units linked by **a-1,4 glycosidic bonds.** This serves to lower blood glucose levels.

2. **Glycogen Degradation.** During hypoglycemia (e.g., fasting), exercise, or other stressful situations, hepatocytes degrade glycogen using the enzymes **phosphorylase 4:4 transferase,** and α **1,6 glucosidase,** which generates glucose 1-phosphate and glucose in a 10:1 ratio. Glucose 1-phosphate is converted to glucose 6-phosphate using **phosphoglucomutase.** Glucose 6-phosphate is converted to glucose using **glucose 6-phosphatase** (found only in the liver and kidney). Liver glycogen is degraded due to **decrease in the insulin: glucagon ratio** and the **secretion of epinephrine** from the adrenal medulla, which binds to α- and β-adrenergic receptors on the hepatocyte. This serves to raise blood glucose levels. The liver stores ≈80 grams of glycogen, which is enough to maintain blood glucose levels for ≈24 hours at rest, but less time during strenuous exercise.

3. **Monosaccharide Metabolism.** Hepatocytes metabolize glucose, fructose, and galactose.

4. **Gluconeogenesis.** Gluconeogenesis is the production of glucose from noncarbohydrate sources, which are mainly **amino acids, lactate,** and **glycerol.** The two major organs involved in gluconeogenesis are the liver and kidney. The starting substrate for gluconeogenesis is **pyruvate,** whereby the synthesis of one molecule of glucose from 2 molecules of pyruvate requires the expenditure of energy equivalent to **6 molecules of ATP.**

F. **Protein and Amino Acid Metabolism.**
   1. **Synthesis of Proteins.**
   2. **Metabolism of Ammonia (NH_3).** NH_3, which is produced from protein and nucleic acid catabolism, is highly neurotoxic and is therefore converted to nontoxic **urea** in hepatoctyes by the **urea cycle.** ≈30 grams of urea/day is excreted by a healthy adult eating a normal diet.
   3. **Synthesis of the Eleven Nonessential Amino Acids.** Of the 20 amino acids commonly found in proteins, the hepatoctyes can synthesize 11 amino acids (hence the term nonessential), which include: glycine, alanine, asparagine, serine, glutamine, proline, aspartic acid, glutamic acid, cysteine, tyrosine, and arginine. The remaining nine amino acids (essential amino acids) must be consumed in the diet, and include: valine, leucine, isoleucine, threonine, phenylalanine, tryptophan, methionine, histidine, and lysine.

G. **Lipid Metabolism.**
   1. **25-hydroxylation of vitamin D.** Vitamin D sources include dietary intake and production by skin keratinocytes stimulated by ultraviolet light. Vitamin D is hydroxylated by liver hepatocytes to **25-(OH) vitamin D.** 25-(OH)vitamin D is hydroxylated in the kidney to **1,25-(OH)$_2$ vitamin D,** which is the active metabolite that functions as a steroid hormone. 1,25-(OH)$_2$D **stimulates absorption of Ca^{2+} and PO_4^{2-} ions** from the intestinal lumen into the blood, thereby **elevating blood Ca^{2+} and PO_4^{2-} levels.**
   2. **β-Oxidation of Fatty Acids.** Fatty acids are a major source of energy in the human and are oxidized by a process called β-oxidation. Prior to β-oxidation, the fatty acid is activated by forming **fatty acyl CoA** and transported into the mitochondria by a **carnitine carrier system.** β-oxidation occurs in the mitochondria in a series of four steps that produce **FADH$_2$** and **NADH,** whereby two

TABLE 33-1	SYNTHESIS OF PROTEINS BY THE LIVER
Protein	Function
Albumin	The liver synthesizes 3 g/day of albumin, which plays an important role in plasma volume and colloid osmotic pressure of the plasma. The importance of albumin is emphasized in that liver disease and long-term starvation result in generalized edema and ascites.
Components of the complement system	Used in the inflammatory response
Fibrinogen, prothrombin, and factors V, VII, IX, X, XII	Cascade proteins used in blood clotting
VLDL, LDL, HDL	Lipoproteins used in the transport of lipids in the blood
Transferrin	Used in iron transport
Ceruloplasmin	Used in Cu^{2+} transport
Haptoglobin, hemopexin, and many other plasma proteins	Functions vary
α-fetoprotein	Produced by the embryonic liver and regenerating liver, which can be used as an indicator of liver carcinoma; sometimes called "fetal albumin"
α_1-antitrypsin	A serum protease inhibitor. **α_1-antitrypsin deficiency** is an autosomal recessive disorder caused by a missense mutation where methionine 358 is replaced with arginine (i.e., the Pittsburgh variant), which destroys the affinity for elastase and results in pulmonary emphysema. Normally, methionine 358 in the reactive center of α_1-antitrypsin acts as a "bait" for elastase, where elastase is trapped and inactivated. This protects the physiologically important elastic fibers present in the lung from destruction.
IGF-1 and IGF-2	Insulin-like growth factors that are involved in growth hormone-independent tissue growth, in general, increase protein synthesis in chondrocytes at the epiphyseal growth plate and cause linear bone growth (i.e., the pubertal growth spurt)
Angiotensinogen	Is converted to angiotensin II by renin (release from the macula densa cells in the kidney), which plays a role in the regulation of blood pressure.
Retinol-binding protein	Binds retinol (vitamin A)
Apoproteins	Plays a role in lipid transport in the plasma

carbons are cleaved from a fatty acyl CoA and released as **acetyl CoA.** This series of steps is repeated until the fatty acid is completely converted to acetyl CoA. FADH$_2$ and NADH interact with the electron transport chain to produce **ATP.** In the liver, acetyl CoA is converted to **ketone bodies,** which can be oxidized by muscle, kidney, or the brain during starvation.

3. **Synthesis of Fatty Acids.** The synthesis of fatty acids and their esterification to glycerol to form triacylglycerols occurs mainly in the liver. The de novo synthesis of fatty acids from acetyl CoA involves the **fatty acid synthase complex.** Acetyl CoA (derived mainly from glucose) is converted to malonyl CoA using **acetyl CoA carboxylase.**

4. **Production of Ketone Bodies.** The synthesis of ketone bodies (acetoacetate and β-hydroxybutyrate) occurs mainly in the liver whenever fatty acid levels are high in the blood. Acetyl CoA (derived mainly from glucose) forms acetoacetyl CoA, which condenses with another acetyl CoA to form hydroxymethylglutaryl CoA (HMG CoA). HMG CoA is cleaved to form acetyl CoA and acetoacetate using **HMG CoA lyase.** Acetoacetate can be reduced to 3-hydroxybutyrate. Acetoacetate is spontaneously decarboxylated to acetone. The liver cannot utilize ketone bodies because it lacks a thiotransferase enzyme. Therefore, the liver releases ketone bodies into the blood that can be used as fuel in muscle, kidney, and brain.

5. **Synthesis of Cholesterol.** The synthesis of cholesterol occurs mainly in the liver and intestine. Acetyl CoA (derived mainly from glucose) forms acetoacetyl CoA which condenses with another acetyl CoA to form hydroxymethylglutaryl CoA (HMG CoA). HMG CoA is reduced to mevalonic acid using **HMG CoA reductase.**

6. **Synthesis of Lipoproteins (figure 33-1, 33-2).** Lipids (e.g., free cholesterol, cholesterol esters, and triacyglycerols) are insoluble in plasma and therefore are transported in the plasma as **lipoproteins.** Lipoproteins consists of a polar coat (composed of **phospholipids, free cholesterol,** and **apoproteins**) surrounding a central core (composed of **triacylglycerols** and **cholesterol esters**).

   a. **Very Low Density Lipoprotein (VLDL).** Hepatocytes synthesize and release VLDL, which is relatively rich in triacylglycerols (55%), into the plasma. VLDL travels to skeletal muscle and adipose tissue where, the triacylglycerols are hydrolyzed by **lipoprotein lipase** (located on the endothelial cells of capillaries) to **fatty acids** and **glycerol.** The fatty acids are oxidized in skeletal muscle or stored as triacylglycerols in adipose tissue. As the triacylglycerols in VLDL are hydrolyzed, the core of VLDL is reduced, thereby generating intermediate density lipoprotein (IDL).

   b. **Intermediate Density Lipoprotein (IDL).** IDL returns to the liver, binds to LDL or IDL receptors located on hepatocytes, and undergoes lysosomal digestion. IDL may also undergo further hydrolysis of triacylglycerol by lipoprotein lipase or hepatic lipase and thereby be converted to LDL.

   c. **Low Density Lipoprotein (LDL).** LDL, which is rich in cholesterol and cholesterol esters distributes cholesterol to cells throughout the body (i.e., both hepatic and non-hepatic cells) that have specific **LDL receptors.** LDL can also enter macrophages that have **scavenger receptors** which results in the intracellular accumulation of cholesterol and the formation of **foam cells.** LDL is internalized by a normal process called **receptor-mediated endocytosis,** which involves the following steps: 1) Circulating serum LDL ("bad cholesterol") binds to the LDL receptor located on the cell membrane (apoB$_{100}$ is the ligand), and the complex undergoes endocytosis as clathrin-coated vesicles. 2) The clathrin-coated vesicles fuse with **endosomes,** where LDL disassociates from the LDL receptor due to pH↓, and the LDL receptor is recycled to the cell membrane. 3) **Endolysosomes** containing active lysosomal enzymes fuse and digest the LDL to cholesterol. Cholesterol can then be used for the following processes: 1) synthesis of cell membranes 2) synthesis of bile salts in hepatocytes 3) synthesis of steroid hormones in certain endocrine cells 5) inhibition of **3-hydroxy-3-methyglutaryl CoA reductase,** which suppresses de novo cholesterol synthesis, and therefore maintains normal levels of serum cholesterol 6) activates acyl cholesterol acyl transferase (ACAT) which converts cholesterol to cholesterol esters for storage. Since LDL distributes cholesterol to cells throughout the body LDL, LDL is called **"bad cholesterol"** and is the target in lipid lowering therapy. **Familial Hypercholesterolemia** is a genetic disease involving a mutation in the **LDL receptor,** in which patients have greatly elevated levels of serum cholesterol and suffer myocardial infarctions early in life. The mutation in the LDL receptor blocks receptor-mediated endocytosis.

d. **High Density Lipoprotein (HDL).** Hepatocytes synthesize and release HDL, which is relatively poor in triacylglycerols (8%), cholesterol (5%), and cholesterol esters (15%) into the plasma. HDL has various functions, which include: 1) travels to various tissues in the body and acquires free cholesterol with the aid of **apoprotein A-I,** which is a signal transduction protein that mobilizes cholesterol esters from intracellular pools and **cholesterol efflux regulatory protein.** After diffusion of free cholesterol onto HDL, the cholesterol is re-esterified to cholesterol esters by **lecithin-cholesterol acyl transferase (LCAT)** 2) acquires free cholesterol, phospholipids, and apoproteins from chylomicron remnants and IDL 3) transfers some of the re-esterified cholesterol esters to VLDL, IDL, and LDL using **cholesterol ester transfer protein (CETP)** in exchange for triacylglycerols so that cholesterol can be delivered to various tissues for storage or steroid synthesis 4) transfers apo C-II (which activates lipoprotein lipase) and apoE (which is the ligand for IDL receptors) to chylomicrons and VLDL 5) travels back to the liver with its re-esterified cholesterol esters, is endocytosed by hepatocytes where lysosomal enzymes digest the re-esterified cholesterol esters to free cholesterol. The free cholesterol can then be either packaged into VLDL and released into the plasma or excreted in the bile. Since HDL facilitates the flow of excess plasma triacylglycerols and cholesterol back to the liver, HDL is called **"good cholesterol"**.

e. **Chylomicrons.** Enterocytes of the small intestine synthesize and release chylomicrons which are relatively rich in triacylglycerols (85%), cholesterol esters, and phospholipids directly into the lymph, which then enter the plasma. Nascent chylomicrons contain $apoB_{48}$ and then acquire apo C-II (which activates lipoprotein lipase) and apoE (which is the ligand for IDL receptors) from HDL. Chylomicrons travel to skeletal muscle and adipose tissue, where the triacylglycerols are hydrolyzed by **lipoprotein lipase** (located on the endothelial cells of capillaries) to **fatty acids** and **glycerol.** The fatty acids are oxidized in skeletal muscle or stored as triacylglycerols in adipose tissue. The resulting **chylomicron remnants** travel to the liver, and are endocytosed by hepatocytes, where lysosomal enzymes digest the chylomicron remnants to amino acids, fatty acids, and cholesterol, which are re-utilized by the hepatocytes.

H. **Metabolism of Drugs.** The oral bioavailability of drugs is enhanced by making drugs lipophilic. However, the lipophilic nature of drugs prevents clearance by the kidneys. Therefore, drugs must be transformed into hydrophilic compounds that are soluble in aqueous urine. Phase I and II reactions make drugs more hydrophilic. The hepatocytes metabolize drugs by biotransformation which occurs in three stages as indicated below.

1. **Phase I Reactions (Oxidation).** The enzymes that catalyze **cytochrome P_{450}-dependent Phase I reactions** are **hemeprotein monooxygenases** of the **cytochrome P_{450} class** (also called the **microsomal mixed function oxidases**), which catalyze the biotransformation of drugs by hydroxylation, dealkylation, oxidation, desulfuration, and epoxide formation. In addition, there are **cytochrome P_{450}-independent Phase I reactions,** which allow local hydrolysis of ester-containing and amide-containing drugs (e.g., local anesthetics) at their site of administration, and allow the oxidation of amine-containing compounds (e.g., catecholamines, tyramine) using **monoamine oxidase.** Phase I reactions often produce more active metabolites of the administered drug (**prodrug → drug**). Activation of cytochrome p450 by one compound enhances the detoxification of other compounds, which has clinical implications. In **chronic alcoholics** or **newborns,** large amounts of anesthesia are needed (which may be dangerous) because cytochrome p450 has been activated by detoxifying either alcohol or breakdown products of fetal hemoglobin, respectively.

2. **Phase II Reactions (Conjugation).** The enzymes that catalyze Phase II reactions are transfer enzymes that catalyze the biotransformation of drugs by glucuronidation (using **UDP glucuronyl transferase** and **UDP-glucuronic acid** as the glucuronide donor), acetylation, glycine conjugation, sulfate conjugation, glutathione conjugation, and methylation. Phase II reaction metabolites are pharmacologically inactive. Acetoaminophen is inactivated by glucoronidation and sulfation. If these conjugation pathways become saturated, microsomal mixed function oxidases form a toxic metabolite that is inactivated by glutathione conjugation. However, hepatic stores of glutathione are limited. In acetaminophen overdose, toxic metabolites cause liver necrosis and renal tubule damage.

3. **Phase III Reactions (Elimination).** The elimination of Phase I and II biotransformation products from hepatocytes requires active transport using transporters (i.e., ATPase pumps) that pump the products either into the blood for elimination by the kidneys or into the bile for elimination by the GI tract.

I. **Metabolism of Ethanol.** Most ethanol ($\approx$80%) is metabolized to **acetaldehyde and NADH** by hepatocytes using **alcohol dehydrogenase.** The acetaldehyde is oxidized to acetate using **acetaldehyde dehydrogenase.** A majority of the acetate enters the bloodstream and travels to skeletal muscle, where it is converted to acetyl CoA. The acetyl CoA enters the TCA cycle, where it is metabolized to CO_2 and produces ATP. When ethanol consumption is high, $\approx$20% of ethanol is metabolized in the liver by the **microsomal ethanol-oxidizing system (MEOS)** to produce **acetaldehyde.** In chronic alcoholism, much of the tissue damage is believed to result from an excess of acetaldehyde.

J. **Synthesis of Bile Salts.** The hepatocytes synthesize bile salts and release them into bile canaliculi, which are formed by the cell membranes of adjacent hepatocytes and partitioned by a zonula occludens (i.e., a tight junction). Bile salts are synthesized from cholesterol when an α-OH group is added to carbon 7 of cholesterol using **7α-hydroxylase** (the rate limiting step). The double bond of cholesterol is reduced and further hydroxylations occur forming a 3α,7α diol and a 3α,7α,12α triol. The side chain of the 3α,7α diol and a 3α,7α,12α triol is converted to a branched 5-carbon chain with a carboxyl group at the end. This results in the formation of **chenocholate** (from the 3α,7α diol) and **cholate** (from the 3α,7α,12α triol). At pH 6 (the pH of the intestinal lumen), 50% of chenocholate and cholate are in the form of salts (i.e., are ionized and carry a negative charge) and 50% of chenocholate and cholate are in the form of acids (i.e., are protonated at the carboxy group). Chenocholate can conjugate with either glycine or taurine amino acids, forming **glycochenocholate** or **taurochenocholate.** Cholate can also conjugate with either glycine or taurine amino acids, forming **glyco-cholate** or **taurocholate.** At pH 6 (the pH of the intestinal lumen), ≈85% of gly-cochenocholate, taurochenocholate, glycocholate, and taurocholate are in the form of salts (i.e., are ionized and carry a negative charge) and therefore are better detergents than unconjugated bile salts. Chenocholate, cholate, and their conjugates are called **primary bile salts.** In the intestine, primary bile salts are deconjugated and dehydroxylated (at position 7) by intestinal flora to form **lithocholate** and **deoxycholate,** which are called **secondary bile salts.** Secondary bile salts can be reconjugated with glycine or taurine but are never rehydroxylated. The primary and secondary bile salts are reabsorbed by the **ileum** and returned to the liver. The liver recycles ≈95% of bile salts each day; 5% of bile salts are lost in the feces. The total pool of bile salts is recycled 6–8 times/day.

K. **Production and Composition of Bile (Figure 33-3).** Bile is a green-yellow complex mixture of organic and inorganic components that are released into bile canaliculi and travel to the gall bladder by the following route: bile canaliculi→ cholangioles → canals of Hering → bile ductules in the portal triad → right and left hepatic ducts → common hepatic duct → gall bladder. The liver produces ≈**700 mL of bile/day.** The components of bile include the following:

1. **Bile Salts.** Bile salts are the major component of bile and are taken up from the portal blood into hepatocytes using the **Na⁺-conjugated bile salt cotransporter, Na⁺ independent conjugated bile salt transporter, anion-unconjugated bile salt exchanger,** and **diffusion** of unconjugated bile salts. In the hepatocyte cytoplasm, bile salts are bound to **bile salt-binding proteins,** which prevents the disruption of hepatocyte organelles. The bile salts are then released into bile canaliculi using the **biliary acid transporter (BAT).**

2. **Cholesterol.** Cholesterol is released into bile canaliculi using the **MDR1 transporter** (**m**ulti**d**rug **r**esistance).

3. **Lecithin (phosphatidylcholine).** Lecithin is released into bile canaliculi using the **MDR 2 transporter.**

4. **Bilirubin-Glucuronide (Bile pigment).** Bilirubin-glucuronide is released into bile canaliculi using **MOAT** (**m**ultispecific **o**rgan **a**nionic **t**ransporter).

5. **H₂O, Na⁺, Cl⁻, K⁺, Ca²⁺, and HCO₃⁻.** The release of H_2O and electrolytes into bile canaliculi occurs by two mechanisms.

    a. In the **bile salt dependent mechanism,** the active transport of bile salts into bile canaliculi creates an osmotic gradient that allows H_2O to flow into bile canaliculi through the "leaky" zonula occludens whereby various electrolytes follow by solvent drag.

    b. In the **intrahepatic bile duct dependent mechanism,** the epithelial cells lining the intrahepatic bile ducts secrete an aqueous solution that makes up ≈50% of the total volume of bile. The intrahepatic bile ducts are not just merely conduits for bile. This aqueous secretion contains H_2O, Na^+, Cl^-, K^+, and HCO_3^- and is under the control of **secretin,** which is secreted by enteroendocrine S cells in the crypts of Lieberkuhn of the small intestine. In addition, there appears to be a **HCO₃⁻ - Cl⁻ exchanger** located on the cell membrane of the bile canaliculi that contributes to the HCO_3^- content of bile. The intrahepatic bile ducts also absorb H_2O, Na^+, and Cl^-, although secretion predominates.

6. **Secretory IgA.**

7. **Conjugated Drugs and Steroid hormones.** Drugs and steroid hormones that have undergone Phase I and II reactions (see Chapter 33 IH) are released into bile canaliculi using unidentified ATPase pumps for elimination by the GI tract.

L. **Production and Fate of Bilirubin (Figure 33-4).** Bilirubin (water-insoluble) is derived mainly from the breakdown of hemoglobin (heme moiety; i.e., senescent RBCs) by macrophages and in the spleen and Kupffer cells (Heme → biliverdin → bilirubin). ≈15% of bilirubin is derived from the breakdown of other heme-containing proteins (e.g., myoglobin, cytochromes, and catalase). Bilirubin travels in the blood as an **albumin-bilirubin complex** (Note: free bilirubin is toxic to the brain). Bilirubin is endocytosed by hepatocytes and conjugated to glucuronide by **UDP-glucuronyltransferase** in the sER to form **bilirubin-glucuronide** (a water soluble bile pigment), which is released into bile canaliculi using MOAT. Within the distal small intestine and colon, bilirubin-glucuronide is broken down to **free bilirubin** by intestinal bacterial flora. Free bilirubin is reduced to **urobilinogen** and eliminated in feces, reabsorbed, or excreted into the urine. Urobilinogen is oxidized in the urine and feces to form **urobilin** and **stercobilin,** which are responsible for the color of the urine and feces.

1. **Crigler-Najjar disease** is a genetic disease involving UDP-glucuronyltransferase resulting in a failure to conjugate bilirubin.

2. **Dubin-Johnson syndrome** is a familial disease involving failure to release bilirubin-glucuronide into bile canaliculi.

3. **Bilirubin-induced neurotoxicity (BIND).** Neonatal jaundice is the yellowish discoloration of the skin and/or sclerae in newborn infants caused by deposition of bilirubin. Most newborn infants have a total serum bilirubin (TSB) >1 mg/dL and appear clinically jaundiced. Bilirubin is a potential neurotoxin, whereby free bilirubin (i.e., bilirubin not conjugated to albumin) enters the brain (i.e., basal ganglia and brain stem) and causes cell death by apoptosis or necrosis and cause **bilirubin-induced neurotoxicity (BIND).** BIND may present as **acute bilirubin encephalopathy** (a reversible condition), whose clinical signs include: lethargy, hypotonia, poor sucking, high-pitched cry, backward arching of the neck (retrocollis) and trunk (opisthotonus), stupor, and coma. BIND may present as **kernicterus** (a chronic, permanent condition), whose clinical signs include: chorea, ballismus, tremor, upward gaze abnormalities, auditory abnormalities.

II **Clinical Consideration.** **Liver Damage Due to Drugs or Chemicals.** The liver can be damaged by various drugs and chemicals as indicated in Table 33-2.

TABLE 33-2	VARIOUS TYPES OF LIVER DAMAGE DUE TO DRUGS OR CHEMICALS
Morphological Appearance	**Drug/Chemical**
Acute Hepatitis	Isoniazid (10–20% liver damage; acetyl hydrazine is the active metabolite); salicylate, halothane (symptoms occur after 1 week, fever precedes jaundice, and metabolites form via action of P_{450} system); methyldopa (positive Coombs test), phenytoin, and ketoconazole
Chronic Active Hepatitis	Methyldopa, acetaminophen, aspirin, isoniazid, nitrofurantoin, and halothane
Zonal Necrosis	**Zone 1:** Undergo necrosis in poisoning due to: yellow phosphorus, manganese,ferrous sulphate, allyl alcohol, and endotoxin of *Proteus vulgaris* Undergo necrosis due to: chronic hepatitis, primary biliary cirrhosis, bile duct occlusion, and preeclampsia/eclampsia (Note: Hepatic disease is very common in preeclamptic women, and monitoring of platelet count and serum liver enzymes is standard practice.) Hepatocytes are exposed to blood high in nutrients, oxygen, and toxins; synthesize glycogen and plasma proteins actively
	Zone 2: Undergo necrosis due to yellow fever Are exposed to blood with moderate levels of nutrients and oxygen
	Zone 3: Undergo necrosis due to: ischemic injury, right-sided cardiac failure,and bone marrow transplantation Undergo necrosis in poisoning due to: ethanol, carbon tetrachloride, chloroform, L-amanitine, pyrrolizidine alkaloids (bush tea), tannic acid, copper, acetaminophen (free radicals formed; acetylcysteine therapy replaces glutathione to neutralize free radicals) Hepatocytes are exposed to blood low in nutrients, oxygen, and toxins
Intrahepatic Cholestasis	**Non-inflammatory:** oral contraceptives and anabolic steroids
	Inflammatory: erythromycin estolate, amoxicillin-clavulanic acid, chlorpromazine, and thiazides
Fatty Change	**Single droplet:** ethanol, corticosteroids, amiodarone (looks like alcoholic hepatitis)
	Microvesicular: tetracycline, valproic acid
Fibrosis	Methotrexate, hypervitaminosis A, ethanol (Zone 3)
Vascular Lesions	**Budd-Chiari syndrome:** oral contraceptives
	Peliosis hepatis: oral contraceptives, anabolic steroids
	Angiosarcoma: vinyl chloride, arsenic, Thorotrast
Tumors	**Nodular hyperplasia:** azathioprine, anticancer agents
	Benign tumors: oral contraceptives
	Malignant tumors: oral contraceptives
Granulomatous Hepatitis	Allopurinol, hydralazine, sulfonamides, phenylbutazone

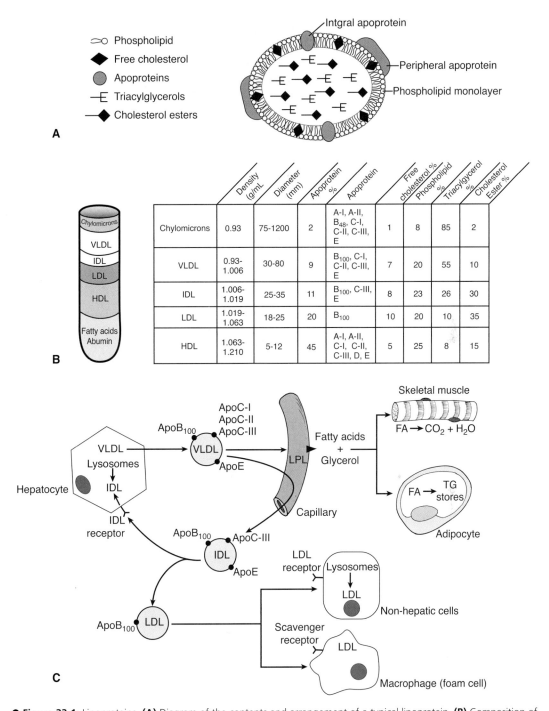

● **Figure 33-1:** Lipoproteins. **(A)** Diagram of the contents and arrangement of a typical lipoprotein. **(B)** Composition of lipoproteins. **(C)** Metabolism of VLDL, IDL, and LDL.
VLDL = very low density lipoprotein; IDL = intermediate density lipoprotein; LDL = low density lipoprotein; FA = fatty acids; TG = triacylglycerol.

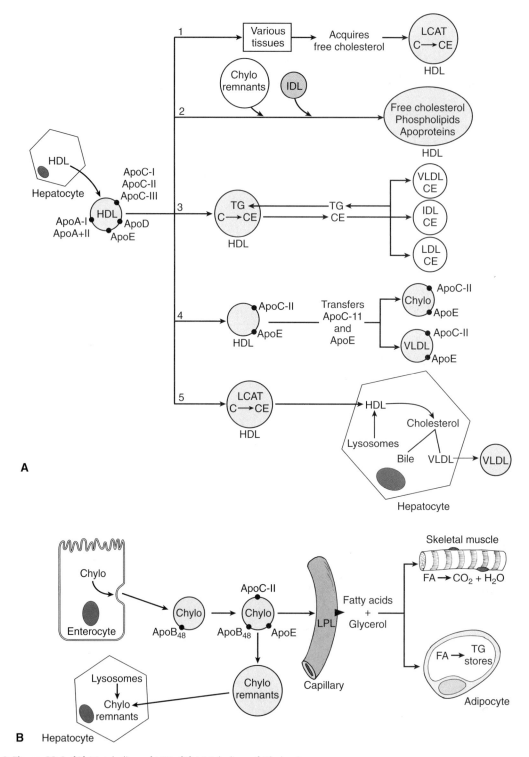

● **Figure 33-2: (A)** Metabolism of HDL. **(B)** Metabolism of Chylomicrons.
C = cholesterol; CE = cholesterol esters; CHYLO = chylomicrons; LCAT = lecithin-cholesterol acyl transferase; FA = fatty acids; TG = triacylglycerol.

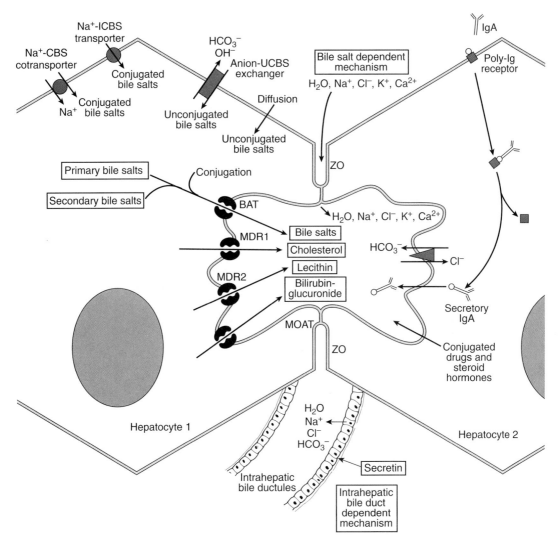

● **Figure 33-3:** Production and Composition of Bile.
ZO = zonula occludens; BAT = biliary acid transporter; MDR1 = multidrug resistance 1 transporter; MDR2 = multidrug resistance 2 transporter; MOAT = multispecific organ anionic transporter; CBS = conjugated bile salt; ICBS = independent conjugated bile salt; UCBS = unconjugated bile salt.

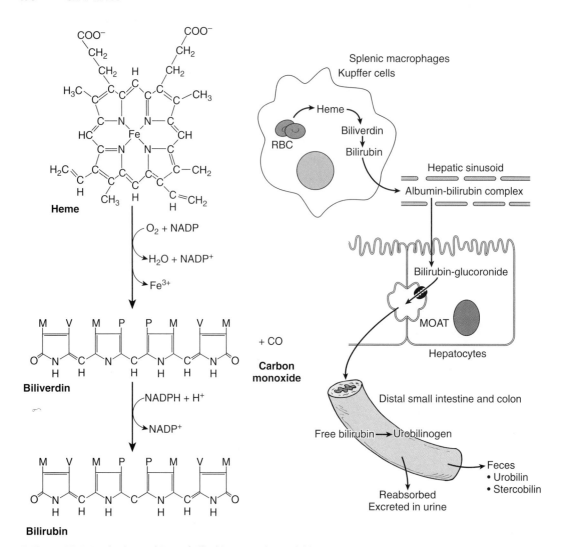

● **Figure 33-4:** Production and Fate of Bilirubin. Heme-hemoglobin

34

Gall Bladder and Extrahepatic Biliary Ducts

I **General Features.** The function of the gall bladder is storage and concentration of bile. The gall bladder is a pear-shaped distensible sac that has the capacity to store ≈**35 mL of bile** (range: 15–60 mL). The gall bladder is divided into the **fundus** (anterior portion), **body,** and the **neck** (posterior portion). A small pouch **(Hartmann's pouch)** may extend from the neck as a sequela to pathological changes and is a common site for gallstones to lodge. The **right and left hepatic ducts** join together after leaving the liver to form the **common hepatic duct.** The common hepatic duct is joined at an acute angle by the **cystic duct** to form the **common bile duct.** The cystic duct drains bile from the gall bladder. The mucosa of the cystic duct is arranged in a spiral fold with a core of smooth muscle known as the **spiral valve (valve of Heister).** The spiral valve keeps the cystic duct constantly open so that bile can flow freely in either direction. The common bile duct passes posterior to the pancreas and ends at the **hepatopancreatic ampulla (ampulla of Vater)** where it joins the **pancreatic duct.** The **sphincter of Oddi** is an area of thickened smooth muscle that surrounds the bile duct as it traverses the ampulla. The gall bladder is innervated by the parasympathetic and sympathetic nervous systems.

II **Concentration of Bile.** The liver produces ≈700 mL of bile/day while the gall bladder can store only ≈35 mL of bile. The discrepancy between the amount of bile produced by the liver and the amount stored by the gall bladder is explained by the ability of the gall bladder to concentrate the bile 5–20 times through absorption of water and electrolytes by the **standing osmotic gradient mechanism.**

III **Bile Release from Gall Bladder to the Small Intestine.**

    A. Stimulation. Gall bladder emptying begins several minutes after the start of a meal. During the cephalic phase of HCl secretion, the sight, smell, taste, and conditioned reflexes involved with food begin gall bladder emptying mediated by **CN X (vagus nerve)** and probably **gastrin.** During the gastric phase of HCl secretion, stomach distention also plays a role in gall bladder emptying mediated by CN X and probably gastrin. During the intestinal phase of HCl secretion, **CCK** is secreted into the blood by the enteroendocrine I-cells in response to amino acids/small peptides and fatty acids/monoglycerides present in the small intestinal lumen. CCK binds to **CCK 1 receptors** located on the smooth muscle cells. The highest rate of gall bladder emptying occurs during the intestinal phase of HCl secretion mostly in response to CCK. CCK causes the contraction of smooth muscle in the wall of the gall bladder and relaxation of the smooth muscle of the sphincter of Oddi. In addition, the relaxation of the smooth muscle of the sphincter of Oddi involves the neurotransmitter **nitric oxide (NO)** released from post-ganglionic parasympathetic neurons.

B. Inhibition. Relaxation of the smooth muscle in the wall of the gall bladder and contraction of the smooth muscle of the sphincter of Oddi are mediated by the **sympathetic nervous system. Somatostatin** has an inhibitory effect on the gall bladder.

Ⅳ Clinical Considerations (Figure 34-1). The term **cholelithiasis** refers to the presence or formation of gallstones either in the gall bladder (called **cholecystolithiasis**) or common bile duct (called **choledocholithiasis**).

A. Gallstones form when bile salts and lecithin are overwhelmed by cholesterol. Most stones consist of **cholesterol (major component), bilirubin, and calcium.** There are three main types of gallstones:

1. **Cholesterol stones** are yellow, large, smooth and composed mainly of cholesterol. These stones are associated with: obesity, Crohn disease, cystic fibrosis, clofibrate, estrogens, rapid weight loss, and the US or Native American population (4F's: female, fat, fertile, over forty).

2. **Pigment (bilirubin) stones** are brown or black, smooth and composed mainly of bilirubin salts. These stones are associated with: chronic RBC hemolysis (e.g., sickle cell anemia or spherocytosis), alcoholic cirrhosis, biliary infection, and the Asian population.

3. **Calcium bilirubinate stones** are associated with infection and/or inflammation of the biliary tree.

B. Gallstone Obstruction. There are three clinically important sites of gallstone obstruction, as follows:

1. **Within the cystic duct.** A stone may transiently lodge within the cystic duct and cause pain (**biliary colic**) within the epigastric region due to the distention of the duct. If a stone becomes entrapped within the cystic duct, bile flow from the gall bladder will be obstructed, resulting in inflammation of the gall bladder (**acute cholecystitis**) and pain will shift to the right hypochondriac region. Bile becomes concentrated and precipitates in the gall bladder, forming a layer of high density material called **"milk of calcium" bile** due to large amount of calcium carbonate. Bile flow from the liver remains open (i.e., **no jaundice**). This may lead to **Mirizzi syndrome,** where impaction of a large gallstone in the cystic duct extrinsically obstructs the nearby common hepatic duct.

2. **Within the common bile duct.** If a stone becomes entrapped within the common bile duct, bile flow from both the gall bladder and liver will be obstructed, resulting in inflammation of the gall bladder and liver. **Jaundice** is frequently observed and is first observed clinically **under the tongue.** The jaundice is moderate and fluctuates since a stone rarely causes complete blockage of the lumen.

3. **At the hepatopancreatic ampulla.** If a stone becomes entrapped at the ampulla, bile flow from both the gall bladder and liver will be obstructed. In addition, the pancreatic duct may be blocked. In this case, **jaundice** and **pancreatitis** are frequently observed.

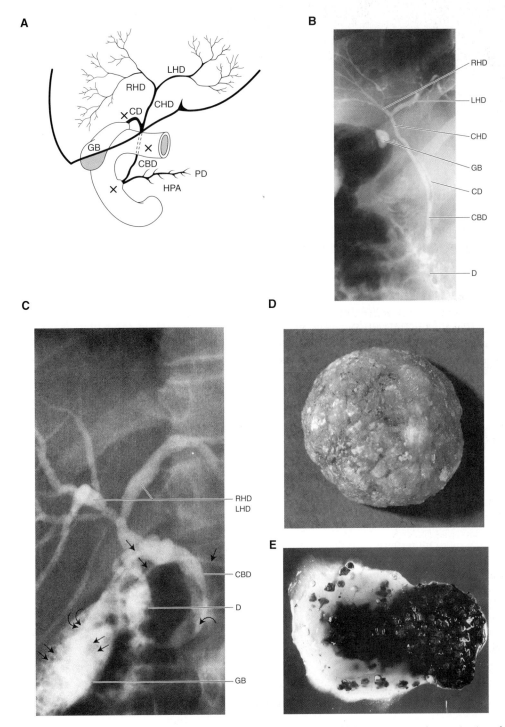

● **Figure 34-1: Gall Bladder Pathology. (A)** Diagram of the gall bladder and biliary tree. Note the termination of the common bile duct (CBD) at the hepatopancreatic ampulla (HPA) along with the pancreatic duct (PD). Note the three main sites (X) of gallstone obstruction. PD = pancreatic duct; CHD = common hepatic duct; CD = cystic duct; LHD = left hepatic duct; RHD = right hepatic duct; GB = gall bladder; D = duodenum; CBD = common bile duct. **(B)** Endoscopic retrograde cholangiograph shows the normal gall bladder and biliary tree. Note that the cystic duct normally lies on the right side of the common hepatic duct and joins it superior to the duodenal cap. **(C)** Endoscopic retrograde cholangiograph shows gallstones within the gallbladder (cholelithiasis; double straight arrows) and within the common bile duct (choledocholithiasis; curved arrow). A nasobiliary drain (straight single arrows) is in place with the tip (double curved arrows) in the gallbladder. **(D)** Photograph shows a solitary cholesterol gallstone. **(E)** Photograph shows pigmented gallstones embedded in a mucus gel.

35

Exocrine Pancreas

I   General Features. In the adult, the pancreas is a retroperitoneal organ that measures 15–20 cm in length and weighs about 85–120 grams. The normal pancreas is tan-pink to yellow in color and uniformly lobulated. A cut section of the pancreas reveals an extensive branching network of ducts extending into the lobules of the pancreas. The pancreas is both an exocrine gland and an endocrine gland. Gross anatomically, the pancreas consists of four parts, as follows: 1) the **head of the pancreas** is the expanded part of the pancreas that lies in the concavity of the C-shaped curve of the duodenum and is firmly attached to the descending and horizontal parts of the duodenum. The **uncinate process** is a projection from the inferior portion of the pancreatic head, 2) the **neck of the pancreas,** 3) the **body of the pancreas,** and 4) the **tail of the pancreas.** The pancreas is innervated by the parasympathetic and sympathetic nervous systems.

II   Pancreatic Secretion (Figure 35-1). The pancreas secretes ≈**1.5 L of fluid/day,** which contains digestive enzymes, cations (Na^+, K^+), anions (Cl^-, HCO_3^-), albumin, and globulins.

A. Digestive Enzymes. The digestive enzymes are secreted by **pancreatic acinar cells** and then enter a network of ducts that deliver the enzymes into the lumen of the small intestine. The digestive enzymes include: **trypsinogen, chymotrypsinogen, proelastase, procarboxypeptidase A, procarboxypeptidase B, pancreatic lipase, colipase, cholesterol ester hydrolase, phospholipase A_2, ribonuclease, deoxyribonuclease,** and **pancreatic amylase.** Several of the digestive enzymes are capable of damaging the pancreas and are therefore secreted in an inactive form (called a **proenzyme**). The proenzymes are activated in the duodenum by **enterokinase** located in the glycocalyx of enterocytes which converts trypsinogen (inactive proenzyme) → trypsin (active enzyme). Trypsin then converts all other inactive proenzymes to their active form. A **trypsin inhibitor** (called the **kazal inhibitor**), and **enzyme Y,** which destroys proenzymes before they are activated, are other means by which the pancreas protects itself from damage.

B. Cl^- and HCO_3^- Secretion. The bulk of the pancreatic juice is a **Na^+, K^+, Cl^-, and HCO_3^- -rich juice (135 mM $NaHCO_3^-$ at pH 8)** produced by the **duct epithelium** of the **intercalated, intralobular,** and **interlobular ducts,** which together with the secretions from the gall bladder and intestine serve to neutralize the gastric HCl in the duodenum. Na^+ and K^+ follow Cl^- into the pancreatic juice by moving through the zonula occludens. Cl^- and HCO_3^- are secreted into the pancreatic juice by various transporter proteins and ion channel proteins, which include:

1. **Na^+-K^+ ATPase** transports Na^+ across the basolateral membrane into the interstitial fluid (i.e., "pumps" Na^+ out of the cell) keeping cytoplasmic $[Na^+]$ low by countertransport with K^+ into the cytoplasm (i.e., "pumps" K^+ into the cell), keeping cytoplasmic $[K^+]$ high.

2. **Na^+-K^+-$2Cl^-$ Cotransporter** transports Na^+ across the basolateral membrane into the cytoplasm by cotransport with K^+ and Cl^- into the cytoplasm which occurs because cytoplasmic $[Na^+]$ is kept low by Na^+-K^+ ATPase.

3. **Na^+-HCO_3^- Cotransporter** transports Na^+ and HCO_3^- across the basolateral membrane into the cytoplasm.

4. **Na^+-H^+ Exchanger** transports Na^+ across the luminal membrane into the cytoplasm by countertransport with H^+ into intestinal fluid. The H^+ are supplied by the reaction $H_2CO_3 \rightarrow H^+ + HCO_3^-$, which is catalyzed by **carbonic anhydrase.**

5. **Cl^- - HCO_3^- Exchanger** transports Cl^- across the luminal membrane into the cytoplasm by countertransport with HCO_3^- into the intestinal fluid. The HCO_3^- is supplied by the reaction $H_2CO_3 \rightarrow H^+ + HCO_3^-$, which is catalyzed by **carbonic anhydrase.**

6. **Cl^- ion-channel protein (cystic fibrosis transmembrane conductance regulator; CFTR;** also found in the upper airways of the lung) transports Cl^- across the luminal membrane into the intestinal fluid by forming hydrophilic pores that allow diffusion of Cl^-. CFTR is usually closed but can be opened by $\uparrow$cAMP elicited by hormones, neurotransmitters, or cholera toxin.

7. **Cl^- ion-channel protein** transports Cl^- across the luminal membrane into the intestinal fluid by forming hydrophilic pores that allow diffusion of Cl^-. This Cl^- ion channel protein is usually closed but can be opened by $\uparrow$cytoplasmic Ca^{2+}.

III **Absorption of HCO_3^-.** The HCO_3^- content of the pancreatic juice is modified by the absorption of HCO_3^- in the main pancreatic duct (duct of Wirsung). HCO_3^- is absorbed into the blood by a **Cl^- - HCO_3^- Exchanger** that transports Cl^- across the basolateral membrane into the cytoplasm by countertransport with HCO_3^- into the blood. In other words, Cl^- is ultimately transported into the pancreatic juice and HCO_3^- is transported out of the pancreatic juice.

IV **Concentration of Anions in Pancreatic Juice versus Flow (Figure 35-2).**
The concentration of Cl^- and HCO_3^- varies with the rate of flow of the pancreatic juice.

A. **Low Flow Rate (Long Contact Time).** When the pancreas is not stimulated by secretin, a low flow rate of pancreatic juices occurs. With a low flow rate, there is more time for absorption of HCO_3^- and exchange for Cl^- by the main pancreatic duct (duct of Wirsung) to occur. Therefore, the concentration of HCO_3^- will be low and the concentration of Cl^- will be high in the pancreatic juice.

B. **High Flow Rate (Short Contact Time).** When the pancreas is stimulated by secretin, a high flow rate of pancreatic juice occurs. With a high flow rate, there is less time for absorption of HCO_3^- and exchange for Cl^- by the main pancreatic duct (duct of Wirsung) to occur. Therefore, the concentration of HCO_3^- will be high and the concentration of Cl^- will be low in the pancreatic juice.

Ⓥ Control of Pancreatic Secretion.

A. **Stimulation.**
   1. **Cholecystokinin (CCK).** CCK is secreted into the bloodstream (endocrine mechanism) by the enteroendocrine I-cells in the intestinal glands (crypts of Lieberkühn). CCK increases pancreatic enzyme secretion (major role) and aqueous/HCO_3^- secretion (weak, but physiologically relevant). CCK plays a role in the intestinal phase of pancreatic secretion.
   2. **Secretin (SEC).** SEC is secreted into the bloodstream (endocrine mechanism) by the enteroendocrine S cells in the intestinal glands (crypts of Lieberkühn). SEC increases aqueous/HCO_3^- secretion from the duct epithelium. When secretin is administered along with CCK or vagal stimulation (acetylcholine), the full postprandial HCO_3^- response is observed, suggesting a synergistic interplay between secretin, CCK, and acetylcholine. SEC plays a role in the intestinal phase of pancreatic secretion.
   3. **Parasympathetic Nervous System. CN X (vagus)** enhances the rate secretion, of pancreatic enzymes and aqueous components of the pancreatic juice. CN X plays a role in the cephalic and gastric phases of pancreatic secretion.

B. **Inhibition.**
   1. **Hyperglycemia** and **hyperaminoacidemia** inhibit exocrine pancreatic secretion, probably through the secondary release of inhibitory hormones like **glucagon** or **somatostatin.**
   2. **Presence of lipid in the colon** inhibits exocrine pancreatic secretion, which may serve as a physiological signal to stop pancreatic secretion after digestion and absorption are completed.
   3. **Peptide YY, PP (pancreatic polypeptide),** and **GLP-1** inhibit exocrine pancreas secretion, although little is known about their mechanism except that they do not work by direct inhibition of pancreatic acinar cells.
   4. **Sympathetic Nervous System.** Postganglionic axons (norepinephrine) from the celiac ganglion inhibit pancreatic secretion probably by reducing the blood flow.

Ⅵ Phases of Pancreatic Secretion.

A. **Cephalic Phase.** The cephalic phase is initiated by **sight, smell, taste,** and **conditioned reflexes.** The cephalic phase accounts for ≈25% of the total pancreatic juice secreted in response to a meal. The cephalic phase is controlled by the **parasympathetic nervous system (CN X).**

B. **Gastric Phase.** The gastric phase is initiated by **stomach distention.** The gastric phase accounts for ≈10% of the total pancreatic juice secreted in response to a meal. The gastric phase is controlled by the **parasympathetic nervous system (CN X)** via a **vagovagal reflex mechanism** involving stretch receptors in the stomach wall.

C. **Intestinal Phase.** The intestinal phase is initiated by the presence of **amino acids (e.g., phenylalanine, valine, methionine), fatty acids in micelles (C18 > C12 > C8 order of potency),** and **monoacylglycerols** in the proximal small intestine. The intestinal phase accounts for 65% of the total pancreatic juice secreted in response to a meal and is the most important phase in humans. The intestinal phase is controlled by **CCK** and **secretin.**

VII Clinical Considerations: Gastrinoma (Zollinger-Ellison Syndrome). A gastrinoma is a malignant tumor of the pancreas consisting of G cells and is generally associated with the MEN I syndrome. A gastrinoma secretes **excess gastrin,** thereby producing hyperacidity (HCl) and peptic ulcer disease. In most cases, a single peptic ulcer is observed but multiple ulcers may also occur. A gastrinoma should always be suspected if a peptic ulcer is found in an unusual site. Clinical findings include: abdominal pain caused by peptic ulcer; diarrhea (malabsorption since enzymes cannot work in an acid pH); markedly increased basal acid output (BAO) test; secretin test is confirmatory (secretin administration results in an elevation of gastrin levels in patients with a gastrinoma); and serum gastrin levels >600pg/mL. Other causes of elevated serum gastrin levels include: use of H_2 blockers (e.g., Tagamet, Zantac, etc.), which decreases HCl production and thereby elevates gastrin; atrophic gastritis, which decreases HCl production (by destruction of parietal cells) and thereby elevates gastrin.

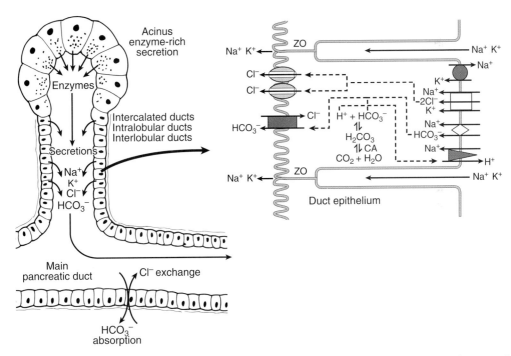

● **Figure 35-1: Pancreatic Secretion. (A)** Diagram of an acinus and duct system shows the secretion of enzymes from the acinus and production of the aqueous component (Na^+, K^+, Cl^-, and HCO_3^-) into the duct network. **(B)** Diagram shows the mechanism of secretion of Cl^- and HCO_3^- by the duct epithelium and the flow of Na^+ and K^+ through the zonula occludens (ZO).

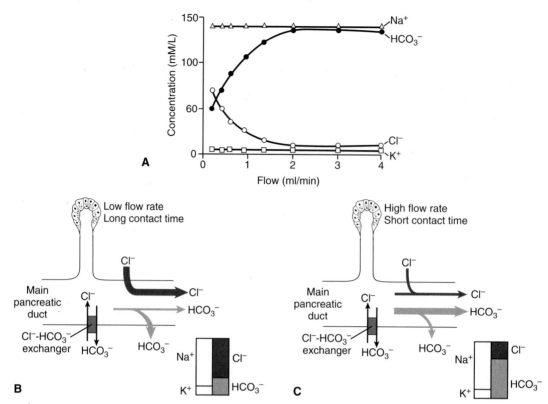

● **Figure 35-2:** Concentration of Anions in Pancreatic Juice versus Flow. **(A)** Graph shows the changes in concentration of Na^+, K^+, Cl^-, and HCO_3^- in the pancreatic juice in relation to the flow rate. **(B)** Low flow rate (long contact time). Diagram shows a relatively high Cl^- concentration and low HCO_3^- concentration of the pancreatic juice due to a Cl^- - HCO_3^- Exchanger present in the main pancreatic duct that transports Cl^- into the pancreatic juice and transports HCO_3^- out of the pancreatic juice. **(C)** High flow rate (short contact time). Diagram shows a relatively low Cl^- concentration and high HCO_3^- concentration of the pancreatic juice because the pancreatic juice has a short contact time with the Cl^-- HCO_3^- Exchanger in the main pancreatic duct.

36

General Principles of Endocrine Physiology

I. Types and Characteristics of Hormones (Table 36-1).

A. Protein and Peptide Hormones. The synthesis of protein/peptide hormones uses **amino acids** as a starting material and begins with the synthesis of a **preprohormone** in the rough endoplasmic reticulum. The synthesis is directed by a specific mRNA. Signal peptides are cleaved from the preprohormone to produce a **prohormone** that is transported to the Golgi. Additional peptide sequences are cleaved from the prohormone, then packaged into secretory granules for later release.

B. Steroid Hormones. The synthesis of steroid hormones uses **cholesterol** as a starting material.

C. Amine Hormones (Epinephrine, Norepinephrine, Dopamine, T_3, T_4). The synthesis of amine hormones uses **tyrosine** as a starting material.

II. Regulation of Hormone Secretion (Figure 36-1A).

A. Negative Feedback. Negative feedback means that some biological function of the hormone inhibits further secretion of the hormone either directly or indirectly. Negative feedback is a very common method used to regulate hormone secretion. In this regard, a number of negative feedback loops have been described.
1. **Ultrashort-loop Feedback.** A hypothalamic releasing factor feeds back to the hypothalamus and inhibits its own release.
2. **Short-loop Feedback.** An adenohypophyseal hormone feeds back to the hypothalamus and inhibits secretion of its hypothalamic releasing factor.
3. **Long-loop Feedback.** A hormone from a peripheral endocrine gland feeds back to the and hypothalamus and adenohypophysis inhibits secretion of its hypothalamic releasing factor and its tropic hormone, respectively.

B. Positive Feedback. Positive feedback means that some biological function of the hormone stimulates further secretion of the hormone. Positive feedback is not a common method used to regulate hormone secretion but when used it leads to an explosive event.

TABLE 36-1	PROPERTIES OF HORMONES			
Property	Protein/Peptide Hormones	Steroid Hormones	Epinephrine Norepinephrine Dopamine	T₄ (Thyroxine)
Negative Feedback Regulations	Yes	Yes	Yes	Yes
Storage of Hormone	1 day	Minimal	Several days	Several weeks
Mechanism of Secretion	Exocytosis of secretory granules	Diffusion through the cell membrane	Exocytosis of secretory granules	Proteolysis of thyroglobulin
Binding to Plasma Proteins	Rarely	Yes; needed for H_2O solubility	No	Yes
Lifespan in Plasma	Minutes	Hours	Seconds ↓lifespan ↑action	Days
Time course of action	Minutes → Hours	Hours → Days	Seconds or less	Days
Receptor	Cell membrane receptors	Cytosolic or Nuclear receptors	Cell Membrane receptors	Nuclear receptors
Mechanism of Receptor Action	Second messenger or protein kinase activity; hormone does not enter the cell	Receptor-hormone complex controls transcription and stability of mRNAs; hormone enters the cell	Second messenger or changes membrane potential; hormone does not enter the cell	Receptor-hormone complex controls transcription and stability of mRNAs; hormone enters the cell

III **Circadian Rhythms of Hormone Secretion (Figure 36-1B).** A central nervous system clock sets the circadian rhythm that affects bodily functions (e.g., body temperature, blood pressure) and diurnal variation in hormone secretion each with its own daily profile.

IV **Regulation of Hormone Receptors (Figure 36-1C).** The response of a target tissue to a hormone is expressed as a **dose-response curve,** in which the magnitude of the response is correlated with the hormone concentration. The **sensitivity** of a target tissue is the hormone concentration that produces 50% of the maximal response. If more hormone is required to produce 50% of the maximal response, then the target tissue has a decreased sensitivity and is **down-regulated.** If less hormone is required to produce 50% of the maximal response, then the target tissue has an increased sensitivity and is **up-regulated.**

A. **Down-Regulation of Hormone Receptors.** Down-regulation is a mechanism by which a hormone decreases the number or affinity of its receptors or the receptors for other hormones in a target tissue.

B. **Up-Regulation of Hormone Receptors.** Up-regulation is a mechanism by which a hormone increases the number or affinity of its receptors or the receptors for other hormones in a target tissue.

V G Protein-Linked Receptors (Figure 36-2).

G protein-linked receptors are proteins that span the cell membrane seven times (**seven pass receptor**) and are linked to **trimeric GTP-binding proteins (called G proteins)** composed of an **α-chain, β-chain**, and **γ-chain.** These receptors activate a chain of cellular events through either the **adenylate cyclase (AC) pathway** (by increasing or decreasing cAMP levels) or the **phospholipase C (PL$_C$) pathway.**

A. **AC Pathway ($\uparrow$ cAMP levels).** When a hormone binds to its receptor, **inactive G$_S$ protein** (which exists as a trimer with GDP bound to the α_S chain) exchanges its GDP for GTP to become **active G$_S$ protein.** This allows the α_S chain to disassociate from the β_S chain and γ_S chain and **stimulate adenylate cyclase to increase cAMP levels.** Active G$_S$ protein is short-lived since the α_S chain has **GTPase activity,** which quickly hydrolyzes GTP to GDP to form inactive G$_S$ protein. cAMP activates the enzyme **cAMP-dependent protein kinase** (or **protein kinase A; PKA**), which catalyzes the **covalent phosphorylation** of serine and threonine within certain intracellular proteins to increase their activity. The enzyme **serine/threonine protein phosphatase** reverses the effects of protein kinase A by dephosphorylating serine and threonine.

B. **AC Pathway ($\downarrow$ cAMP levels).** When a hormone binds to its receptor, **inactive G$_i$ protein** (which exists as a trimer with GDP bound to the α_i chain) exchanges its GDP for GTP to become **active G$_i$ protein.** This allows the α_i chain to disassociate from the β_i chain and γ_i chain and **inhibit adenylate cyclase to decrease cAMP levels.** The β_i and γ_i complex stimulates a K^+ channel protein (probably K_{IR}) so that the channel opens and K^+ flows out of the cell, causing a hyperpolarization of the cell (probably the main effect).

C. **PL$_C$ Pathway.** When a hormone binds to its receptor, **inactive G$_q$ protein** (which exists as a trimer with GDP bound to the α chain) exchanges its GDP for GTP to become **active G$_q$ protein.** Active G$_q$ protein activates **phospholipase C,** which cleaves **phosphatidylinositol biphosphate (PIP$_2$)** into **inositol triphosphate (IP$_3$)** and **diacylglycerol (DAG).** IP$_3$ causes the **release of Ca^{++} from the endoplasmic reticulum,** which activates the enzyme **Ca^{++}/calmodulin-dependent protein kinase (or CaM-kinase),** which catalyzes the **covalent phosphorylation** of serine and threonine within certain intracellular proteins to increase their activity. DAG activates the enzyme **protein kinase C (PKC),** which catalyzes the **covalent phosphorylation** of serine and threonine within certain intracellular proteins to increase their activity.

VI Enzyme-Linked Receptors.

All enzyme-linked receptors are composed structurally of single or multiple polypeptides that span the cell membrane once (**one-pass transmembrane receptors**). These receptors are unique in that their cytoplasmic domain has **intrinsic enzyme activity** or **associates directly with an enzyme.** The various types of enzyme-linked receptors include:

A. **Receptor Guanylate Cyclase.** When the appropriate signal binds to receptor guanylate cyclase, its intrinsic enzyme guanylate cyclase activity produces cGMP. cGMP activates **cGMP-dependent protein kinase (protein kinase G; PKG),** which catalyzes the **covalent phosphorylation** of serine and threonine within certain intracellular proteins to increase their activity.

B. Receptor Tyrosine Phosphatase. When the appropriate signal binds to a receptor tyrosine phosphatase, its intrinsic tyrosine phosphatase will catalyze the **dephosphorylation** of tyrosine within certain intracellular proteins to increase their activity.

C. Receptor Serine/Threonine Kinase. When the appropriate signal binds to a receptor serine/threonine kinase, its intrinsic serine/threonine kinase activity will catalyze the **covalent phosphorylation** of serine and threonine within certain intracellular proteins to increase their activity.

D. Tyrosine Kinase-associated Receptor. When the appropriate signal binds to a tyrosine kinase-associated receptor, the tyrosine kinase that is associated with the receptor will catalyze the **covalent phosphorylation** of tyrosine within certain intracellular proteins to increase their activity. One important tyrosine kinase that is associated with the receptor is the Src protein. Src protein is a tyrosine kinase that is the gene product of the **src proto-oncogene.**

E. Receptor Tyrosine Kinase (Figure 36-3). When the appropriate signal binds to a receptor tyrosine kinase, its intrinsic tyrosine kinase activity will catalyze the **autophosphorylation** of tyrosine (producing **phosphotyrosine**) within the receptor. There is a vast array of intracellular proteins that bind to the phosphotyrosine residues, all of which share a sequence homology (called SH$_2$ domain) and are called **SH$_2$-domain proteins.** The SH$_2$-domain protein interacts with **Sos protein (son-of-sevenless).** The Sos protein activates **Ras protein** by causing Ras protein to bind GTP. Ras protein is a monomeric G protein that is the gene product of the **ras proto-oncogene.** The activated Ras protein activates **Raf protein kinase.** The activated Raf protein kinase activates **mitogen-activated protein kinase (MAP kinase)** by covalent phosphorylation of tyrosine and threonine. The activated MAP kinase leaves the cytoplasm and enters the nucleus where it phosphorylates gene regulatory proteins that then cause **gene transcription.**

VII ## Steroid Hormone Receptors (Figure 36-4). Steroid hormone receptors are composed structurally of a polypeptide with a zinc atom that is bound to four cysteine amino acids, which falls into the classification of a **zinc finger protein.** A zinc finger protein has a **hormone-binding region** and a **DNA-binding region** that activates gene transcription. An inactive steroid hormone receptor is found in the cytoplasm, where it is bound to **heat shock proteins (hsp 90 and hsp 56).** When a steroid hormone diffuses across the cell membrane and binds to the hormone-binding region of the receptor, hsp 90 and hsp 56 are released and the DNA-binding region is exposed. Subsequently, the steroid hormone-receptor complex is transported into the nucleus, where it binds to DNA and activates the transcription of a small number of specific genes within approximately 30 minutes (**primary response**). The gene products of the primary response activate other genes to produce a **secondary response.** Steroid hormone receptors are actually gene regulatory proteins.

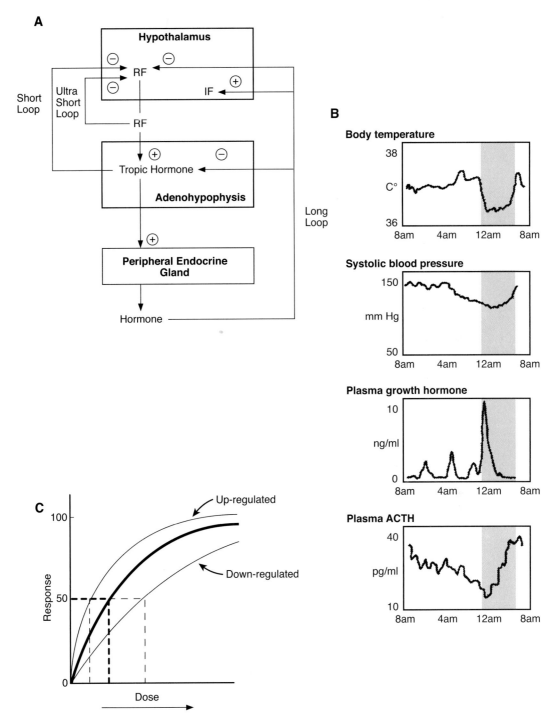

● **Figure 36-1: General Hormone Principles. (A)** Diagram shows the ultra-short loop, short-loop, and long-loop feedback regulation of hormone secretion. **(B)** Diagram shows circadian rhythm of body temperature, systolic blood pressure, growth hormone, and ACTH. **(C)** Diagram shows the down-regulation and up-regulation of hormone receptors.

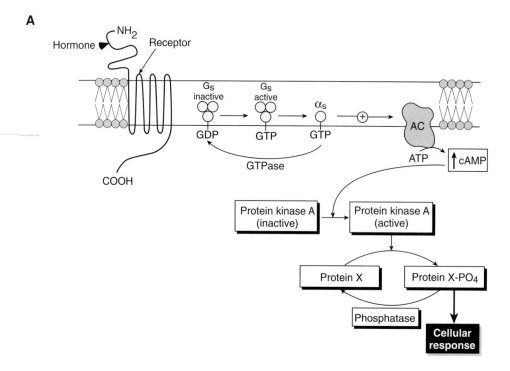

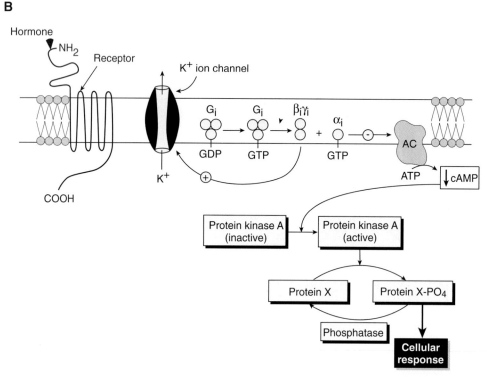

● **Figure 36-2: Diagram of G Protein-Linked Receptor Action. (A)** Adenylate Cyclase Pathway (increase cAMP levels). **(B)** Adenylate Cyclase Pathway (decrease cAMP levels). **(C)** Phospholipase C Pathway
AC = adenylate cyclase; SER = smooth endoplasmic reticulum; PL$_C$ = phospholipase C; CaM = Ca^{2+}/calmodulin-dependent protein kinase; IP$_3$ = inositol triphosphate; DAG = diacylglycerol; PIP$_2$ = phosphatidylinositol biphosphate.

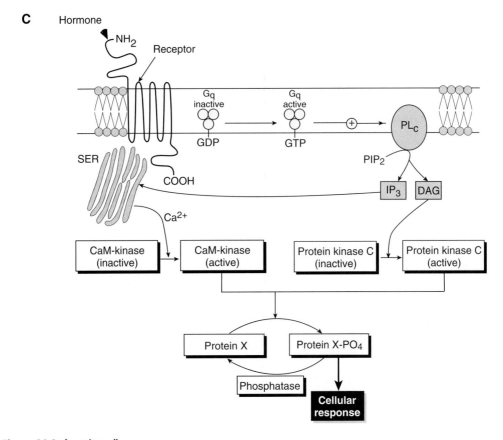

● Figure 36-2: *(continued)*

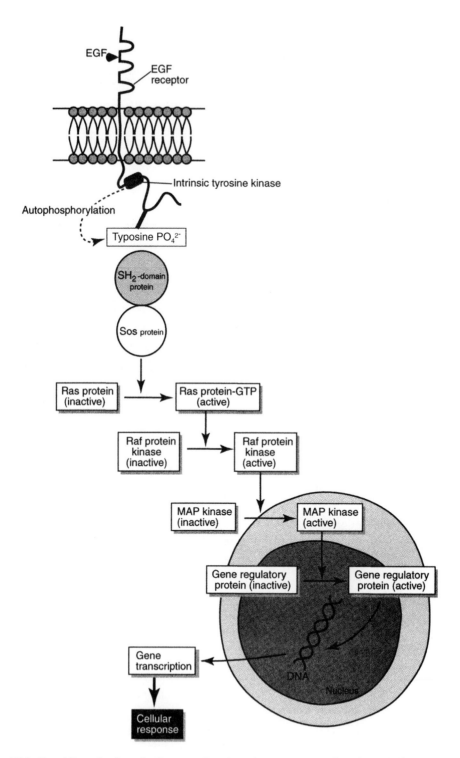

● **Figure 36-3: Signal Transduction of a Receptor Tyrosine Kinase.** EGF = epidermal growth factor; Sos = son-of-sevenless; Ras = rat sarcoma; MAP = mitogen-activated protein; SH_2 = sequence homology; DNA = deoxyribonucleic acid.

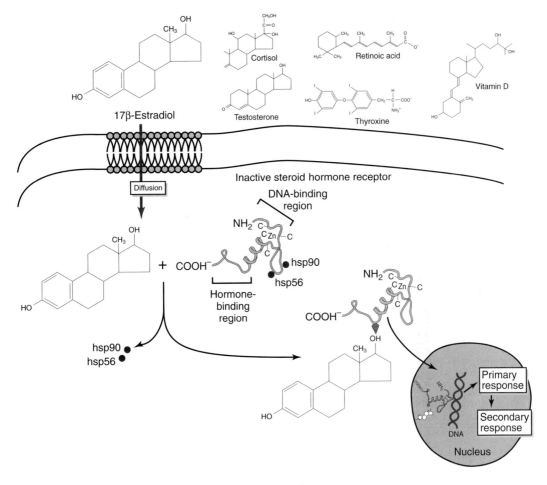

● **Figure 36-4: Steroid Hormone Action.** C = cysteine; Zn = zinc.

37

Hypophysis

I   **General Features.** The hypophysis (also called the pituitary gland)is about $10 \times 13 \times 6$ mm in size, weighs about 0.5 grams, and lies in the cavity of the sphenoid bone called the **sella tursica** (an important radiographic landmark). The hypothalamus and the hypophysis form an integrated neuroendocrine network called the **hypothalamo-hypophyseal system.** The hypothalamus consists of clusters of neurons called **neuroendocrine cells.** Some neuroendocrine cells of the hypothalamus secrete **releasing factors (RFs)** and **inhibiting factors (IFs)** that affect the adenohypophysis. Other neuroendocrine cells of the hypothalamus project long axons to the neurohypophysis where they secrete **oxytocin** and **anti-diuretic hormone (ADH).**

II   **The Adenohypophysis.** The adenohypophysis has three subdivisions, called the **pars distalis, pars tuberalis,** and **pars intermedia.** The pars distalis contains the hormone-secreting cells called the **somatotrophs, mammotrophs, thyrotrophs, corticotrophs,** and **gonadotrophs.**

III   **Growth Hormone (GH).** GH (21,700kDa) is secreted by **somatotrophs** in a pulsatile fashion under the control of hypothalamic factors, **growth hormone-releasing factor (GHRF)** and **growth hormone inhibiting factor (somatostatin).** GH binds to the **GH receptor,** which is a **tyrosine kinase-associated receptor.** The functions of GH include the following:

A. **Effects on Skeletal Muscle.** GH decreases glucose uptake and increases protein synthesis.

B. **Effects on Adipose Tissue.** GH decreases glucose uptake and increases lipolysis.

C. **Effects on Hepatocytes.** GH increases gluconeogenesis, increases glycogen degradation, and stimulates release of **IGF-1 (insulin-like growth factor; somatomedin C)** from hepatocytes.

D. **Actions of IGF-1.** IGF-1 binds to the **IGF receptor** which is a **receptor tyrosine kinase** (similar to the insulin receptor). IGF-1 increases protein synthesis and stimulates mitosis in chondrocytes at the epiphyseal growth plate and therefore causes **linear bone**

growth (pubertal growth spurt). IGF-1 also increases protein synthesis and mitosis in various organs and therefore causes **organ growth.**

IV **Prolactin (PRL).** PRL (22,500kDa) is secreted by **mammotrophs** under the control of the hypothalamic factors **thyrotropin-releasing factor (TRF)** and **prolactin-inhibiting factor (dopamine).** PRL binds to the **PRL receptor,** which is a **tyrosine kinase-associated receptor.** The functions of PRL include the following:

A. **Effects on the Mammary Gland (Breast).** PRL promotes milk secretion in a lactating woman and growth of mammary gland during pregnancy (along with estrogens).

B. **Effects on the Ovary.** PRL inhibits release of gonadotropin releasing factor (GnRF) and thereby prevents ovulation in women.

C. **Effects on the Testes.** PRL inhibits release of GnRF and thereby prevents spermatogenesis in men.

V **Thyroid-Stimulating Hormone (TSH).** TSH (28,000 kDa) is secreted by **thyrotrophs** under the control of hypothalamic factor **thyrotropin-releasing factor (TRF).** TSH binds to the **TSH receptor,** which is a **G protein-linked receptor ($\uparrow$cAMP).** The functions of TSH include the following:

A. **Effects on the Thyroid Gland.** TSH stimulates triiodothyronine (T_3) and thyroxine (T_4) secretion from thyroid follicular cells.

VI **Adenocorticotropic Hormone (ACTH).** ACTH (4,000 kDa) is secreted by **corticotrophs** under the control of hypothalamic factor **corticotropin-releasing factor (CRF).** ACTH binds to the **ACTH receptor,** which is a **G protein-linked receptor ($\uparrow$cAMP).** ACTH is derived from a large precursor protein called **pro-opiomelanocortin (POMC).** POMC is cleaved into ACTH and **β-lipotrophic hormone (β-LPH).** β-LPH is further cleaved into **γ-LPH** and **β-endorphin.** γ-LPH may give rise to **β-melanocyte-simulating hormone (β-MSH),** which explains the hyperpigmentation observed in Addison disease. The functions of ACTH include the following:

A. **Effects on the Adrenal Cortex.** ACTH stimulates the enzyme desmolase that converts cholesterol → pregnenolone, a key step in the synthesis of adrenocortical steroids. ACTH also stimulates the zona fasciculata and zona reticularis to secrete cortisol, androstenedione, and DHEA.

VII **Follicle–Stimulating Hormone (FSH).** FSH (28,000 kDa) is secreted by **gonadotrophs** under the control of hypothalamic factor **gonadotropin-releasing factor (GnRF).** FSH binds to the **FSH receptor,** which is a **G protein-linked receptor ($\uparrow$cAMP).** The functions of FSH include the following:

A. **Effects on the Ovary.** FSH promotes the growth of secondary follicles → Graafian follicles, stimulates estradiol secretion by granulosa cells of the follicle, and stimulates estradiol and progesterone secretion by the granulosa lutein cells of the corpus luteum.

B. Effects on the Testes. FSH maintains spermatogenesis and stimulates synthesis of androgen-binding protein (ABP) in Sertoli cells.

VIII Leutinizing Hormone (LH).

LH (28,300 kDa) is secreted by gonadotrophs under the control of hypothalamic factor **gonadotropin-releasing factor (GnRF)**. LH binds to the **LH receptor,** which is a **G protein-linked receptor ($\uparrow$cAMP).** The functions of LH include the following:

A. Effects on the Ovary. LH promotes ovulation (LH surge), formation of the corpus luteum (leutinization), stimulates androstenedione secretion by theca interna cells of the follicle, and stimulates androstenedione and progesterone secretion by theca lutein cells of the corpus luteum.

B. Effects on the Testes. LH stimulates testosterone secretion from Leydig cells.

IX Hormonal Secretion

from the adenohypophysis is controlled by hypothalamic neurons and the hypophyseal portal system.

A. Hypothalamic neurons. Neuronal cell bodies are located in the **arcuate nucleus, medial preoptic nucleus**, and **paraventricular nucleus** of the hypothalamus. The cell bodies synthesize **releasing factors (RFs)** and **inhibiting factors (IFs).** Axons project to the **median eminence,** where axon terminals secrete RFs and IFs into the primary capillaries of the hypophyseal portal system. RFs and IFs control hormone secretion from the adenohypophysis and include the following: **growth hormone-releasing factor (GHRF), growth hormone-inhibiting factor (somatostatin), prolactin-inhibiting factor (dopamine), thyrotropin-releasing factor (TRF), corticotropin-releasing factor (CRF), and gonadotropin-releasing factor (GnRF).**

B. The hypophyseal portal system has three components:
1. **Primary capillaries** (fenestrated) are formed by the superior hypophyseal artery. They are located in the median eminence and are the site where RFs and IFs are secreted into the bloodstream.
2. **Portal venules** are located in the pars tuberalis. They transport RFs and IFs to the pars distalis.
3. **Secondary capillaries** (fenestrated) are located in the pars distalis. They are the site where RFs and IFs leave the bloodstream to stimulate or inhibit endocrine cells of the adenohypophysis.

X The Neurohypophysis.

The neurohypophysis contains unmyelinated axons and their axon terminals whose neuronal cell bodies (i.e., neuroendocrine cells) are located in the **supraoptic nucleus** and **paraventricular nucleus** of the hypothalamus. The neuroendocrine cells synthesize **oxytocin** and **antidiuretic hormone (ADH)**, which are packaged into neurosecretory vesicles. Axon terminals secrete oxytocin and ADH into a capillary network.

XI **Oxytocin (OXY).** OXY (9 amino acids) is secreted by neuronal axon terminals into the blood. OXY binds to the **OXY receptor,** which is a **G protein-linked receptor ($\uparrow$IP$_3$ + DAG).** The functions of OXY include the following:

A. **Effects on the Mammary Gland (Breast).** OXY is secreted in response to suckling of the baby. OXY stimulates myoepithelial cells in the mammary gland to contract thereby causing milk letdown (ejection).

B. **Effects on the Uterus.** OXY stimulates smooth muscle cells of the myometrium to contract, thereby causing uterine contractions during childbirth.

XII **Antidiuretic Hormone (ADH).** ADH (9 amino acids) is secreted by neuronal axon terminals into the blood. ADH binds to the **V$_1$ (vasopressin) receptor** which is a **G protein-linked receptor ($\uparrow$IP$_3$ + DAG)** or the **V$_2$ receptor,** which is a **G protein-linked receptor ($\uparrow$cAMP).** The functions of ADH include the following:

A. **Effects on the Kidneys.** ADH increases H$_2$O reabsorption from tubular fluid $\rightarrow$ plasma by the principal cells of the cortical and medullary collecting ducts (via the V$_2$ receptor) and thereby decreases H$_2$O excretion in the urine.

B. **Effects on Blood Vessels.** ADH stimulates smooth muscle cells of blood vessels to contract (via the V$_1$ receptor), thereby causing vasoconstriction.

XIII **Clinical Considerations.**

A. **Growth Disorders.**
    1. **Non-Hypophyseal Origin. Achondroplasia (AC)** is the most prevalent form of dwarfism. AC is an autosomal dominant genetic disorder caused by a mutation in the gene for **fibroblast growth factor receptor 3 (FGFR3)** on chromosome 4p16. Pathological changes are observed at the epiphyseal growth plate, where the zones of proliferation and hypertrophy are narrow and disorganized. Horizontal struts of bone eventually grow into the growth plate and "seal" the bone, thereby preventing bone growth. These individuals are short in stature with shortening of the arms and legs along with a disproportionately long trunk. Mental function is not affected. Chances of achondroplasia increase with increasing paternal age.
    2. **Hypophyseal Origin (Table 37-1).**
        a. **Dwarfism.** A minority of dwarfs are true hypophyseal dwarfs; this may be caused by a variety of defects involving either the absence of GH and IGF-1, or the absence of the GH receptor and IGF-1, or the absence of the IGF-1 receptor on the background of $\uparrow$GH and IGF-1 levels.
        b. **Gigantism and Acromegaly.** A GH-secreting adenoma or an oversecretion of GHRF from the hypothalamus cause gigantism (in children or adolescents before the epiphyseal growth plate closes) or acromegaly (in the adult). Clinical findings in acromegaly include: overgrowth of the mandible and maxilla; thickened nose; enlarged hands, feet, head, and viscera; headaches; paresthesias; arthralgias; muscle weakness; hypertension; diabetes; and renal stones.

TABLE 37-1		GROWTH DISORDERS OF HYPOPHYSEAL ORIGIN				
	Normal	Hypopituitary Dwarfism	Laron Dwarfism	End-organ resistance Dwarfism	Gigantism Acromegaly	Gigantism Acromegaly
Hypothalamus Hypophysis						↑↑GHRF
	GH ⊕↓	X	GH	GH	↑↑GH	↑↑GH
Liver	GHr	GHr	X	GHr	GHr	GHr
	IGF-I ⊕↓	X	X	IGF-I	↑↑IGF-I	↑↑IGF-I
Peripheral tissue	IGFr	IGFr	IGFr	X	IGFr	IGFr
	+ GH	− GH	+ GH	+ GH	↑GH	↑↑GHRF
	+ GHr	+ GHr	− GHr	+ GHr	+ GHr	↑↑GH
	+ IGF-I	− IGF-I	− IGF-I	+ IGF-I	↑IGF-I	+ GHr
	+ IGFr	+ IGFr	+ IGFr	− IGFr	+ IGFr	↑↑IGF-I
						+ IGFr

B. Sheehan Syndrome. The Sheehan syndrome is a type of hypopituitarism caused by ischemic necrosis of the gland, commonly due to hypotension induced by postpartum hemorrhage. The hypophysis enlarges during pregnancy, which makes the gland vulnerable to a reduction in blood. Clinical findings include: amennorhea, hypothyroidism, and inadequate adrenal function.

C. Prolactinoma. A prolactinoma (a prolactin (PRL)-secreting adenoma) is the most common secretory neoplasm of the adenohypophysis. Clinical findings in women include: amenorrhea, galactorrhea, and infertility (the consistently high PRL levels inhibit the LH surge necessary for ovulation). Clinical findings in men include: decreased libido and erectile dysfunction. Prolactinomas (microadenomas) may be treated with bromocriptine (a dopamine agonist), which inhibits PRL secretion. Prolactinomas (macroadenoma) may require surgery and/or radiation treatment.

D. Syndrome of inappropriate ADH secretion (SIADH). SIADH is caused by pulmonary disorders (e.g., small cell carcinoma with ectopic secretion of ADH, tuberculosis), drugs (e.g., chlorpropamide, cyclophosphamide, morphine, carbamazepine, oxytocin), and central nervous system disorders [e.g., tumor, infection, hypopituitarism (or the loss of the inhibitory effect of cortisol on ADH)]. SIADH is characterized by excessively increased H_2O reabsorption (tubular fluid → plasma) and, therefore, excessively decreased H_2O excretion in the urine. This results in a dilutional hyponatremia (low serum Na+) and a great increase in total body water. Eventually, the effective arterial blood volume is increased, leading to an inhibition of the renin-angiotensin system; hence, no aldosterone is secreted. This leads to decreased Na+ reabsorption, increased loss of urea, and increased loss of uric acid. The trial of hyponatremia, low serum BUN (blood urea nitrogen), and hypouricemia is virtually pathognomonic for SIADH.

E. **Diabetes Insipidus (DI).** DI is due to a **deficiency of ADH** (anti-diuretic hormone) and the resulting decreased H_2O reabsorption from tubular fluid → plasma by the principal cells of the cortical and medullary collecting ducts. DI is the only significant disease condition associated with the neurohypophysis. DI is caused by unknown idiopathic events; sporadic or familial mutations in the ADH-neurophysin II gene, the V_1 or V_2 (vasopressin) receptor gene, or ADH-sensitive H_2O channel genes; a craniopharyngioma, which may compress the neurohypophysis; trauma; or post-hypophysectomy. Clinical findings include: inability to concentrate urine leading to chronic water diuresis and polydipsia.

XIV Summary Table of Hormones of the Hypophysis (Table 37-2).

TABLE 37-2		HORMONES OF THE HYPOPHYSIS	
Hypothalamic Factor	Cell	Hormone/Receptor	Function
GHRF **Somatostatin**	Somatotrophs	GH/ tyrosine kinase-associated receptor	Muscle: GH decreases glucose uptake and increases protein synthesis Adiposetissue: GH decreases glucose uptake and increases lipolysis
			Hepatocytes: GH increases gluconeogenesis, increases glycogen degradation, and stimulates release of IGF-1 (somatomedin C).
			Actions of IGF-1: IGF-1 increases protein synthesis and stimulates mitosis in chondrocytes at the epiphyseal growth plate and therefore causes linear bone growth (pubertal growth spurt); IGF-1 increases protein synthesis and mitosis of various organs (organ growth)
TRF **Dopamine**	Mammotrophs	PRL/tyrosine kinase-associated receptor	Mammary Gland: PRL promotes milk secretion in a lactating woman and growth of mammary gland during pregnancy
			Ovary: PRL inhibits release of GnRF and thereby prevents ovulation (in women) or spermatogenesis (in men)
TRF	Thyrotrophs	TSH/ G protein-linked receptor	Thyroid Gland: TSH stimulates T_3 and T_4 secretion from thyroid follicular cells
CRF	Corticotrophs	ACTH/ G protein-linked receptor [is derived from a large precursor called proopiomelanocortin]	Adrenal Cortex: ACTH stimulates the enzyme desmolase that converts cholesterol → pregnenolone, a key step in the synthesis of adrenocortical steroids; ACTH stimulates the zona fasciculata and zona reticularis to secrete cortisol, androstenedione, and DHEA

TABLE 37-2   *(continued)*

Hypothalamic Factor	Cell	Hormone/Receptor	Function
GnRF	Gonadotrophs	FSH/G protein-linked receptor	Ovary: FSH promotes the growth of secondary follicles → Graafian follicles, stimulates estradiol secretion by granulosa cells of the follicle, and stimulates estradiol and progesterone secretion by the granulosa lutein cells of the corpus luteum.
			Testes: FSH maintains spermatogenesis and stimulates synthesis of ABP in Sertoli cells
		LH/G protein-linked receptor	Ovary: LH promotes ovulation (LH surge), formation of corpus luteum (luteinization), stimulates androstenedione secretion by theca interna cells of the follicle, and stimulates androstenedione and progesterone secretion by theca lutein cells of the corpus luteum.
			Testes: LH stimulates testosterone secretion from Leydig cells
————	Neuroendocrine cells in the SO and PV	OXY/G protein-linked receptor	Mammary Gland: OXY stimulates myoepithelial cells in the mammary gland to contract thereby causing milk letdown (ejection)
			Uterus: OXY stimulates smooth muscle cells of the myometrium to contract thereby causing uterine contractions during childbirth
————	Neuroendocrine cells in the SO and PV	ADH/G protein-linked receptor	Kidney: ADH increases H_2O reabsorption from tubular fluid → plasma by the principal cells of the cortical and medullary collecting ducts (via the V_2 receptor) and thereby decreases H_2O excretion in the urine
			Blood Vessels: ADH stimulates smooth muscle cells of blood vessels to contract (via the V_1 receptor) thereby causing vasoconstriction

GHRF = growth hormone releasing factor; TRF = thyrotropin releasing factor; CRF = corticotropin releasing factor; GnRF = gonadotropin releasing factor; GH = growth hormone; PRL = prolactin; TSH = thyroid-stimulating hormone; ACTH = adrenocroticotropin; FSH = follicle stimulating hormone; LH = leutinizing hormone; DHEA = dihydroepiandrosterone; OXY = oxytocine; ADH = anti-diuretic hormone; SO = supraoptic nucleus; PV = paraventricular nucleus; V = vasopressin; IGF-1 = insulin-like growth factor-1 or somatomedin C.

38

Thyroid

① General Features. The normal adult thyroid gland is red-brown in color and butterfly-shaped with 2 bulky lateral lobes connected by a thin isthmus. Each lateral lobe is about 2–2.5 cm wide, 5–6 cm long, and 2 cm thick. The normal adult thyroid gland weighs about 15–25 grams. The **thyroid follicles** are the functional unit of the thyroid gland. The thyroid follicles are bounded by **follicular cells** and **parafollicular cells.** The follicular cells secrete **triiodothyronine (T_3)** and **thyroxine (T_4).** The parafollicular cells secrete **calcitonin.** The follicles are filled with a **colloid** that consists of iodinated thyroglobulin.

② Transport of T_3 and T_4 in the Blood.

A. T_3. 46% of T_3 is bound to TBG (thyroid-binding globulin) and 53% of T_3 is bound to albumin. TBG has the highest binding affinity, but lowest binding capacity. Albumin has the lowest binding affinity, but the highest binding capacity. This means that ≈0.2% of T_3 circulates in the free state. The serum T_3 assay measures total T_3 (bound + free).

B. T_4. 67% of T_4 is bound to TBG, 20% is bound to thyroxine-binding prealbumin, and 13% is bound to albumin. This means that ≈0.02% of T_4 circulates in the free state. The serum T_4 assay measures total T_4 (bound + free).

③ Functions of T_3 and T_4. The functions of T_3 and T_4 include the following:

A. Effects on the CNS.
   1. Fetal Brain. T_3 and T_4 play a role in the maturation of the brain during fetal development. **Congenital hypothryroidism (cretinism)** occurs when a thyroid deficiency exists during the early fetal period due to either a severe lack of dietary iodine, thyroid agenesis, or mutations involving the biosynthesis of thyroid hormone. This condition causes impaired skeletal growth and mental retardation. This condition is characterized by: coarse facial features, a low-set hair line, sparse eyebrows, wide-set eyes, periorbital puffiness, a flat broad nose, an enlarged, protuberant tongue, a hoarse cry, umbilical hernia, dry and cold extremities, dry, rough skin (myxedema), and mottled skin. It is important to note that the majority of infants with congenital hypothyroidism have no physical stigmata. This has led to screening of all newborns in the United States and in most other developed countries for depressed thyroxin or elevated thyroid-stimulating hormone levels because there is only a brief perinatal window when replacement therapy can reverse the pathology.

2. **Adult Brain.** T_3 and T_4 play a role in normal adult mentation and increase the response to central catecholamines.

B. **Effects on the Sympathetic Nervous System.** T_3 and T_4 up-regulate β_1-adrenergic receptors in the heart.

C. **Effects on Peripheral Tissues.** T_3 and T_4 increase O_2 consumption and BMR (basal metabolic rate) in all peripheral tissues, except the adult brain, testes, ovaries, uterus, lymph nodes, and spleen). This underlies the role of T_3 and T_4 in temperature regulation. T_3 and T_4 also increase the synthesis of Na^+-K^+ ATPase and consequently increase O_2 consumption related to Na^+-K^+ ATPase pump activity.

D. **Effects on the Heart.** T_3 and T_4 increase cardiac output (CO), increase systolic blood pressure, and decrease diastolic blood pressure.

E. **Effects on the Lung.** T_3 and T_4 increase the ventilation rate in the lung.

F. **Effects on the GI Tract.** T_3 and T_4 increase glucose absorption and increase eating.

G. **Effects on Metabolism.** T_3 and T_4 increase gluconeogenesis, glucose oxidation, glycogen degradation, lipolysis, and protein synthesis. The overall effect of T_3 and T_4 is catabolic.

H. **Effects on Bone.** T_3 and T_4 promote **bone formation** by acting synergistically with growth hormone and IGF-1. T_3 and T_4 promote **bone maturation** as a result of ossification and fusion of growth plates. T_3 and T_4 are required for the attainment of adult height.

IV **Parafollicular Cells** secrete **calcitonin,** which acts directly on osteoclasts to decrease bone resorption, thereby lowering blood Ca^{2+} levels. Calcitonin binds to the calcitonin receptor, which is a G-protein-linked receptor.

V **Clinical Considerations (Figure 38-1).**

A. **Hyperthyroidism.** Clinical signs of hyperthyroidism include: increased metabolic rate, weight loss, negative nitrogen balance, increased heat production, increased cardiac output, dyspnea, tremor, weakness, exophthalmus, and goiter.
1. **Graves Disease (GD)** is hyperthyroidism caused by a diffuse, hyperplastic (toxic) goiter. GD is relatively common in women. GD is an autoimmune disease that produces **TSH receptor–stimulating autoantibodies.** Clinical characteristics include: ophthalmopathy (lid stare, eye bulging), heat intolerance, nervousness, irritability, and weight loss in the presence of a good appetite.
2. **Secondary Hyperthyroidism** is relatively uncommon and may be caused by a TSH adenoma in the adenohypophysis.

B. **Hypothyroidism.** Clinical signs of hypothyroidism include: decreased metabolic rate, weight gain, positive nitrogen balance, decreased heat production, decreased cardiac output, hypoventilation, lethargy, mental slowness, drooping eyelids, myxedema, growth and mental retardation (perinatal), and goiter.

1. **Hashimoto Thyroiditis (HT)** is the most common cause of goitrous hypothyroidism. HT is relatively common in middle-aged women. HT is an autoimmune disease that produces **thyroid peroxidase autoantibodies.** Clinical characteristics include: goiter and hypothyroidism. In some variants of Hashimoto thyroiditis, only hypothyroidism and no goiter exists.

2. **Primary Hypothyroidism (PH)** is most commonly idiopathic, whereby **TSH receptor–blocking autoantibodies** are present. Clinical characteristics include: low blood pressure, low heart rate, low respiratory rate, reduced body temperature, and myxedema (peripheral nonpitting edema).

3. **Secondary Hypothyroidism** is relatively uncommon and caused by a deficiency in the adenohypophysis (low TSH secretion) or hypothalamus [low thyrotropin-releasing factor (TRF) secretion].

C. **Estrogen Effect.** The use of oral contraceptive pills, pregnancy, or the use of diethylstilbestrol for treatment of prostatic cancer increases synthesis of TBG. In pregnancy, an increase in TBG would temporarily decrease free T_4. In response to this decrease in T_4, TSH secretion from the adenohypophysis would increase until free T_4 is returned to normal. When the new equilibrium is reached, bound T_4 is elevated but **free T_4 is normal.** However, the serum T_4 would be elevated because the serum T_4 assay measures total T_4 (bound + free). Pregnancy is not a hyperthyroid state because hyperthyroidism is characterized by elevated free T_4 and in pregnancy free T_4 is normal.

D. **Diffuse Nontoxic (simple) Goiter** is an enlargement of the entire thyroid gland in a diffuse manner without producing nodules. A simple goiter occurs most commonly in particular geographic areas (called **endemic goiter**), most often caused by deficiency of iodine in the diet. Wherever endemic goiter is prevalent, endemic **cretinism** occurs. A severe iodine deficiency during fetal development results in growth retardation and severe mental retardation.

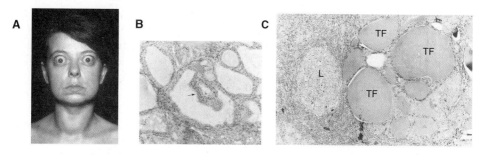

D   Laboratory Findings Used for Diagnosis of Thyroid Disorders

Disorder	Mechanisms	Total T₄*	T₃RU (TBG)**	FTI†	TSH	I¹³¹
Graves Disease	Production of TSH receptor-stimulating autoantibodies	High	High (Low)	High	Undetectable	High
Secondary Hyperthyroidism	TSH adenoma	High	High (Low)	High	High	High
Factitious Thyrotoxicosis	Excessive exogenous thyroid hormone intake	High	High (Low)	High	Low	Low
Thyroiditis	Inflammation of bacterial or viral origin	High	High (Low)	High	Low	Low
Hashimoto thyroiditis	Production of thyroid peroxidase autoantibodies	Low	Low (High)	Low	High	Low
Primary hypothyroidism	Production of TSH receptor-blocking antibodies	Low	Low (High)	Low	Very High	Low
Secondary hypothyroidism	Low TSH secretion by adenohypophysis or low TRF secretion by the hypothalamus	Low	Low (High)	Low	Low	Low
Increased TBG (increased estrogen)	Oral contraceptives, pregnancy, DES therapy for prostate cancer	High	Low (High)	Normal	Normal	Normal
Decreased TBG (increased androgens)	Steroid abuse	Low	High (Low)	Normal	Normal	Normal

DES = diethylstilbestrol; T_3 = triiodothyronine; T_4 = thyroxine; TRF = thyrotropin-releasing factor; TSH = thyroid-stimulating hormone; TBG = thyroid binding globulin
*Total T_4 measures both bound and free T_4
**The T_3 resin uptake (T_3RU) test is not a measure of serum T3 levels; rather, it measures the percentage of free T_4. This test evaluates TBG levels via a competition assay between a resin and TBG for radioactive T_3. If TBG levels are low, then more radioactive T_3 will bind to the resin. TBG has an inverse relationship to T_3RU.
† Free thyroxine (T4) Index (FTI) is a measure of free T_4. It is calculated by multiplying the total T_4 x T_3RU. FTI is rapidly becoming obsolete as major medical centers are using assays that directly measure free T_4.
I^{131}= radioactive iodine I^{131} uptake

● **Figure 38-1: Clinical Considerations. (A)** Photograph shows a woman with Graves disease (hyperthyroidism) demonstrating exophthalmos and a mass in the neck (goiter). **(B)** LM of Graves disease (GD). Graves disease is caused by a diffuse, hyperplastic goiter. The follicular cells are increased in number (hyperplasia) and arranged as a simple tall columnar epithelium. In addition, the follicular cells can form buds that encroach into the colloidal material (arrow). **(C)** LM of Hashimoto thyroiditis (HT). HT is characterized by a high lymphocytic infiltration that may form lymphoid follicles with germinal centers (L). Normal thyroid follicles (TF) also are observed. **(D)** Table shows the laboratory findings used for diagnosis of thyroid disorders.

39

Parathyroid Glands/ Calcium Homeostasis

I General Features. The parathyroid glands are yellow to orange tan (depending on the amount of stromal fat) and measure 3–6mm in length, 2–4 mm in width, and 0.5–2.0 mm in thickness. In 90%–97% of cases, there are four parathyroid glands (in the remaining cases, 2–12 parathyroid glands have been reported). The weight of the parathyroid glands is an important parameter in histopathologic assessment. All parathyroid glands (or parts of parathyroid glands) must be carefully weighed. Each parathyroid gland weighs about **35–40 mg.** The total parathyroid weight ranges from **120–140 mg.** The parathyroid glands contain **chief cells** and **oxyphil cells.** The chief cells express a **Ca^{2+}-sensing receptor** which is a G protein-linked receptor that responds to low plasma Ca^{2+} by stimulating adenylate cyclase ($\uparrow$cAMP) and inhibiting phospholipase C ($\downarrow$IP$_3$), thereby causing **parathyroid hormone (PTH)** secretion. PTH binds in peripheral tissues to the **PTH receptor** which is a G-protein-linked receptor ($\uparrow$cAMP). The oxyphil cells are distinctly eosinophilic because of the numerous mitochondria within the cytoplasm, but they have no known function.

II Functions of PTH (Figure 39-1A). The functions of PTH include the following:

A. Effects on Kidney. PTH increases kidney reabsorption of Ca^{2+} from the tubular fluid $\rightarrow$ plasma by the distal convoluted tubule (DCT) and collecting duct (CD), thereby elevating blood Ca^{2+} levels. PTH also increases the synthesis of 1α-hydroxylase by the proximal convoluted tubule (PCT), thereby elevating blood 1,25-dihydroxyvitamin D [1,25-(OH)$_2$ vitamin D] levels.

B. Effects on Bone. PTH acts directly on osteoblasts to secrete **macrophage colony-stimulating factor (M-CSF)** and to express a cell surface protein called **RANKL.** M-CSF stimulates monocytes to differentiate into macrophages and express a cell surface receptor called **RANK.** RANKL (on the osteoblast) and RANK (on the macrophage) interact and cause the differentiation of macrophages into osteoclasts. Osteoclasts increase bone resorption, thereby elevating blood Ca^{2+} levels.

III Calcium Homeostasis. The body regulates blood Ca^{2+} levels closely because hypocalcemia results in tetanic convulsions and death.

A. GI Tract. Dietary Ca^{2+} intake averages $\approx$1000 mg/day, of which 400 mg (40%) is absorbed by the GI tract. However, 300 mg are returned to the GI tract lumen via GI secretions. Therefore, the typical net Ca^{2+} absorption/day is ≈ 100 mg or $\approx 10\%$ of the dietary intake. The amount of ingested dietary Ca^{2+} absorbed by the GI epithelium from the intestinal lumen $\rightarrow$ plasma is controlled by **1,25-$(OH)_2$ vitamin D.**

B. **Plasma Calcium.** Plasma calcium exists in three forms: **ionized calcium** (Ca^{2+}; 45%; the active plasma fraction), **calcium complexed with anions** (e.g., $CaPO_4$ or citrate; 15%), and **calcium reversibly bound to plasma proteins,** which is profoundly affected by plasma pH (40%). The equilibrium between ionized calcium and protein-bound calcium depends on blood pH. Acidosis increases ionized calcium and decreases protein-bound calcium. Alkalosis decreases ionized calcium and increases protein-bound calcium. In most physiological conditions, plasma concentration of Ca^{2+} ($[P]_{Ca2+}$) changes very little. The normal plasma concentration of Ca^{2+} is 5 mEq/L (**$[P]_{Ca2+}$ = 5 mEq/L**).

C. **Kidneys.** The kidneys maintain a stable balance of total body Ca^{2+}. Ca^{2+} (not bound to proteins) is freely-filtered from the glomerular capillaries $\rightarrow$ Bowman's space and then is reabsorbed by particular segments of the nephron. The proximal convoluted tubule (PCT) reabsorbs **80%** of the filtered Ca^{2+} by diffusion via the paracellular route across the zonula occludens. The distal straight tubule (DST) reabsorbs **10%** of the filtered Ca^{2+} by diffusion via the paracellular route across the zonula occludens. The distal convoluted tubule (DCT; PTH-sensitive) reabsorbs **5%** of the filtered Ca^{2+} via carrier (transporter) proteins and ion channel proteins. The collecting duct (CD; PTH-sensitive) reabsorbs **5%** of the filtered Ca^{2+} via carrier (transporter) proteins and ion channel proteins.

D. **Bone.** About 99% of total body Ca^{2+} resides in bone. Since bone is constantly resorbed and reformed, bone provides a huge source of Ca^{2+} to increase plasma concentration of Ca^{2+} or a huge sink for Ca^{2+} to decrease plasma concentration of Ca^{2+}.

IV Other Hormones Involved in Calcium Homeostasis (Figure 39-1).

A. **1,25-$(OH)_2$ vitamin D.** Vitamin D sources include dietary intake and production by skin keratinocytes stimulated by ultraviolet light. Vitamin D is hydroxylated by liver hepatocytes to **25-(OH) vitamin D.** 25-(OH) vitamin D is hydroxylated by the PCT to **1,25-$(OH)_2$ vitamin D,** the active metabolite that functions similar to a steroid hormone. The plasma concentration of 1,25 $(OH)_2$ vitamin D is controlled by PTH, which increases the synthesis of 1α-hydroxylase used in the second hydroxylation step in the kidney. The functions of 1,25-$(OH)_2$ vitamin include the following:
   1. **Effects on the GI Tract.** 1,25-$(OH)_2$ vitamin D mainly stimulates absorption of Ca^{2+} and PO^{2-} ions from the intestinal lumen into the blood by inducing the synthesis of **vitamin D-dependent Ca^{2+} binding protein (calbindin D-28K),** thereby elevating blood Ca^{2+} and PO^{2-} levels.
   2. **Effects on Bone.** 1,25-$(OH)_2$ vitamin D also acts directly on osteoblasts to secrete IL-1, which stimulates osteoclasts to increase bone resorption, thereby elevating blood Ca^{2+} levels.

B. **Calcitonin.** The parafollicular cells of the thyroid gland express a Ca^{2+}-sensing receptor (similar to the chief cells) that responds to high plasma Ca^{2+}, thereby causing calcitonin secretion. The physiological role of calcitonin in humans is uncertain because neither thyroidectomy nor thyroid tumors result in a serious alteration in Ca^{2+} homeostasis. The functions of calcitonin include the following:
   1. **Effects on Bone.** Calcitonin acts directly on osteoclasts to decrease bone resorption, thereby lowering blood Ca^{2+} levels.

CLINICAL CONSIDERATIONS (Table 39-1).

A. Primary hypoparathyroidism (e.g., accidental surgical removal, DiGeorge syndrome, autoimmune destruction) is characterized by the absence of PTH, leading to **hypocalcemia.** Chronic renal failure and vitamin D deficiency also lead to hypocalcemia. Clinical findings include: carpopedal spasm, laryngospasm, **Chvostek sign** (tapping facial nerve elicits spasm of facial muscles), **Trousseau phenomenon** (elated blood pressure cuff on arm elicits carpel tunnel spasm), calcification of basal ganglia, cataracts, and tetany. Seizures and cardiac arrest may occur in severe cases.

B. Pseudohypoparathyroidism is a rare condition characterized by abnormal PTH receptors, leading to **hypocalcemia,** although there are high PTH levels.

C. Primary Hyperparathyroidism (e.g., adenoma, hyperplasia, associated with MEN sydromes) is characterized by excessive secretion of PTH, leading to **hypercalcemia.** Clinical findings include: osteitis fibrosa cystica (bone softening and painful fractures), urinary calculi, abdominal pain (due to constipation, pancreatitis, or biliary stones), depression/lethargy, and cardiac arrhythmias. Think "painful bones, kidney stones, belly groans, mental moans".

D. Malignant Tumors (e.g., lung, breast, or ovarian carcinomas) may secrete a PTH-related protein, leading to **hypercalcemia.**

E. Osteomalacia (in adults) and **rickets** (in children). Osteomalacia and rickets are characterized by **lack of minerals within osteoid,** which occurs as a result of **vitamin D deficiency.** Physical signs of osteomalacia in adults include: bowed legs, increased tendency to fracture, and scoliotic deformity of the vertebral column. Physical signs of rickets in non-ambulatory children include: craniotabes (elastic recoil of the skull upon compression), "rachitic rosary" (excess osteoid at the costochondral junction), and "pigeon-breast deformity" (anterior protrusion of sternum).

TABLE 39-1	LABORATORY FINDINGS USED FOR DIAGNOSIS OF PARATHYROID DISORDERS		
Disorder	**Calcium**	**Phosphorus**	**PTH**
Hypocalcemia			
Primary Hypoparathyroidism	Low	High	Low
Pseudohypoparathyroidism	Low	High	Normal →High
Secondary Hypoparathyroidism (Malabsorption)	Low	Low	High
Secondary Hypoparathyroidism (Renal Failure)	Low	High	High
Hypoalbuminemia	Low (Normal ionized calcium)	Normal	Normal
Alkalosis	Normal (Decreased ionized calcium)	Normal	High
Hypercalcemia			
Primary Hyperparathyroidism	High	Low	High
Malignant Tumors	High	Low	Low

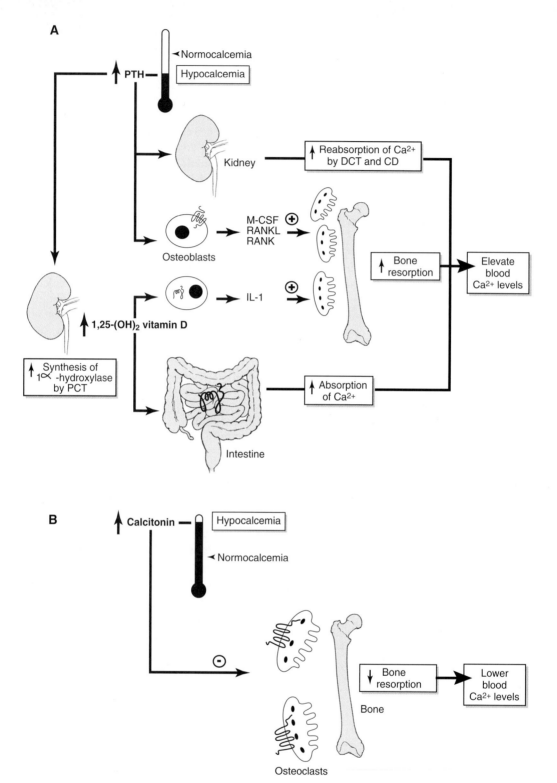

● **Figure 39-1: Calcium Homeostasis. (A)** Blood calcium levels can be depicted on a thermometer such that when blood calcium levels are too low, PTH is released. PTH and 1,25-(OH_2) vitamin D regulate blood calcium levels by acting on the kidney, bone, and intestine to elevate blood calcium levels. **(B)** Blood calcium levels can be depicted on a thermometer such that when blood calcium levels are too high, calcitonin is released. Calcitonin regulates blood calcium levels by acting on bone to lower blood calcium levels. M-CSF = macrophage colony-stimulating factor; RANKL = RANK ligand; RANK = receptor for activation of nuclear factor kappa B; DCT = distal convoluted tubule; CD = collecting duct; PCT = proximal convoluted tubule; IL-1 = interleukin-1.

40

Adrenal Gland

① General Features. The adrenal glands are paired organs that lie near the superior pole of the kidneys, embedded in adipose tissue. The right adrenal gland is **pyramid-shaped.** The left adrenal gland is **half-moon shaped.**

② Adrenal Cortex. Cortical cells of the adrenal gland synthesize and secrete steroid hormones under the influence of **CRF** and **ACTH.** ACTH stimulates the enzyme desmolase that converts cholesterol → pregnenolone, a key step in the synthesis of all adrenocortical steroids. Cortical cells have abundant **smooth endoplasmic reticulum (sER), mitochondria with tubular cristae,** and **lipid droplets,** which are characteristic of all steroid-secreting cells. The adrenal cortex is divided into 3 distinct histological zones.

A. **Zona Glomerulosa (ZG).** The ZG is a narrow, inconstant band of cortex located immediately below the capsule and constitutes **15%** of the cortical volume. ZG cells are arranged in a glomerular-like fashion. ZG cells synthesize and secrete **aldosterone (ALD).** ZG cells lack the enzyme 17α-hydroxylase and therefore cannot synthesize cortisol, androstenedione, or DHEA. ALD is controlled by CRF and ACTH, but is also separately controlled by the **renin-angiotensin system** and **K^+. Angiotensin II** stimulates the conversion of corticosterone → ALD, whereas **hyperkalemia** stimulates ALD secretion. ALD has a **half-life of 20 minutes** as it is metabolized by the liver and excreted as a glucuronide. Urine levels of **aldosterone 3-glucuronide** are used for diagnostic purposes. The functions of ALD include the following:
   1. **Effects on Kidney.** ALD **increases Na^+ reabsorption** from tubular fluid → plasma (H_2O water) by the principal cells of the cortical collecting ducts. ALD **increases K^+ secretion** from plasma → tubular fluid by the principal cells of the cortical collecting ducts. ALD **increases H^+ secretion** from plasma → tubular fluid by the Type A intercalated cells of the cortical collecting ducts.
   2. **Effect on the Colon.** ALD increases Na^+ absorption by enterocytes.
   3. **Effect on Eccrine Sweat Glands.** ALD increases Na^+ reabsorption from the excretory ducts.
   4. **Effects on Salivary Glands.** ALD increases Na^+ reabsorption from the excretory ducts. ALD increases K^+ secretion from the excretory ducts.

B. **Zona Fasciculata (ZF).** The ZF is a broad band of cortex that lies between the ZG and ZR and constitutes **78%** of the cortical volume. ZF cells are arranged in 2-cell wide vertical cords perpendicular to the capsule. ZF cells synthesize and secrete **cortisol.**

The secretion of cortisol is controlled by **CRF** and **ACTH**. Abnormally high levels of ACTH (e.g., adenoma of adenohypophysis) cause hypertrophy of the ZF. Abnormally low levels of ACTH (e.g., hypophysectomy) cause atrophy of the ZF. 5% of circulating cortisol is in the free form. The remaining 95% of circulating cortisol is bound to **corticosteroid-binding protein** (high affinity, low capacity) and **albumin** (low affinity, high capacity). Cortisol has a **half-life of 70 minutes** as it is metabolized by the liver and excreted in the urine as a glucuronide. Urine levels of **17-hydroxycorticoids** are used for diagnostic purposes. The functions of cortisol include the following:

1. **Effects on Metabolism.**
    a. Cortisol decreases glucose utilization and insulin sensitivity of muscle and adipose tissue.
    b. Cortisol stimulates lipolysis in adipose tissue, which forms glycerol (used by the liver as substrate for gluconeogenesis) and fatty acids (which are metabolized by the liver for energy).
    c. Cortisol stimulates protein catabolism in muscle, which forms amino acids that are used by the liver as substrate for gluconeogenesis.
    d. Cortisol stimulates gluconeogenesis and glycogen synthesis in the liver. Overall the most important metabolic effect of cortisol is the conversion of fat and muscle protein to glycogen. Cortisol is called a glucocorticoid because one of its long-term effects is to increase blood glucose (hyperglycemia).
2. **Effects on Bone.** Cortisol inhibits bone formation by reducing the synthesis of type I collagen and decreasing the absorption of Ca^{2+} by the GI tract by blocking the action of 1,25-(OH_2) vitamin D. This results in osteoporosis.
3. **Effects on Inflammation.** Cortisol inhibits the inflammation response (i.e., anti-inflammatory) at high concentrations by inhibition of: **phospholipase A_2,** which releases arachidonic acid (a precursor for many immune mediators, like PGE_2) through the synthesis of **lipocortin;** and, **histamine** and **serotonin release** from mast cells.
4. **Effects on the Immune System.** Cortisol inhibits **IL-2 production,** thereby preventing proliferation of T lymphocytes.
5. **Effects on the Fetus.** Cortisol promotes fetal development and stimulates surfactant production in the fetus.
6. **Effects on the CNS.** Cortisol modulates emotional tone and wakefulness probably by acting on the hippocampus, which has cortisol receptors.
7. **Effects on Arterioles.** Cortisol up-regulates α_1-adrenergic receptors on arterioles, thereby increasing their sensitivity to the vasoconstrictor effect of norepinephrine.

C. **Zona Reticularis (ZR).** The ZR is a narrow band of cortex that lies between the ZF and the medulla, and constitutes **7%** of the cortical volume. ZR cells are arranged in an anastomosing network of cords and contain large amounts of lipofuscin pigment. ZR cells synthesize and secrete **dehydroepiandrosterone (DHEA)** and **androstene-dione.** The secretion of DHEA and androstenedione is controlled by **CRF** and **ACTH.** Although DHEA and androstenedione are weak androgens, they are converted to testosterone by peripheral tissues. DHEA and androstenedione are metabolized by the liver to 17-ketosteroids. Urine levels of **17-ketosteroids** are used for diagnostic purposes. The functions of DHEA and androstenedione include the following:

1. **Effects in Women.** The conversion of DHEA and androstenedione → testosterone is a main source of testosterone. During puberty, DHEA and androstenedione also may serve as substrates for conversion to estrogen.
2. **Effects in Men.** The conversion of DHEA and androstenedione → testosterone is of little biological significance because the testes produce most of the testosterone.

III **Adrenal Medulla.** The adrenal medulla contains **chromaffin cells,** which are **modified postganglionic sympathetic neurons.** Preganglionic sympathetic axons (via splanchnic nerves) synapse on chromaffin cells, and upon stimulation cause chromaffin cells to secrete catecholamines: **epinephrine** (90% of the output) and **norepinephrine** (10% of the output). **Epinephrine-containing cells** comprise a majority of the chromaffin cells in the medulla and contain small, homogeneous, light-staining granules. All of the circulating epinephrine in the blood is derived from the adrenal medulla. Epinephrine binds to α- and β-adrenergic receptors, which are G-protein-linked receptors. Epinephrine has a **half-life of 1–3 minutes** as it is metabolized by the liver and excreted in the urine as **free epinephrine** or **metanephrine. Urinary levels of free epinephrine** are used for diagnostic purposes in problems of adrenal medulla function. **Norepinephrine-containing cells** comprise a minority of the chromaffin cells in the medulla and contain large, electron-dense core granules. The majority of circulating norepinephrine in the blood is derived from the postganglionic sympathetic neurons and brain, with the secretion from the adrenal medulla contributing only a minor portion. Norepinephrine binds to α- and β-adrenergic receptors, which are G-protein-linked receptors. Norepinephrine has a **half-life of 1–3 minutes,** as it is metabolized by the liver and excreted in the urine as **free norepinephrine, normetanephrine, vanillylmandelic acid (VMA), or 3-methoxy-4-hydroxyphenyglycol (MOPEG). Urinary levels of VMA and MOPEG** are used for diagnostic purposes in problems of the sympathetic nervous system. The functions of epinephrine include the following:

A. **Effects on Metabolism.**
  1. Epinephrine increases gluconeogenesis and increases glycogen degradation in the liver.
  2. Epinephrine increases free fatty acid mobilization in adipose tissue.
  3. Epinephrine increases glycogen degradation and decreases release of amino acids in skeletal muscle.

B. **Effects on Heart.** Epinephrine accelerates the SA node (increases heart rate; positive chronotropism). Epinephrine increases contractility of cardiac muscle (positive inotropism).

C. **Effects on the GI Tract.** Epinephrine relaxes smooth muscle in GI tract wall causing a decrease in gut motility and gut tone. Epinephrine contracts the internal anal sphincter.

D. **Effect on the Lungs.** Epinephrine relaxes bronchial smooth muscle in lung causing bronchodilation.

E. **Effects on Blood Vessels.** Epinephrine contracts smooth muscle in skin and visceral blood vessels. Epinephrine relaxes smooth muscle in skeletal muscle blood vessels.

F. **Effects on the Eyes.** Epinephrine contracts the dilator pupillae muscle, causing dilation of pupil (mydriasis).

IV **Clinical Considerations (Figure 40-1 and Table 40-1).**

A. **Primary Hyperaldosteronism.** Primary hyperaldosteronism is caused by elevated levels of aldosterone due most commonly to an aldosterone-secreting adenoma (**Conn syndrome**) within the ZG. Clinical findings include: hypertension, hypernatremia due to increased Na$^+$ reabsorption, weight gain due to water retention, and hypokalemia due to increased K^+ secretion. This condition is treated by **surgery and/or spironolactone,** which is an aldosterone receptor antagonist and therefore an effective antihypertensive and diuretic agent.

B. **Cushing Syndrome.** Cushing syndrome is most commonly caused by administration of **large doses of steroids** for treatment of primary disease. If not iatrogenic, elevated levels of cortisol (i.e., hypercortisolism) are caused by an **ACTH-secreting adenoma** within the adenohypophysis (75% of the cases; strictly termed **Cushing disease**) or **adrenal cortical adenoma** (25% of the cases). Clinical findings include: mild hypertension, impaired glucose tolerance, acne, hirsutism, oligomenorrhea, men complain of impotence and loss of libido, osteoporosis with back pain and buffalo hump, central obesity, moon facies, and purple skin striae (bruise easily). This condition is treated by surgery or **aminoglutethimide, metyrapone, and ketoconazole.**

C. **Congenital Adrenal Hyperplasia.** Congenital adrenal hyperplasia is caused most commonly by mutations in genes for enzymes involved in adrenocortical steroid biosynthesis (e.g., **21-hydroxylase deficiency, 11b-hydroxylase deficiency**). In 21-hydroxylase deficiency (90% of all cases), there is virtually no synthesis of the aldosterone or cortisol, so that intermediates are funneled into androgen biosynthesis, thereby elevating androgen levels. Clinical findings include: elevated levels of androgens lead to virilization of a female fetus ranging from mild clitoral enlargement to complete labioscrotal fusion with a phalloid organ (female pseudohermaphroditism); in the male fetus, macrogenitosomia occurs; ↑adrenal androgens; ↑urinary 17-ketosteroids;↓cortisol and ↓ALD levels; ↑17-progesterone and ↑progesterone levels; ↑ACTH because negative feedback to the adenohypophysis by cortisol does not occur; hyperplasia of ZF and ZR because of ↑ACTH; early acceleration of linear growth; early appearance of pubic and axillary hair. Since cortisol cannot be synthesized, negative feedback to the adenohypophysis does not occur, so ACTH continues to stimulate the adrenal cortex resulting in adrenal hyperplasia. Since aldosterone cannot be synthesized, the patient presents with **hyponatremia ("salt-wasting")** with adjoining **dehydration** and **hyperkalemia.** Treatment includes: immediate infusion of intravenous saline, long-term steroid hormone replacement both cortisol and mineralocorticoids (9α-fludrocortisone), and surgical reconstruction of the genitalia depending on the severity.

D. **Primary Adrenal Insufficiency (Addison Disease).** Addison disease is commonly caused by autoimmune destruction of the adrenal cortex. Clinical findings include: fatigue, anorexia, nausea, weight loss, hypotension, skin hyperpigmentation due to increased melanocyte-stimulating hormone (MSH) caused by an increase in ACTH secretion, hyponatremia, and hyperkalemia (may lead to fatal cardiac arrhythmias). This condition is managed by steroid replacement therapy.

E. **Secondary Adrenal Insufficiency.** Secondary adrenal insufficiency is caused by a disorder of the hypothalamus or adenohypophysis that reduces the secretion of ACTH. It is clinically very similar to Addison disease, except there is no hyperpigmentation of the skin.

F. **Pheochromocytoma.** Pheochromocytoma is a relatively rare (usually not malignant) catecholamine-producing tumor (both epinephrine and norepinephrine) of the adrenal medulla. Pheochromocytoma occurs mainly in adults and is generally found in the region of the adrenal gland but also is found in extra-adrenal sites. It occurs within families as part of the MEN Type II syndrome. Clinical findings include: persistent or paroxysmal hypertension, anxiety, tremor, profuse sweating, pallor, chest pain, and abdominal pain. Laboratory findings include: increased urine VMA and metanephrine levels, inability to suppress catecholamines with clonidine, and hyperglycemia. Pheochromocytoma is treated by surgery or phenoxybenzamine (an α-adrenergic antagonist).

G. Neuroblastoma. Neuroblastoma is a common extracranial neoplasm containing primitive neuroblasts of neural crest origin. Neuroblastomas occur mainly in children. They are found in extra-adrenal sites usually along the sympathetic chain ganglia (60%) or within the adrenal medulla (40%). They metastasize widely. Clinical findings include: opsoclonus (rapid, irregular movements of the eye in horizontal and vertical directions; "dancing eyes"). Laboratory findings include: a neuroblastoma contains small cells arranged in Homer-Wright pseudorosettes; increased urine VMA and metanephrine levels. Neuroblastoma is treated by surgery, radiation, and chemotherapy.

TABLE 40-1			LABORATORY FINDINGS USED FOR DIAGNOSIS OF ADRENAL DISORDERS				
			Plasma Levels				
Clinical Condition	**Dex***	**ALD**	**Cortisol**	**Androgens**	**ACTH**	**Other**	
Primary Hyperaldosteronism (Conn Syndrome)		High					
Cushing Syndrome							
Normal patient	+		Normal		Normal		
ACTH adenoma	+		High		High		
Adrenal adenoma	−		High		Low		
Congenital Adrenal Hyperplasia							
21-hydroxylase deficiency		Low	Low	High	High	Salt Loss with volume depletion	
11β-hydroxylase deficiency		Low	Low	High	High	Salt retention with hypertension	
Addison Disease (Primary Adrenal Insufficiency)		Low	Low	Low	High		
Secondary Adrenal Insufficiency		Normal	Low	Low	Low		

*Dex = **high dose dexamethasone suppression test.** This test is based on the ability of dexamethasone (a synthetic glucocorticoid) to inhibit ACTH and cortisol secretion. If the adenohypophysis–adrenal cortex axis is normal, dexamethasone will suppress ACTH and cortisol secretion and the test is considered positive (i.e, suppression occurred).

ALD = aldosterone; ACTH = adrenocorticotropin.

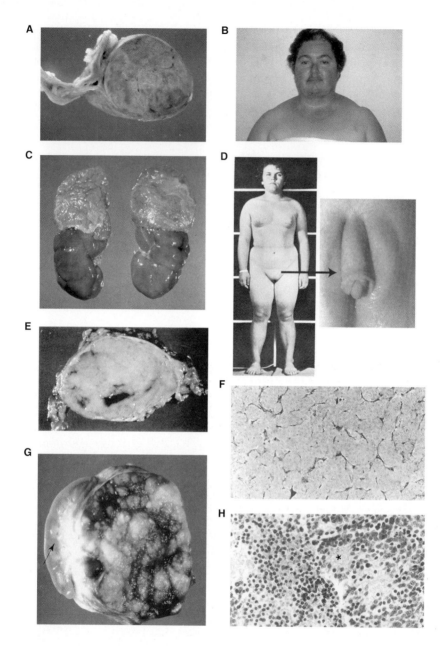

● **Figure 40-1: (A,B)** Cushing Syndrome. (A) Photograph of an adrenal adenoma (cut surface) shows mottled yellow appearance with a rim of compressed normal adrenal tissue. (B) Photograph shows a woman with an ACTH-secreting pituitary adenoma with a moon face, buffalo hump, and increased facial hair. **(C,D)** Congenital Adrenal Hyperplasia. (C) Photograph shows the markedly enlarged adrenal glands from a 7 week old infant who died of severe salt-wasting congenital adrenal hyperplasia. (D) Photograph shows a patient (XX genotype) with female pseudointersexuality due to congenital adrenal hyperplasia. Masculinization of female external genitalia is apparent with fusion of the labia majora and enlarged clitoris. **(E,F)** Pheochromocytoma. (E) Gross photograph of a pheochromocytoma. Pheochromocytomas vary in size from 3–5cm in diameter. They are gray-white to pink-tan in color. Exposure of the cut surface often results in darkening of the surface due to formation of yellow-brown adenochrome pigment. (F) LM of a pheochromocytoma. A pheochromocytoma generally appears as a diffuse or nodular hyperplasia. The neoplastic cells are abundant cytoplasms with small centrally located nuclei. The neoplastic cells are separated into clusters by a slender stroma and numerous capillaries. **(G,H)** and Neuroblastoma (G) Gross photograph of a neuroblastoma. Neuroblastomas vary in size from 1cm to filling the entire abdomen. They are generally soft and white to gray-pink in color. As the size increases, the tumors become hemorrhagic, and undergo calcification and cyst formation. Note the nodular appearance of this tumor with the kidney apparent on the left border (arrow). (H) LM of a neuroblastoma, which is commonly composed of small, primitive-looking cells with dark nuclei and scant cytoplasm. The cells generally are arranged as solid sheets, and some cells arrange around a central fibrillar area, forming Homer-Wright pseudorosettes (asterisk).

41

Endocrine Pancreas

General Features. The endocrine pancreas comprises only 2% of the entire pancreas and consists of the **islets of Langerhans** that are scattered throughout the pancreas. The islets of Langerhans consists mainly of the following cell types:

A. **Alpha (α) cells** (20% of the islet) secrete **glucagon** (29 amino acids; 3.5 kDa) in response to hypoglycemia, which will elevate blood glucose, free fatty acid, and ketone levels. Glucagon binds to the **glucagon receptor** which is a **G-protein linked receptor ($\uparrow$cAMP)** present on hepatocytes and adipocytes. Glucagon is derived from a large precursor protein called **preproglucagon** which is processed to **glucagon** and **glucagon-related polypeptide (GRPP).** About 30–40% of glucagon within the blood is derived from pancreatic α cells and the remainder is derived from L cells within the small intestine called **glycentin (a large peptide that contains glucagon).**

B. **Beta (β) cells** (75% of the islet) secrete **insulin** [51 amino acids consisting of **chain A** (21 amino acids) and **chain B** (30 amino acids) held together by **disulfide bonds;** 6 kDa] in response to hyperglycemia which will lower blood glucose, free fatty acid, and ketone levels. Insulin binds to the **insulin receptor,** which is a **receptor tyrosine kinase** present on hepatocytes, skeletal muscle cells, and adipocytes. Insulin is derived from a large precursor protein called **preproinsulin** whose gene is present on chromosome 11. Preproinsulin is converted to proinsulin by removal of the **signal sequence** in the rER. **Proinsulin** (86 amino acids; 9kDa; consists of the **C-peptide** connecting chain A and chain B together) is transferred to the Golgi where it is package into secretory granules. Within secretory granules, proinsulin is cleaved by a protease to release the C peptide (35 amino acids) from insulin. Within the secretory granule, insulin organizes as a **hexamer** associated with **Zn^{2+}.** Insulin secretion is triggered when glucose enters the β cell via **glucose transporter 2 (GLUT2). Glucokinase** is the glucose sensor in the β cell that phosphorylates glucose $\rightarrow$ glucose-6-phosphate and generates ATP. ATP closes an **ATP-sensitive K^+ ion channel** and depolarizes the β cell resulting in an opening of a **Ca^{2+} ion channel** ($\uparrow$intracellular Ca^{2+}) which stimulates insulin secretion.

C. **Delta (δ) cells** (5% of the islet) secrete **somatostatin** (14 amino acids), which inhibits hormone secretion from nearby cells in a paracrine manner. Somatostatin binds to the **somatostatin receptor,** which is a **G-protein linked receptor ($\downarrow$cAMP + open a K^+ ion channel).**

Functions of Glucagon. The functions of glucagon include the following:

A. Effects on the Liver.
1. Glucagon increases glycogen degradation ($\uparrow$glycogen phosphorylase activity).
2. Glucagon increases gluconeogenesis ($\uparrow$fructose 1,6 bisphosphatase activity and $\downarrow$pyruvate kinase activity).

B. Effects on Adipose Tissue.
1. Glucagon increases lipolysis ($\uparrow$hormone-sensitive lipase activity) forming free fatty acids and glycerol.
2. Glucagon increases β-oxidation of free fatty acids. Ketoacids (β-hydroxybutyrate and acetoacetate are produced from acetyl CoA.

C. Effect on Urea Production. Glucagon increases urea production. Amino acids are used for gluconeogenesis and the resulting amino groups are incorporated into urea.

D. Net Effect of Glucagon. Glucagon increases plasma glucose, free fatty acids, glycerol, ketoacids, and urea.

Functions of Insulin. The functions of insulin include the following:

A. Effects on the Liver.
1. Insulin increases glycogen synthesis ($\uparrow$glycogen synthase activity).
2. Insulin increases glycolysis ($\uparrow$phosphofructokinase activity and $\downarrow$pyruvate dehydrogenase activity)
3. Insulin increases fatty acid synthesis
4. Insulin inhibits ketoacid formation

B. Effects on Adipose Tissue.
1. Insulin increases glucose uptake by GLUT 4
2. Insulin increases triacylglycerol synthesis (i.e., fat deposition)
3. Inhibits lipolysis

C. Effects of Skeletal Muscle.
1. Insulin increases glucose uptake by GLUT 4
2. Insulin increases glycogen synthesis ($\uparrow$glycogen synthase activity).
3. Insulin increases glycolysis ($\uparrow$phosphofructokinase activity and $\downarrow$pyruvate dehydrogenase activity)

D. Effects on Peripheral Cells. Insulin increases amino acid uptake into cells, thereby increasing protein synthesis (i.e., anabolic)

E. Net Effect of Insulin. Insulin decreases plasma glucose, free fatty acids, glycerol, ketoacids, and amino acids

Insulin Receptor and Signal Transduction. The insulin receptor is found on insulin-sensitive tissues like liver hepatocytes, adipocytes, and skeletal muscle. The insulin receptor is a tetramer with two α subunits and two β subunits. The β subunits have tyrosine kinase activity. The number of insulin receptors is up-regulated in starvation and down-regulated in obesity.

V **Regulation of Glucagon and Insulin Secretion (Figure 41-2).** Blood glucose is the primary regulator of both glucagon and insulin secretion. Decreased blood glucose levels (e.g., during a fast) increase glucagon secretion and decrease insulin secretion. Increased blood glucose levels (e.g., after a meal) decrease glucagon secretion and increase insulin secretion.

VI **Diabetes in General.** Although diabetes is characterized by hyperglycemia, a certain level of blood glucose must be maintained or convulsion, coma, and death result. A **glucose tolerance test** demonstrates the inability of a diabetic to properly handle a glucose load. The measurement of **hemoglobin A1C** (nonenzymatic glycosylation of amino groups on hemoglobin) is a good index of blood glucose levels during an 8–12 week interval prior to measurement (the target for diabetes in control is <7%).

A. **Type 1 diabetes** is marked by **autoantibodies** and an **insulitis reaction** that results in the **destruction of pancreatic beta cells.** Clinical findings include: hyperglycemia, ketoacidosis, and exogenous insulin dependence. Long term clinical effects include: neuropathy, retinopathy leading to blindness, and nephropathy leading to kidney failure.

B. **Type 2 diabetes** is marked by **insulin resistance of peripheral tissues** and **abnormal beta cell function.** It is often detected during routine screening by detection of hyperglycemia or by patient complaints of polyuria. Before the onset of frank symptoms, individuals pass through phases which include: i) hyperinsulinemia is present and euglycemia is maintained ii) hyperinsulinemia is present but postprandial hyperglycemia is observed iii) insulin secretion declines in the face of persistent insulin resistance of peripheral tissues.

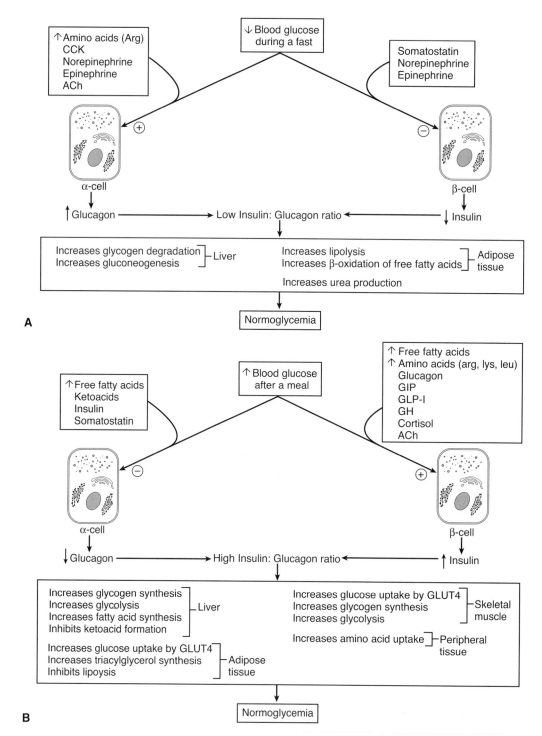

● **Figure 41-1:** Regulation of Glucagon and Insulin Secretion. **(A)** Low Blood Glucose Levels **(B)** High Blood Glucose Levels. CCK = cholecystokinin; ACh = acetylcholine; NE = norepinephrine released from postganglionic sympathetic axons; E = epinephrine released from the adrenal medulla; arg = arginine; lys = lysine; leu = leucine; GIP = gastric inhibitory peptide of glucose insulinotropic peptide; GLP-1 = glucagon-like peptide; GH = growth hormone.

42

Female Endocrinology

I   Ovaries (Figure 42-1A).   The ovaries are almond-shaped structures located posterior to the broad ligament. The ovaries are covered by a surface epithelium (simple cuboidal) called the **germinal epithelium,** with a subjacent connective tissue layer called the **tunica albuginea.** The ovaries are divided into a **cortex** and **medulla.** The cortex contains follicles in various stages of development, which include the: **primordial follicle, primary follicle, secondary follicle,** and **Graafian follicle.** Follicles are composed of an **oocyte** (i.e., the female egg), **thecal cells,** and **follicular (granulosa) cells.**

A. Secondary Follicles and Graafian Follicles. The cells responsible for steroid hormone production in the secondary and Graafian follicles are the **thecal interna cells** and **granulosa cells.**

1. **Theca Interna Cells.** The theca interna cells possess **LH receptors.** In response to LH, theca interna cells synthesize **androstenedione** which is transferred to granulosa cells.

2. **Granulosa Cells.** The granulosa cells possess **LH receptors** and **FSH receptors.** In response to FSH, granulosa cells **convert androstenedione (received from the theca interna cells) to testosterone.** The testosterone is then converted to **estradiol** by the enzyme **aromatase.** The estradiol produced by the secondary and Graafian follicles induces the **proliferative (follicular) phase of the menstrual cycle.**

B. Corpus Luteum (Figure 42-1B). The corpus luteum is a temporary endocrine gland formed within the ovary whose formation is **LH dependent.** After ovulation, the wall of the Graafian follicle collapses and becomes extensively infolded. The theca interna cells and granulosa cells hypertrophy, develop smooth endoplasmic reticulum (sER), and accumulate lipid droplets (a process called **luteinization**), thereby becoming **lutein cells**. If fertilization occurs, the corpus luteum enlarges and becomes the predominant source of steroids needed to sustain pregnancy for approximately **8 weeks.** Thereafter, the placenta becomes the major source of the steroids required. If fertilization does not occur, the corpus luteum regresses and forms a **corpus albicans.** The cells responsible for steroid hormone production in the corpus luteum are the **thecal lutein cells** and **granulosa lutein cells.**

1. **Theca Lutein Cells.** The theca lutein cells possess **LH receptors.** In response to LH, theca lutein cells synthesize **androstenedione,** which is transferred to granulosa lutein cells and **progesterone.** The progesterone produced by the theca lutein cells induces the **secretory (luteal) phase of the menstrual cycle.**

2. **Granulosa lutein Cells.** The granulosa lutein cells possess **LH receptors** and **FSH receptors.** In response to FSH, granulosa lutein cells **convert androstenedione (received from the theca lutein cells) to testosterone.** The testosterone is then converted to **estradiol** by the enzyme **aromatase.** In response to FSH, granulosa lutein cells also synthesize **progesterone.** The estradiol and progesterone produced by the granulosa lutein cells induce the **secretory (luteal) phase of the menstrual cycle.**

Placenta: Endocrinology of Pregnancy (Figure 41-C).

A. **Human Chorionic Gonadotropin (hCG).** hCG is a glycoprotein hormone produced by the **placenta (i.e., syncytiotrophoblast)** which stimulates the production of progesterone by the corpus luteum (i.e., maintains corpus luteum function). HCG can be assayed in **maternal blood at day 8** or **maternal urine at day 10,** which is the basis of the early pregnancy test kits purchased over the counter.

B. **Human Placental Lactogen (hPL)** is a protein hormone produced by the **placenta** that induces lipolysis thereby elevating free fatty acid levels in the mother. It is considered the "growth hormone" of the latter half of pregnancy. HPL can be assayed in **maternal blood at week 6.** hPL levels vary with placental mass (i.e., may indicate a multiple pregnancy) and rapidly disappear from maternal blood after delivery.

C. **Prolactin (PRL)** is a protein hormone produced by the **maternal adenohypophysis, fetal adenohypophysis,** and **placenta,** which prepares the mammary glands for lactation. PRL can be assayed in **maternal blood throughout pregnancy** or in **amniotic fluid.** Near term, PRL levels rise to a maximum of about 100ng/ml (normal nonpregnant PRL levels range between 8–25 ng/ml).

D. **Progesterone** is a steroid hormone produced by the **corpus luteum** until week 8 and then by the **placenta** until birth.

E. **Estrone, Estradiol, and Estriol.** These steroid hormones are produced by a complex series of steps involving the **maternal liver, placenta, fetal adrenal gland,** and **fetal liver. Estrone** is a fairly weak estrogen. **Estradiol** is the most potent estrogen. **Estriol** is a very weak estrogen but is produced in very high amounts during pregnancy. Estriol can be assayed in **maternal blood** (shows a distinct diurnal variation with peak amounts early in the morning) and **maternal urine** (24 hour urine sample shows no diurnal variation). Maternal urinary levels of estriol have long been recognized as a **reliable index of fetal-placental function,** since estriol production is dependent on a normal functioning fetal adrenal cortex, fetal liver, and placenta.

Menstrual Cycle (Figure 42-2). The menstrual cycle is a series of phases that repeats ideally every 28 days.

A. **The Menstrual Phase (Days 1–4)** is characterized by the **necrosis and shedding** of the functional layer of the endometrium.

B. **The Proliferative (follicular) Phase (Days 4–15)** is characterized by the **regeneration** of the functional layer of the endometrium from the devastating effects of the menstrual phase. This phase is controlled by **estradiol** secreted by the granulosa cells of the secondary and Graafian follicle. Estradiol causes a negative feedback inhibition of FSH and LH from the adenohypophysis during this phase.

C. **The Ovulatory Phase (Days 14–16)** is characterized by **ovulation** of the secondary oocyte arrested in metaphase of meiosis II that coincides with **peak levels of LH (LH surge).** A burst of estradiol causes a positive feedback stimulation of FSH and LH (LH surge) at the end of the proliferative phase. Estradiol decreases just after ovulation but then rises again during the secretory phase.

D. **The Secretory (luteal) Phase (Days 15–25)** is characterized by the **secretory activity** of the endometrial glands. This phase is controlled by **progesterone** secreted by the theca lutein cells and granulosa lutein cells of the corpus luteum. This phase is also controlled by **estradiol** secreted by the granulosa lutein cells. Progesterone causes a negative feedback inhibition of FSH and LH from the adenohypophysis and also of GRF from the hypothalamus during this phase. Progesterone **increases the basal body temperature** by affecting the hypothalmic thermoregulatory center.

E. **The Premenstrual Phase (Days 25–28)** is characterized by **ischemia** due to reduced blood flow to the endometrium. This phase is controlled by the **reduction in progesterone and estradiol** as the corpus luteum involutes.

IV **Transport of Estradiol and Progesterone.** 1–2% of circulating estradiol is in the free form. The remaining 98–99% of circulating estradiol is bound to liver-derived **sex steroid-binding globulin** (38%) or **albumin** (60%). 1–2% of circulating progesterone is in the free form. The remaining 98–99% of circulating progesterone is bound to **corticosteroid-binding globulin** (18%) or **albumin** (80%).

V **Functions of Estradiol.** The functions of estradiol include the following:

A. **Effects on the Female Reproductive System.** Estradiol induces the proliferative (follicular) phase of the menstrual cycle; causes maturation and maintenance of the uterine tubes (increases cilia formation and increases contractility of the smooth muscle), uterus (increases growth and contractility of the smooth muscle), cervix (stimulates a watery secretion), and vagina (induces epithelial proliferation); causes the development of the breasts (stimulates development of the duct system and adipose tissue); causes the development of female secondary sex characteristics; maintains the endometrium during pregnancy; lowers uterine threshold to contractile stimuli during pregnancy; blocks the action of prolactin (PRL) on the breast.

B. **Effects on the Adenohypophysis.** Estradiol causes negative feedback inhibition of FSH and LH. A burst of estradiol at the end of the proliferative phase causes a positive feedback stimulation of FSH and LH (LH surge). Estradiol stimulates PRL secretion.

C. **Effects on Bone.** Estradiol stimulates and terminates the pubertal growth spurt. Estradiol inhibits bone resorption.

VI **Functions of Progesterone.** The functions of progesterone include the following:

A. **Effects on the Female Reproductive System.** Progesterone induces the secretory (luteal) phase of the menstrual cycle; causes maturation and maintenance of the uterine tubes (increases epithelial secretory activity and decreases contractility of the smooth muscle), uterus (decreases contractility of the smooth muscle), cervix (stimulates a viscous secretion), and vagina (induces epithelial differentiation); prepares the endometrium for implantation (nidation); causes the development of the breasts (induces formation of secretory alveoli); maintains the endometrium during pregnancy; raises uterine threshold to contractile stimuli during pregnancy.

B. Effects on the Adenohypophysis. Progesterone causes negative feedback inhibition of FSH and LH.

C. Effects on Body Temperature. Progesterone increases basal body temperature.

D. Effect on the Fetal Adrenal Cortex. Progesterone is used by the fetal adrenal cortex as a precursor for corticosteroid and mineralocorticoid synthesis.

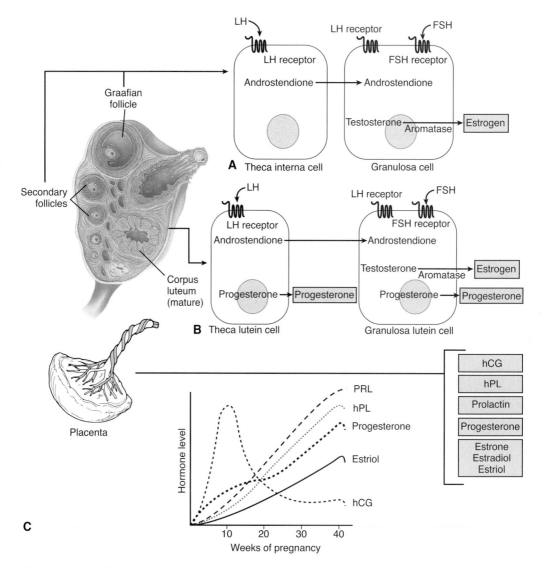

● **Figure 42-1: Female Hormonal Output.** The diagram of the entire ovary shows the cycle of ovarian follicle maturation, luteinization, and residual scarring forming a corpus albicans. **(A)** The secondary follicles and Graafian follicle contain theca interna cells and granulosa cells, which ultimately produce estrogen. **(B)** The corpus luteum contains theca lutein cells and granulosa lutein cells, which ultimately produce estrogen and progesterone. **(C)** The placenta produces hCG, hPL, prolactin, progesterone, and estrogens at various levels during pregnancy as indicated in the graph.

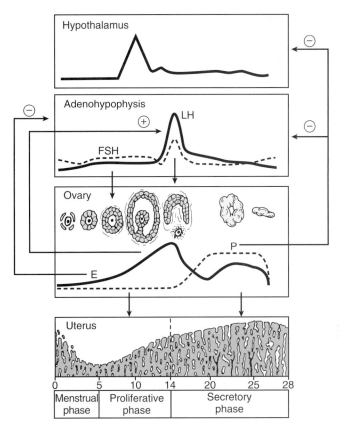

● **Figure 42-2: Hormonal control of the menstrual cycle.** The hypothalamus secretes gonadotropin-releasing factor (GRF). In response to GnRH, the adenohypophysis secretes follicle-stimulating hormone (FSH) and luteinizing hormone (LH). In response to FSH, the development of a secondary follicle to a Graafian follicle is stimulated in the ovary. The granulosa cells within the secondary follicle and Graafian follicle secrete estradiol (E). In response to estradiol, the endometrium of the uterus enters the proliferative phase. In response to LH (LH surge), ovulation occurs. After ovulation, the corpus luteum secretes progesterone (P) and estradiol. In response to progesterone and estradiol, the endometrium of the uterus enters the secretory phase. **Female infertility** is usually treated with **clomiphene (Clomid, Serophene).** Clomiphene is a selective estrogen receptor modulator (SERM) used to induce ovulation. Clomiphene acts as an estrogen receptor antagonist in the hypothalamus and adenohypophysis, and as a partial agonist in the ovaries. The antagonistic activity in the hypothalamus and adenohypophysis prevents estrogen feedback inhibition and thereby increases FSH and LH secretion so that ovulation occurs.

43

Male Endocrinology

Testes (Figures 43-1). The testes (plural) are paired, ovoid organs located in the scrotum that contain the **seminiferous tubules** and the **Leydig (interstitial) cells.**

A. **Seminiferous Tubules.** The seminiferous tubules are lined by a complex stratified epithelium (called **germinal epithelium**) consisting of two basic cell types: **Sertoli cells** and **spermatogenic cells.**
1. **Sertoli cells.** Sertoli cells are columnar cells with unusually ruffled apical and lateral surfaces due to the fact that these surfaces surround the developing spermatogenic cells. The functions of Sertoli cells include:
   a. Provide mechanical and nutritional support for developing spermatogenic cells.
   b. Phagocytose excess cytoplasm discarded by spermatids.
   c. Form the **blood-testes barrier** through **tight junctions** on their lateral surfaces.
   d. Secrete **inhibin** that inhibits release of FSH from adenohypophysis.
   e. Secrete **MIF (Mullerian inhibitory factor)** during fetal development that inhibits development of the paramesonephric duct in a genotypic XY fetus.
   f. Synthesize **androgen-binding protein (ABP)** that binds testosterone and acts as a local testosterone sink so that high levels of testosterone are present in the seminiferous tubules, which is necessary for spermatogenesis to occur.
   g. Possess **FSH receptors** (G-protein-linked receptor) so that FSH from the adenohypophysis stimulates spermatogenesis and synthesis of ABP.
2. **Spermatogenic cells.** Spermatogenic cells are the male germ cells that are undergoing the transformation from Type A spermatogonia → sperm.

B. **Leydig Cells.** The Leydig cells (or interstitial cells) of the testes are located in the loose connective tissue between the seminiferous tubules. Leydig cells have an elaborate smooth endoplasmic reticulum (sER), lipid droplets, mitochondria with tubular cristae, and highly-refractive, rod-shaped crystals called crystals of Reinke. The functions of the Leydig cells include:
1. Synthesize **testosterone.** Testosterone is transferred to the Sertoli cells and enters the bloodstream. Testosterone gives rise to two other potent androgens via the following pathways:

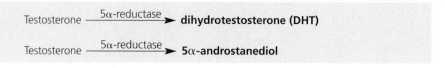

Testosterone $\xrightarrow{\text{5}\alpha\text{-reductase}}$ **dihydrotestosterone (DHT)**

Testosterone $\xrightarrow{\text{5}\alpha\text{-reductase}}$ **5α-androstanediol**

2. Possess **LH receptors** (G-protein-linked receptor) so that LH from the adeno-hypophysis stimulates testosterone secretion. LH in males is usually released in 90-minute frequency pulses, although this is variable between subjects, time of day, and seasons of the year. The LH pulses are maintained by GRF pulses from the hypothalamus.

II   Transport of Testosterone.   1–2% of circulating testosterone is in the free form. The remaining 98–99% of circulating testosterone is bound to liver-derived **sex steroid-binding globulin** or **albumin.**

III   Functions of Testosterone.   The functions of testosterone include the following:

A. **Effects in the Embryo.** Testosterone causes the prenatal differentiation of the mesonephric duct (Wolffian duct) into the epididymis, ductus deferens, seminal vesicles, and ejaculatory duct. Although no direct evidence is available in humans, animal studies indicate that testosterone sexually differentiates the fetal brain.

B. **Effects on the Male Reproductive System.** Testosterone is transferred to Sertoli cells where testosterone binds to androgen-binding protein (ABP) to maintain spermatogenesis (production of sperm). Testosterone stimulates the growth of the penis and seminal vesicles.

C. **Effects on Bone.** Testosterone increases growth hormone (GH) secretion, which increases IGF-1 from the liver and thereby stimulates the epiphyseal growth plate resulting in the pubertal growth spurt. At the end of puberty, testosterone promotes the closure of the epiphyseal growth plate.

D. **Effects on Muscle.** Testosterone increases protein synthesis in skeletal muscle thereby increasing the muscle mass.

E. **Effects on the Kidney.** Testosterone stimulates the secretion of erythropoietin by the kidneys thereby increasing red blood cell production.

F. **Effects on the Liver.** Testosterone increases very low density lipoprotein (VLDL), increases low density lipoprotein (LDL), and decreases high density lipoprotein (HDL).

G. **Effects on the Larynx.** Testosterone causes a deepening of the voice.

H. **Effects on Behavior.** Testosterone increases libido.

I. **Effects on the Hypothalamus and Adenohypophysis.** Testosterone causes a negative feedback inhibition of gonadotropin releasing factor (GRF) from the hypothalamus and LH from the adenohypophysis.

IV   Functions of Dihydrotestosterone (DHT).

A. **Effects on the Embryo.** DHT causes the prenatal differentiation of penis, scrotum, urethra, and prostate gland.

B. Effects on the Male Reproductive System. DHT stimulates the growth of the penis and seminal vesicles. DHT also stimulates the growth of the prostate gland.

C. Effects on Hair. DHT directs the hair distribution during puberty (e.g., beard, chest hair). DHT is also involved in male pattern baldness.

D. Effects on Sebaceous Glands. DHT increases sebaceous gland activity.

Ⓥ Clinical Considerations.

A. Benign Prostatic Hypertrophy (BPH). BPH is characterized by hypertrophy of the **transitional (periurethral) zone,** which generally involves the lateral and middle lobes. BPH compresses the prostatic urethra and obstructs urine flow. The hypertrophy may be due to increased sensitivity of prostate to **DHT (dihydrotestosterone).** BPH is NOT pre-malignant. Clinical signs include: increased frequency of urination, nocturia, difficulty starting and stopping urination, sense of incomplete emptying of bladder. Treatment may include: 5α-reductase inhibitors [e.g. **finasteride (Proscar)**] to block conversion of T → DHT, and/or α-adrenergic antagonists (e.g., **terazosin, prazosin, doxazosin**) to inhibit prostate gland secretion.

B. Prostatic carcinoma (PC). PC is most commonly found in the **peripheral zone,** which generally involves the posterior lobes (which can be palpated upon a digital rectal exam). Since PC begins in the peripheral zone, by the time urethral blockage occurs (i.e., patient complains of difficulty in urination) the carcinoma is in an advanced stage. **Prostatic intraepithelial neoplasia (PIN)** is frequently associated with PC. Serum **PSA levels** are diagnostic. Metastasis to bone (e.g., lumbar vertebrae, pelvis) is frequent. Treatment may include: **Leuprolide (Lupron)** which is a GNRH agonist that inhibits the release of FSH and LH when administered in a continuous fashion thereby inhibiting secretion of testosterone, **Cyproteron (Androcur)** or **Flutamide (Eulexin),** which are androgen receptor antagonists, radiation and/or prostatectomy.

C. Male pseudointersexuality (MP) Figure 43-2A. MP occurs when an individual has only testicular tissue histologically and various stages of stunted development of the male external genitalia. These individuals have a **46, XY genotype.** MP is most often observed clinically in association with a condition in which the fetus produces a **lack of androgens (and MIF).** This is caused most commonly by mutations in genes for androgen steroid biosynthesis (e.g., **5α-reductase 2 deficiency** or **17β-hydroxysteroid dehydrogenase).** Normally, 5α-reductase 2 catalyzes the conversion of testosterone → dihydrotestosterone and 17β HSD 3 catalyzes the conversion of androstenedione → testosterone. An increased **T:DHT ratio** is diagnostic (Normal=5; 5α-reductase 2 deficiency = 20–60). The reduced levels of androgens lead to the **feminization of a male fetus.** MP produces the following clinical findings: underdevelopment of the penis and scrotum (microphallus, hypospadias, and bifid scrotum) and prostate gland. The epididymis, ductus deferens, seminal vesicle, and ejaculatory duct are normal. These clinical findings have led to inference that DHT is essential in the development of the penis and scrotum (external genitalia) and prostate gland in genotypic XY fetus. At puberty, these individuals demonstrate a striking virilization.

D. **Complete Androgen Insensitivity (CAIS; or Testicular feminization syndrome)**
    Figure 43-2B. CAIS occurs when a fetus with a 46, XY genotype develops testes and
    female external genitalia with a rudimentary vagina; uterus and uterine tubes are gener-
    ally absent. The testes may be found in the labia majora and are surgically removed to
    circumvent malignant tumor formation. These individuals present as normal-appearing
    females, and their psychosocial orientation is female despite their genotype. The most
    common cause is a mutation in the gene for the **androgen receptor.** Even though the
    developing male fetus is exposed to normal levels of androgens, the lack of androgen
    receptors renders the phallus, urogenital folds, and labioscrotal swellings unresponsive
    to androgens.

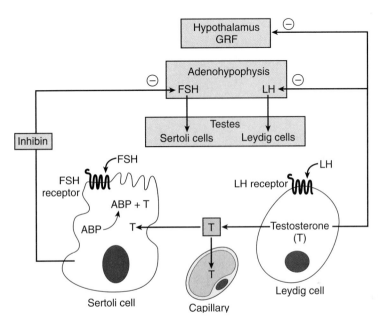

● **Figure 43-1: Male Hormonal Output.** The Leydig cell synthesizes testosterone, which then is either transferred to
the Sertoli cell or enters the bloodstream. Testosterone binds to androgen binding protein (ABP) so that high levels of
testosterone are present in the seminiferous tubules, which is necessary for spermatogenesis to occur. Testosterone and
inhibin both participate in negative feedback inhibition. GRF = gonadotropin releasing factor; FSH = follicle-stimulating
hormone; LH = luteinizing hormone; T = testosterone.

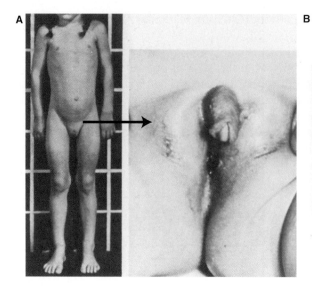

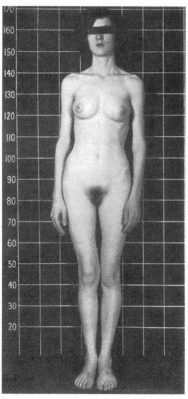

● **Figure 43-2: Endocrine Disorders. (A)** A patient (XY genotype) with male pseudointersexuality. Stunted development of male external genitalia is apparent. The stunted external genitalia fooled parents and physician into thinking that this XY infant was a girl. In fact, this child was raised as a girl (note pigtails). As this child neared puberty, testosterone levels increased and clitoral enlargement ensued. This alarmed the parents and the child was brought in for clinical evaluation. **(B)** A patient (XY genotype) with complete androgen insensitivity (CAIS or testicular feminization). Complete feminization of male external genitalia is apparent.

Credits

Figure 1-1: Modified from Costanzo LS; BRS Physiology; 4th ed; LWW. Baltimore, 2007, page 11, figure 1-6.

Figure 2-1: B. From Dudek RW; HY Histology; 3rd ed, LWW, Baltimore; 2004, page 63, Figure 8-1B. C. From Dudek RW; HY Histology; 3rd ed, LWW; Baltimore; 2004, page 63, Figure 8-1B D. From Dudek RW; HY Histology; 3rd ed, LWW; Baltimore; 2004, page 63, Figure 8-1C.

Figure 2-2: Dudek RW; HY Histology; 3rd ed, LWW; Baltimore; 2004, page 65, Figure 8-2.

Figure 3-1: Dudek RW; HY Histology; 3rd ed; LWW; Baltimore; 2004; page 67, figure 8-3.

Figure 4-1A and B: Dudek RW; HY Histology, LWW, Baltimore, 2006, page 90, figure 10-1.

Figure 4-2: Dudek RW; HY Histology, LWW, Baltimore, 2006, page 92, figure 10-2.

Table 23-1: Dudek RW; HY Kidney; 1st ed; LWW; Baltimore; 2007; page 109; Table 5-4.

Figure 27-1B and C: Reprinted with permission from Longnecker JC, High Yield Acid-Base, LWW, Baltimore, 1998 page 15, Figure 2-2 and Figure 2-3.

Figure 29-1: A: Reprinted with permission from Costanzo LS; BRS Physiology, 3rd ed, LWW, Baltimore, 2003, page 228, figure 6-5. C; From Sternberg SS; Histology for Pathologists; 2nd ed, LWW, Baltimore, 1997, page 467, figure 10B.D: From Ross MH, Pawlina W; Histology A Text and Atlas; 5th ed; LWW, Baltimore, 2006, page 557, Plate 51; Figure 1. E: From Sternberg SS; Histology for Pathologists; 2nd ed, LWW, Baltimore, 1997, page 475, figure 22.F: From Sternberg SS; Histology for Pathologists; 2nd ed, LWW, Baltimore, 1997, page 476, figure 23A.

Figure 30-1: A: Redrawn from Johnson L; Gastrointestinal Physiology; 6th ed; St. Louis, Mosby, 2000. B: From Bullock J, Boyle J III, Wang MB; NMS Physiology; 4th ed; LWW, Baltimore, 2001 page 525, figure 42-3. C: Redrawn from Pasley JN; USMLE Road Map Physiology; Lange; New York, 2003 page 119, figure 5-3.

Figure 30-2B: Modified from Dudek RW; HY Histology; 3rd ed; LWW; Baltimore; 2004; page 137, figure 15-2. Also see page 136, figure 15-1 for a digitized figure of the parietal cell.

Figure 30-3: A: Reprinted with permission from Erkonen WE, Smith WL; Radiology 101 the basics and fundamental of imaging; 2nd ed; LWW, Baltimore, 2005 page 113, figure 3-51. B: From Erkonen WE, Smith WL; Radiology 101 the basics and fundamental of imaging; 2nd ed; LWW, Baltimore, 2005 page 113, figure 3-52.

Figure 31-3: A: Redrawn from Costanzo L; Physiology; 3rd ed; Saunders Elsevier, Philadelphia, 2006, page 370, figure 8-31.

Figure 32-1: B: Taken with permission from from Kamath PS, Phillips SF, OConnor MK, et al: Colonic capacitance and transit in man: modulation by luminal contents and drugs. Gut 1990; 31:443.C: Redrawn from Despopoulos A and Silbernagl S; Color Atlas of Physiology, 5th ed; Thieme Stuttgart and New York, 2003, page 265, figure A.

Figure 34-1: A: Reprinted with permission from Dudek RW; HY Gross Anatomy, 2nd ed; LWW, Baltimore, 2002, page 72, figure 9-2A.B; From Moore KL, Dalley AF; Clinically oriented Anatomy; 5th ed, LWW, Baltimore, 2006 page 346, figure 2.82B. C: From Erkonen WE, Smith WL; Radiology 101 the basics and fundamental of imaging; 2nd ed; LWW, Baltimore, 2005 page 94, figure 3-24. D: From Yamada T et al; Atlas of Gastroenterology, 2nd ed, Philadelphia, LWW, 1999, page 474, figure 52-1B. E: From Yamada T et al; Atlas of Gastroenterology, 2nd ed, Philadelphia, LWW, 1999, page 475, figure 52-4.

Figure 36-1: Data taken from Schwartz MJ; Adv. Int. Med.; 38:81, 1994.

Figure 36-2: From Dudek RW; HY Cell and Molecular Biology; 2nd ed; LWW, Baltimore, 2006, page 13, Figure 1-3.

Figure 36-3: From Dudek RW; HY Cell and Molecular Biology; 2nd ed; LWW, Baltimore, 2006, page 20, Figure 1-4.

Figure 38-1: A: From Rubin E and Farber JL; Pathology, 3rd ed, LWW, Baltimore, 1999, page 1167, figure 21-13. B: From Dudek RW; HY Histology; 3rd ed; LWW; Baltimore; 2004, page 197, figure 23-2D. Courtesy of Dr. RW Dudek. C: From Dudek RW; HY Histology; 3rd ed; LWW; Baltimore; 2004, page 197, figure 23-2C. From Dudek RW; HY Histology; 3rd ed; LWW; Baltimore; 2004, page 197, figure 23-2D.

Figure 39-1: Modified from Dudek RW; HY Histology; 3rd ed; LWW; Baltimore; 2004, page 200, figure 24-1.

Figure 40-1: Reprinted with permission from Rubin E and Farber JL; Pathology; 3rd ed; LWW; 1999; page 1193, figure 21-34, 21-37 and 21-31B. From Dudek RW, Fix J; BRS Embryology; 3rd ed; LWW, Baltimore, 2005, page 163, figure 15-5A. Original source: Courtesy of Dr. J. Kitchin, Department of Obstetrics and Gynecology, University of Virginia. From Dudek RW; HY Histology; 3rd ed; LWW; Baltimore, 2004, page 212, figure 25-5A. From Dudek RW; HY Histology; 3rd ed; LWW; Baltimore, 2004, page 212, figure 25-5B. From Dudek RW; HY Histology; 3rd ed; LWW; Baltimore, 2004, page 212, figure 25-5C. Reprinted with permission from Sternberg SS: Diagnostic Surgical Pathology, Vol. 1, 3rd ed. Philadelphia: Lippincott Williams & Wilkins, 1999, p. 609, fig. 33. From Dudek RW; HY Histology; 3rd ed; LWW; Baltimore, 2004, page 212, figure 25-5D.

Figure 42-1: A: Picture of ovary from: Dudek RW; HY Histology; 3rd ed; LWW; Baltimore; 2004; page 214; figure 26-1. Original

Index

Note: Page numbers in *italics* denote figures; those followed by a t denote tables.

Osmoreceptors, 99
Osmosis, 4–5
Osmotic diarrhea, 151
Osmotic pressure, 4
Osteomalacia, 207
Ovary (ovaries), 219–220
    follicle-stimulating hormone effects on, 195–196
    follicles of, 219, 222
    luteinizing hormone effects on, 196
    prolactin effects on, 195
Overhydration, 77, 78
Ovulation, 221, 223
Oxidation-reduction reactions, 1
Oxygen
    arterial, 64
    decrease in, 61, 61t, 62–63, 64
    diffusion of, 59
    impaired diffusion of, 62
    increase in, 61, 61t, 64
    partial pressure of, 58, 58t, 65
    transport of, 64
Oxyhemoglobin saturation, 30
Oxytocin, 197, 200t

P wave, 26, 31, 35
Pancreas
    endocrine, 215–217
        cells of, 215
            glucagon of, 215, 216, 217
            insulin of, 215, 216, 217
            somatostatin of, 215
        exocrine, 180–183, 184
            bicarbonate secretion by, 180–181, 184
            chloride secretion by, 180–181, 184
            enzymes of, 180, 184
            regulation of, 182
            secretory phases of, 182–183
Pancreatic enzymes, 146–147, 180, 184
Pancreatic juice, 180–181, 184
Pancreatic polypeptide, 182
Pancuronium, 11
Pantothenic acid, absorption of, 147
Para-aminohippuric acid
    clearance of, 80
    renal handling of, 86, 88t
Parallel circulation, 43, 45
Parasympathetic nervous system
    in cardiac function, 23–24, 26, 46, 49, 50
    in gallbladder function, 178
    in gastrin secretion, 136
    in gastrointestinal function, 124
    in hydrochloric acid secretion, 135
    in large intestine motility, 155
    in pancreatic function, 182
    in small intestine motility, 142
Parathyroid glands, 205–206
    cells of, 205
    disorders of, 207, 207t
Parathyroid hormone, 108, 109, 205, 208
Partial pressures
    carbon dioxide, 58, 58t, 66, 116, 119, 120
    oxygen, 58, 58t, 65
Penicillin, renal handling of, 86, 88t
Pepsinogen, 134
Peptide hormones, 185, 185t-186t
Peptide PP, 182
Peptide YY, 182
Peristalsis
    esophageal, 128
    gastric, 132–133
    large intestine, 155–156
    reverse, 128
    small intestine, 142–143, 152
Peritubular capillaries, 84
Permeability, 3
pH

ammonium ion secretion and, 116–117
    calcium regulation and, 109
    exercise-related change in, 73
    hydrogen ion secretion and, 116
    potassium regulation and, 104
Pheochromocytoma, 212–213, 213t
Phosphate
    renal handling of, 107, 107t
    urinary excretion of, 109
Phosphatidylcholine, 1
Phosphatidylethanolamine, 1
Phosphatidylserine, 1
Phospholipase A$_2$, 1
Phospholipase C, 1, 187, 191
Pink puffers, 69
Pituitary gland, 194–200, 199t-200t
    adrenocorticotropic hormone secretion by, 195, 199t
    estradiol effects on, 220
    follicle-stimulating hormone secretion by, 195–196, 200t
    growth hormone secretion by, 194–195, 199t
    luteinizing hormone secretion by, 196, 200t
    progesterone effects on, 222
    prolactin secretion by, 195, 199t
    regulation of, 196
    testosterone effects on, 225
    thyroid-stimulating hormone secretion by, 195, 199t
Placenta, 220, 222
Plasma, 74
    calcium in, 108
    measurement of, 75, 78
Plasma osmolarity, 99
Plasma volume
    decrease in, 99–100
    increase in, 100
    regulation of, 99
Pneumoconioses, 70
Pneumothorax, 54
Poiseuille equation, 42
Poiseuille law, 58–59
Polycythemia vera, 66
Polypeptides, renal handling of, 85–86, 88t
Positive feedback, 186
Potassium
    aldosterone effects on, 103–104
    deficiency of, 105
    dietary, 105
    diuretic effects on, 104
    excess of, 105
    large intestine secretion of, 158–159, 161
    pancreatic secretion of, 180–181
    regulation of, 105
    renal handling of, 101–102, 102t
    small intestine absorption of, 150, 154
    sodium effects on, 104
    urinary excretion of, 103–104
PR interval, 26
Pregnancy, 220, 222
Preload, 28
Preprohormone, 185
Pressure diuresis, 49, 99
Pressure natriuresis, 49, 99
Progesterone, 220, 221–222, 222, 223
Prohormone, 185
Prolactin, 199t, 220, 222
Prolactinoma, 198
Prostacyclin, 1
Prostaglandins, 1
Prostate gland
    benign hypertrophy of, 226
    carcinoma of, 226
Protein(s)
    carrier, 2
    cell membrane, 2
    hepatic metabolism of, 165, 166t
    ion channel, 2
    renal handling of, 85, 88t